MDCT: A Practical Approach

S. Saini • G.D. Rubin • M.K. Kalra (Eds)

MDCT
A Practical Approach

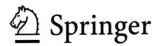

Springer

Sanjay Saini
Department of Radiology
Emory University School of Medicine
Emory University Hospital
Atlanta, GA, USA

Geoffrey D. Rubin
Department of Radiology
Stanford University School of Medicine
Stanford, CA, USA

Mannudeep K. Kalra
Department of Radiology
Emory University School of Medicine
Emory University Hospital
Atlanta, GA, USA

Library of Congress Control Number: 20060920922

ISBN-10 88-470-0412-8 Springer Milan Berlin Heidelberg New York
ISBN-13 978-88-470-0412-2 Springer Milan Berlin Heidelberg New York

Springer is a part of Springer Science+Business Media
springer.com
© Springer-Verlag Italia 2006

Cover design: Simona Colombo, Milan
Typesetting: Compostudio, Cernusco s/N (Milan)
Printing and binding: Arti Grafiche Nidasio, Assago (Milan)
Printed in Italy

Preface

Multidetector-row computed tomography (MDCT) is currently the most rapidly evolving imaging technology. Within a decade of its commercial introduction, MDCT has become an indispensable imaging modality in routine clinical practice. Continuing improvements in MDCT technology make it easier, quicker and safer to detect and diagnose disease. Unfortunately the rapidity with which upgrades occur may sometimes make it difficult for radiologists to keep up to date. This has been the underlying motivation for this textbook on the technical aspects and clinical applications of state-of-the-art MDCT scanners. The book contains chapters prepared by recognized experts in the field of MDCT that describe the various clinical applications of MDCT in different regions of the body. Moreover, in describing the practical aspects of CT technology, this book also addresses concerns over radiation dose and contrast media safety and administration issues. The book contains numerous figures and tables and practical tips for MDCT scanning along with comprehensive details of scanning techniques, contrast medium administration techniques, image post-processing, study indications, and diagnostic applications.

This book has been prepared not only for the benefit of radiologists but also with the interests of radiology fellows and residents, radiology technologists, and medical physicists in mind. In order to organize this book for readers of different radiology sub-specialities or interests, the contents are divided into five sections, beginning with the physics and techniques of MDCT and extending to describe the important applications of MDCT pertaining to imaging of the abdomen, head and neck, cardiovascular system, and trauma.

Section I begins with "A Practical Approach to MDCT", co-authored by Dr. Mannudeep K. Kalra and Professor Sanjay Saini. This chapter describes the history and growth of MDCT technology and outlines the fundamentals of MDCT physics and strategies for setting up effective scanning protocols. In the subsequent chapter, Dr. Kyongtae T. Bae provides an in-depth description of the "Principles of Contrast Medium Delivery and Scan Timing in MDCT" for state-of-the-art MDCT scanners. This chapter outlines the numerous factors associated with contrast medium delivery and scan timing and emphasizes the need to adjust scan timing on the basis of both patient-related factors (body weight, cardiac ouput) and contrast injection parameters (duration and rate of injection, iodine concentration). The modifications to protocol design that are necessary for optimized contrast enhancement in MDCT are discussed, along with clinical considerations for CT angiography (CTA) and hepatic imaging. In the third chapter of this section Professor Richard Solomon shares his immense experience in "Contrast-Induced Nephropathy: Managing At-Risk Patients". Currently an area of much controversy among the radiological and cardiological communities, this chapter aims to address all of the issues related to contrast-induced nephropathy and to bring some perspective to the debate. In the final chapter of this section, Dr. Kalra highlights the increasing concern over "MDCT Radiation Dose", providing valuable insight into the risks associated with radiation exposure in MDCT and presenting useful practical tips for reducing the overall radiation dose. In all, section I provides a concise overview of the technical fundamentals of modern MDCT scanners.

Section II focuses primarily on MDCT of the abdomen, highlighting important practical approaches to MDCT imaging of the liver, hepatobiliary system, pancreas and spleen, as well as for MDCT angiography of the mesenteric and renal vasculature. In the first chapter of the section entitled "Dual-Phase Liver MDCT", Drs. Dushyant V. Sahani and Anandkumar H. Singh provide a detailed description of scanning protocols, contrast media administration techniques, and clinical applications of dual-phase MDCT protocol for detecting and characterization of focal liver lesions. MDCT imaging of focal liver lesions is again addressed in the second chapter of this section prepared by Drs. Sebastian T. Schindera and Rendon C. Nelson. Entitled "Hepatobiliary Imaging by Multidetector Computed Tomography (MDCT)" this chapter also provides a comprehensive review of MDCT applications in the biliary system. In the third chapter entitled "Soft Organ MDCT Imaging: Pancreas and Spleen", Drs. Sahani and Shah describe the role of modern MDCT for evaluation of pancreatic and splenic lesions. The authors cover important technical components and clinical indications for scanning patients with suspected or known pancreatic or splenic pathology. The final chapter of Section II addresses the role of MDCT angiography in patients referred for evaluation of the renal and mesenteric vasculature. Entitled "Mesenteric and Renal CT Angiography", Drs. Lisa L. Wang, Christine O. Menias and Kyongtae T. Bae discuss common indications for which MDCT scanning of the abdominal vasculature is appropriate and provide practical approaches for staging and surgical management of tumors, evaluation for renal donor transplantation, work-up of renovascular hypertension, and assessment of mesenteric ischemia and inflammatory bowel disease.

Section III comprises four chapters dedicated to MDCT of the cardiovascular system, which represents the fastest-growing application for MDCT scanning. The section begins with a chapter on "Imaging Protocols for Cardiac CT" by Drs. Frank J. Rybicki and Tarang Sheth. With the help of several exquisite images, the authors expound the key considerations for planning effective scanning protocols for cardiac MDCT angiography and illustrate the key applications for MDCT angiography in the coronary arteries. In the second chapter of the section entitled "MDCT Angiography of the Thoracic Aorta", Drs. Geoffrey D. Rubin and Mannudeep K. Kalra highlight the value of state-of-the-art MDCT scanners and comprehensively discuss scanning techniques and clinical applications of MDCT aortography. Specifically, the improved temporal and isotropic resolution achievable on the most recent MDCT scanners enable volumetric acquisitions that provide clear anatomic delineation of thoracic aorta, its tortuous branches, and adjacent aneurysms and pseudo aneurysms. With the help of relevant two- and three-dimensional images the authors demonstrate conclusively that MDCT angiography has clear advantages over conventional aortography for evaluation of the thoracic aorta. An important application of MDCT in the emergency setting is presented in the third chapter of the section entitled "Pulmonary Embolism Imaging with MDCT". In this chapter Drs. Joseph J. Kavanagh, Douglas R. Lake, and Philip Costello describe the many advantages of MDCT when compared with other available imaging modalities in the detection of pulmonary embolism. Principal among these advantages are the rapidity of the procedure and the possibility to detect and diagnose additional complications which may contribute to the patient's overall clinical presentation, such as congestive heart failure, pneumonia, interstitial lung disease, aortic dissection, malignancy and pleural disease. The final chapter of this section, again by Drs. Rubin and Kalra, describes the role of MDCT angiography in non-invasive imaging of peripheral vascular disease. Entitled "MDCT Angiography of Peripheral Arterial Disease", the chapter presents the scanning parameters, contrast medium administration features, image post-processing techniques, and many clinical applications (intermittent claudication, acute and chronic lower-limb ischemia, trauma, vascular mapping) of MDCT angiography in imaging of the lower extremities.

Section IV extends the clinical role of MDCT to include applications in the head and neck. In the first of two chapters in this section, entitled "CT Angiography of the Neck and Brain", Dr. David S. Enterline discusses critical aspects of MDCT angiography in assessing neck and brain vasculature and provides several interesting cases to illustrate the full value of MDCT angiography in this setting. The second chapter by Drs. Sanjay K. Shetty and Michael H. Lev, entitled "MDCT Perfusion in Acute Stroke" focuses on applications of MDCT perfusion imaging in the evaluation of patients with acute stroke. The chapter is enhanced by the inclusion of effective scanning protocols and by detailed assessment of the value of CT perfusion relative to other techniques such as magnetic resonance perfusion.

The final section of the book, Section V, addresses the increasing use of MDCT in imaging of acute trauma. The two chapters included in the section consider the role of MDCT in assessing abdominal trauma and musculoskeletal trauma, respectively. In "MDCT of Abdominal Trauma" Dr. Robert A. Halvorsen gives practical advice on the use and interpretation of MDCT in patients with abdominal trauma. In particular, the varied manifestations of bleeding are emphasized while common mistakes and pitfalls in interpretation are also discussed. In the second chapter of the section and final chapter of the book, Drs. Sunit Sebastian and Hamid Salamipour outline the "Role of MDCT in the Evaluation of Musculoskeletal Trauma", focussing on the various techniques and applications of MDCT and the specific value of 3-D reformations in the evaluation of orthopedic trauma.

The book concludes with a detailed appendix that presents optimized scanning protocols for MDCT imaging in a variety of indications.

In summary, *MDCT: A Practical Approach* provides a comprehensive evaluation of the technical developments and rapidly evolving clinical applications of MDCT in routine practice. We believe this textbook will guide radiology personnel and further propel development in the field of MDCT.

Sanjay Saini, M.D.
Geoffrey D. Rubin, M.D.
Mannudeep K. Kalra, M.D.

Contents

SECTION IV - MDCT of Head and Neck

SECTION V - MDCT of Trauma

Contributors

Kyongtae Ty Bae
Washington University
School of Medicine
St. Louis, MO, USA

Philip Costello
Division of Thoracic Imaging
Department of Radiology
Medical University of South Carolina,
Charleston, SC, USA

David S. Enterline
Divisions of Neuroradiology and
Interventional Neuroradiology
Duke University Medical Center
Durham, NC, USA

Robert A. Halvorsen
Department of Radiology
MCV Hospitals/VCU Medical Center
Richmond, VA, USA

Mannudeep K. Kalra
Department of Radiology
Emory University School of Medicine
Emory University Hospital
Atlanta, GA, USA

Joseph J. Kavanagh
Division of Thoracic Imaging
Department of Radiology
Medical University of South Carolina,
Charleston, SC, USA

Douglas R. Lake
Division of Thoracic Imaging
Department of Radiology
Medical University of South Carolina,
Charleston, SC, USA

Michael H. Lev
Director, Emergency Neuroradiology and
Neurovascular Lab
Massachusetts General Hospital
Boston, MA, USA

Christine O. Menias
Washington University
School of Medicine
St. Louis, MO, USA

Rendon C. Nelson
Division of Abdominal Imaging
Duke University Medical Center
Durham, NC, USA

Geoffrey D. Rubin
Stanford University School of Medicine
Department of Radiology
Stanford, CA, USA

Frank J. Rybicki
Cardiovascular Imaging Section
Applied Imaging Science Laboratory
Brigham & Women's Hospital Radiology
Harvard Medical School
Boston, MA, USA

Sanjay Saini
Department of Radiology
Emory University School of Medicine
Emory University Hospital
Atlanta, GA, USA

Dushyant V. Sahani
Department of Abdominal Imaging and
Intervention
Massachusetts General Hospital
Boston, MA, USA

Hamid Salamipour
Department of Radiology
Massachusetts General Hospital
Boston, MA, USA

Sebastian T. Schindera
Division of Abdominal Imaging
Duke University Medical Center
Durham, NC, USA

Zarine K. Shah
Department of Abdominal Imaging and
Intervention
Massachusetts General Hospital
Boston, MA, USA

Tarang Sheth
Department of Diagnostic Imaging
Trillium Health Centre
Mississauga, ON, Canada

Sanjay K. Shetty
Division of Musculoskeletal Radiology
Department of Radiology
Massachusetts General Hospital
Boston, MA, USA

Sunit Sebastian
Department of Radiology
Emory University School of Medicine
Atlanta, GA, USA

Anandkumar H. Singh
Abdominal Imaging
Massachusetts General Hospital
Depatment of Abdominal Imaging
Boston, MA, USA

Richard Solomon
Chief, Division of Nephrology
University of Vermont College of
Medicine
Burlington, VT, USA

Lisa L. Wang
Washington University
School of Medicine
St. Louis, MO, USA

SECTION I

Physics and Techniques of MDCT

I.1

A Practical Approach to MDCT

Mannudeep K. Kalra and Sanjay Saini

Introduction

Over the past 8 years, computed tomography (CT) technology has developed tremendously with the introduction of multidetector-row CT (MDCT) scanners to the clinical radiology practice [1]. Use of CT scanning has increased immensely over the last decade with introduction of newer applications. Demand for better technology continues to propel vendors to develop further innovations in very short time periods. As a result, it has become difficult for many radiologists, physicists, and technologists to keep up with the pace of development. This chapter outlines growth patterns in MDCT application and use and the history of CT technology and describes the fundamentals of MDCT technology.

MDCT: Explosive Growth Patterns

It is estimated that there are more than 25,000 CT scanners in the world, and since 1998, worldwide CT sales have doubled. In 2002, the CT market was reported to be worth in excess of US$2.6 billion [1]. A recent survey indicates that every year, about 90 million CT examinations are performed globally, which corresponds to a frequency of 16 CT examinations per 1,000 inhabitants [1, 2]. According to the 2000–2001 Nationwide Evaluation of X-ray Trends (NEXT) – a survey of patient radiation exposure from CT, performed under the auspices of the United States Food and Drug Administration – approximately 58 million (± 9 million) CT studies are performed annually in 7,800 CT facilities in the United States [1]. As regards CT applications, during 1991–2002, vascular and cardiac applications of CT showed highest growth rates (over 140%), followed by much smaller increments in abdominal, pelvic, thoracic, and head and neck applications (7–27%).

MDCT: Chronology of Technological Advances

• **1971**: The Nobel laureate Sir Godfrey Neobold Hounsfield at the Electrical and Musical Industries, London, a British electronics and music company, developed the first conventional CT scanner. It took 15 h to scan the first patient using this CT instrument and 5 min to acquire each image.

• **1971–1976**: During this period, four generations of conventional CT scanners were developed, and the scan time for each image dropped manifolds to 1–2 s. These conventional scanners revolved a single X-ray tube and detector array on a gantry assembly around the patient. Following each revolution, the X-ray tube and/or detector array returned to their initial position to "unwind" their attached wires and prepare for the next revolution after table movement.

• **Early 1990s**: Just as magnetic resonance imaging (MRI) threatened to make in-roads into several "CT applications," introduction of slip-ring or spiral or helical CT technology marked the beginning of a resurgence of CT scanning in clinical practice. Helical scanning obviated the need for wires and hence the "unwinding" time by using innovative slip-rings on the gantry assembly. An increase in temporal resolution (decrease in scan time) to subsecond durations and acquisition of contiguous volumetric scan data with helical CT scanners improved dynamic contrast-enhanced studies and three-dimensional (3-D) rendering of axial source data.

• **Late 1990s to 2005**: During this period, different vendors offered MDCT scanners with several different slice options from 2, 4, 6, 8, 10, 16, 32, 40, and 64 slices per revolution. The addition of multiple detector rows to the detector array of helical

CT scanners in the scanning direction or Z-axis allowed acquisition of more than one image per revolution of X-ray tube and detector array around the patient and led to development of multidetector or multisection, multichannel, multislice, or multidetector-row helical CT scanners. MDCT scanners offer several advantages over the prior helical and nonhelical CT scanners. In addition, there are several differences in the hardware and software components of single-slice helical CT and MDCT scanners. Depending on the detector configuration, MDCT scanners have multiple detector rows in the scanning direction or Z-axis. The number of detector rows in MDCT scanners can be less than the number of slices reconstructed per rotation (Siemens Sensation 64 with double Z-sampling), equal to the number of slices per rotation (LightSpeed VCT, General Electric Healthcare Technologies), or more than the number of reconstructed slices (LightSpeed QXi, General Electric Healthcare Technologies). For most MDCT scanners, the smallest reconstructed slice thickness is equal to the thickness of an individual detector row. For example, with 64*0.625 detector configuration (LightSpeed VCT), minimum slice thickness is 0.625 although it is possible to generate images with 1.25-, 2.5-, 3.75-, 5-, and 10-mm slice thickness also. However, one vendor (Siemens Medical Solutions) provides scanners that can acquire 0.4-mm slices with 0.6-mm detector width, due to double Z-sampling that occurs due to dynamic, online motion of the focal spot (Z-flying focal spot) and X-ray beam projections over adjoining detector rows.

Compared with single-slice CT, MDCT permits image reconstruction at various slice thicknesses different from the one chosen prior to the scan. Also, MDCT scanners allow faster scan times (330–350 milliseconds), wider scan coverage, and thinner section thickness. Higher temporal resolution helps in vascular and cardiac scanning, better utilization of contrast medium injection bolus, as well as scanning of uncooperative, breathless, or pediatric patients (less need for sedation or shorter duration of sedation). Wider scan coverage with MDCT scanners helps in vascular studies over longer regions, such as chest, abdomen, pelvis for aortic aneurysms or dissection workup, and peripheral CT angiography from origins of renal arteries to feet. Along with wider coverage, MDCT can also acquire "isotropic" scan data, which helps create exquisite 3-D or orthogonal multiplanar images. In addition, due to the wider detector configuration and use of cone-shaped X-ray, more complex cone-beam reconstruction techniques are used for MDCT compared with single-slice CT scanners. These cone-beam reconstruction techniques help reduce streak artifacts, particularly at the site of inhomogeneous objects in the scanning direction, such as ribs.

- **2005**: At 330–350 ms gantry revolution time, MDCT scanners are approaching the engineering limits of the gantry to withstand the mechanical forces from gantry components, so further improvements in scan time appear challenging. For cardiac or coronary CT angiography studies, however, a higher temporal resolution may imply better quality examinations in patients with higher or irregular heart rates. In this respect, dual-source MDCT scanners (Siemens Medical Solutions), with two X-ray tubes (both 80 kW) and two detector arrays (both with 64-slice acquisition per rotation with double Z-axis sampling), may prove beneficial by decreasing single-segment reconstruction scan time to 83 ms [3, 4]. However, patient studies are needed to validate the findings of initial phantom studies. Another recent innovation in MDCT technology is introduction of "sandwich" detector array (Philips Medical Systems), which can enable acquisition of images with characteristics of dual-energy spectra. The dual-source MDCT can also acquire dual kilovoltage (kVp) or energy image data when different kVp are selected for the two sources. However, rigorous studies will be required to assess the clinical potential of dual-energy CT scanning.

MDCT: Practical Approach to Building Scan Protocols

Several important considerations apply when building an "optimum" scanning protocol (Table 1). An "optimum" scanning protocol may be defined as one that provides adequate diagnostic information with an appropriate amount of contrast media and as low as reasonably achievable radiation dose (Table 2). Important aspects of a diagnostic CT study that must be considered while making a protocol are summarised in Figure 1 and include [5]:

- **Diagnostic indication**: Will help determine the number of phases (one or more, arterial, venous, delayed), scan area of interest, need for contrast (oral and/or rectal and/or intravenous), contrast administration protocol, scanning parameters, and appropriate radiation dose required to generate images to answer the diagnostic query. Development of specific scanning protocols for different clinical indications can help in optimizing workflow and managing radiation dose [6, 7].

- **Scan area of interest and scan direction**: It is important to predetermine the appropriate region of interest based on clinical indication [6, 8], for example, scanning of regions such as abdomen only, abdomen-pelvis, or chest-abdomen-pelvis. Concerns have been raised about "overextending" the scan area of interest, as faster MDCT scanners require very little extra time to cover extended scan

Table 1. Important scanning parameters and contrast considerations that must be addressed during development of scanning protocols for a given diagnostic indication

CT scanning parameters	Contrast consideration
Scan area of interest	Contrast versus noncontrast
Scan direction	Route
Localizer radiograph	Concentration
Scan duration	Volume
Gantry revolution time	Rate of injection
Table speed, beam pitch, beam collimation	Trigger-fixed, automatic tracking, or test bolus
Reconstructed section thickness	
Extent of overlap	
Reconstruction algorithms	
Tube potential	
Tube current and automatic exposure control	
Radiation dose	

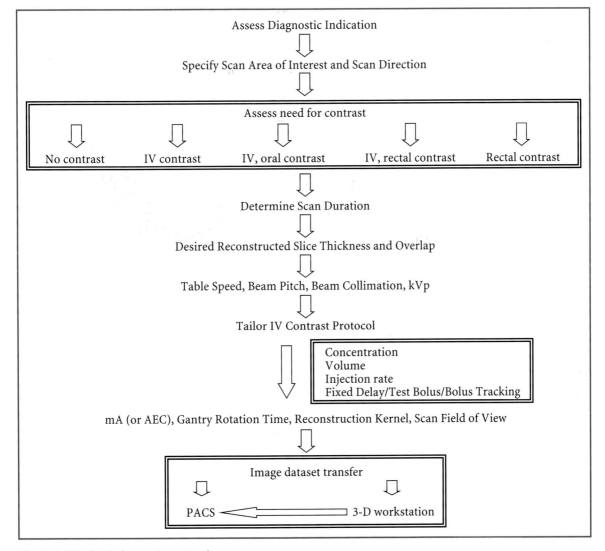

Fig. 1. Building blocks for scanning protocols

Table 2. Salient features of multidetector-row computed tomography (MDCT) scanners

Features	Details
X-ray tube	80–100 kW
	Higher tube current output (up to 800 mA)
	Less issues with tube cooling
	Z-flying focal spot (double Z-sampling)[a]
X-ray filters	Prepatient beam filters – to improve dose efficiency
	Bowtie filters – to reduce dose (especially cardiac applications)
Detector array:	> one detector row in scanning direction (Z-axis)
	Effective detector widths: may be constant or variable
	Effective detector row width (64-MDCT): 0.5, 0.6, or 0.625 mm
	Most scanners: effective detector width = section width
	Double Z-sampling: effective detector width $\geq$ section width[a]
DAS:	Represents data acquisition system or data channels
	Determines slice profiles (number of slices per rotation)
	Example: 4 data channels: 16 detector rows for 4-slice MDCT
	64 data channels: 64 detector rows for 64-slice MDCT
Detector configuration	Describes number of data channels and effective detector row width
	Example: 16×1.25 mm = 16 data channels; 1.25-mm row width
Beam collimation	Refers to X-ray beam width
	Cone-shaped beam leads to "overbeaming" (penumbra effect)
	= number of data channels × effective detector row width
	Example: 16-slice MDCT
	a. 16 data channels × 1.25-mm row width = 20 mm
	b. 16 data channels × 0.625-mm row width = 10 mm
	Radiation dose: b > a
Beam pitch	Table speed in mm per gantry revolution/beam collimation in mm
	Smaller effect on image quality for MDCT than for SSCT
	> 1: nonoverlapping, interspersed acquisition
	= 1: nonoverlapping, contiguous acquisition
	< 1: overlapping acquisition
	Low-contrast lesions (liver): prefer beam pitch <1
	High contrast lesions (CT colography): prefer beam pitch >1
Table speed	Closely related to beam pitch and beam collimation
	Usually described as table travel in mm per gantry revolution
	For mm/second: multiply with number of revolutions per second
	Compared with SSCT, MDCT provides higher table speed, allows faster scanning for thinner sections with dose savings

[a] Siemens 64-slice MDCT
MDCT multidetector-row computed tomography
SSCT single-slice CT

length. Determination of scan area of interest or scan length (which also depends upon patient length or height) can help to determine scanning parameters, scan duration, and contrast administration protocol. Scan direction is an important determinant of vascular contrast enhancement. In general, direction of scanning is similar to the direction of blood flow in the area of interest in order to follow the contrast flow column (for example, pe-ripheral MDCT angiography – craniocaudal) with few exceptions (for example, MDCT angiography of pulmonary embolism to avoid streaks from contrast in systemic veins – caudocranial).

- **Localizer radiograph:** With availability of automatic exposure control techniques and bow-tie filters (a hardware component of the scanner), it is important to emphasize to technologists that patients must be centered appropriately in the scanner. Acquisition of localizer radiograph with miscentering of patient in the gantry isocenter can lead to erroneous calculation of tube current with use of automatic exposure control technique, and this can affect resulting image quality [9, 10]. Likewise, localizer radiograph length must also include the entire scan area of interest, as some automatic exposure control techniques (Z-axis and XYZ-axis modulation) require these radiographs to estimate tube current [9].

- **Contrast consideration:** This aspect of scanning protocol is discussed elsewhere in the textbook.

- **Scan duration:** State-of-the-art MDCT scanners cover most routine CT studies of chest, abdomen and/or pelvis in a single breath hold, fast acquisition (less than 15 s). Further reduction in scan duration with MDCT will also be helpful to avoid or reduce need for sedation in uncooperative patients or children. Estimation of scan duration with MDCT scanning is most critical for catching the peak contrast enhancement over the scan length. Thus, estimation of scan duration can help optimize contrast media injection duration. Scan duration depends on several factors, such as gantry revolution time, table speed, and pitch, as well as scan area(s) of interest.

- **Gantry revolution time:** In general, the shortest gantry revolution time (such as 0.4–0.5 s) must be used for most CT studies. An exception to this rule is CT evaluation of a large patient, where use of longer gantry rotation time helps increase total tube current – time product [milliampere second (mAs)].

- **Table speed, beam pitch, and beam collimation:** For MDCT scanners, change in these parameters affects scan duration and radiation dose more than image quality. However, there are some exceptions to this rule. In the liver, use of higher pitch (>1:1 beam pitch) and faster table speed has been shown to be inferior to lower pitch and slower table speed for detection of small metastatic lesions [11]. Conversely, in high-contrast situations, such as CT colography and CT angiography, use of higher pitch (>1:1 beam pitch) and faster table speed does not affect image quality [2].

From scan length and scan duration, table speed can be estimated. For example, a 350-mm scan length for abdomen-pelvis in 10 s can be covered with a table speed of 35 mm/s or 17.5 mm per gantry revolution (at 0.5-s gantry revolution time). For a given MDCT scanner, desired table speed can then be achieved by selecting beam pitch, number of data channels, effective detector-row width, and gantry revolution speed. Thus, for an 8-slice

MDCT scanner, a table speed of 35 mm/s can be achieved with 0.875:1 beam pitch, 8 data channels with 2.5-mm effective detector-row width (detector configuration of 8*2.5 mm = 20 mm beam collimation), and 0.5-s gantry revolution time. When selecting the detector configuration and beam pitch – most notably, the effective detector-row width – one must take into account the required reconstructed section thickness. For example, if 1.25-mm section thickness is required for an 8-slice MDCT scanner, one must select 8*1.25-mm detector configuration (effective detector-row width = 1.25 mm) and not 8*2.5-mm detector configuration (effective detector-row width = 2.5mm). This becomes redundant for MDCT scanners with matrix array detector configuration, such as 64*0.625 mm (LightSpeed VCT) since users select the same detector configuration (64* 0.625 mm) to obtain any section thickness (0.625, 1.25, 2.5, 3.75, or 5 mm).

- **Reconstructed section thickness:** Compared with single detector-row CT scanners, MDCT ($\geq$4-slice scanners) allows acquisition of thinner section thickness in shorter duration and with less radiation exposure. However, an increase in indications for thinner sections with MDCT scanners can lead to overall increase in radiation dose contributions from these scanners. In such circumstances, radiation dose can be reduced by acquiring thicker sections and reconstructing thinner images from the volumetric raw data. Thinner sections have more noise content but higher spatial resolution and less partial volume averaging so that greater noise can be tolerated. Whereas thinner sections can now be acquired in a short duration, this also poses interpretation and archiving challenges to radiologists and their departments. Therefore, scanning protocols must define use of thinner sections- for interpretation or three-dimensional postprocessing on PACS or dedicated, stand-alone, image postprocessing workstations.

In general, for most routine abdominal CT studies, a section thickness of 2.5–5 mm is preferred for diagnostic interpretation. For these studies, multiplanar reconstructions can be performed at the scanner console from thinner reconstructions or directly from the volumetric raw data. Thinner sections are generally acquired for imaging of other regions of the body, including CT angiography studies of the abdomen.

- **Extent of overlap:** With isotropic scan data from most modern MDCT scanners, need for overlapping intersection distance is limited and can be avoided.

- **Reconstruction algorithms:** Reconstruction algorithms are an important component of scanning protocols. Selection of higher spatial resolution kernels (or sharper kernels) is necessary for viewing bones and lungs but can lead to unacceptably noisy images for soft tissues. Therefore, appropriate algorithms must be selected for specific regions of interest. A softer kernel (or a kernel with lower spatial resolution) provides smoother images and can help in decreasing noise content for low-contrast lesions, lower-dose studies, obese patients, or thinner sections.

- **Tube potential:** Most CT studies in adults are performed at 120 kVp. Tube potential (kVp) has a complex relationship with image noise, CT attenuation values (contrast), and radiation dose. A decrease in kVp increases noise and decreases radiation dose if other parameters are held constant but leads to higher attenuation values (except for water) and image contrast irrespective of other scanning parameters. The latter can help reduce the volume of intravenous contrast media administered for CT scanning. Low kVp CT can help in dose and contrast media volume reduction. Low kVp CT studies are especially well suited for high-contrast regions of interests, such as chest CT and CT angiography. To avoid inadvertently high image noise with low kVp CT studies, tube current may be raised. Several pediatric CT examinations can also be performed at lower kVp in order to reduce associated dose. However, kVp reduction in obese or large patients must be avoided to ensure adequate signal-to-noise ratio for acceptable diagnostic interpretation.

- **Tube current:** Unlike kVp, a change in tube current [milliampere (mA)] does not affect image contrast or CT attenuation values. However, reduction in mA is the most common method of reducing radiation dose. Either fixed tube current or automatic exposure control techniques can be used for maintaining adequate image quality and for managing radiation dose associated with MDCT [9, 12]. These techniques have been discussed in details in the chapter on radiation dose. Automatic exposure control techniques can help optimize tube current and dose irrespective of other scanning parameters. As automatic exposure control techniques allow dose optimization during each gantry revolution (XY-axes) and from one to the next gantry revolution (Z-axis), it may be more dose-efficient to use automatic exposure control over fixed tube current protocols [10, 13].

- **Radiation-dose consideration:** This aspect of scanning protocols is described comprehensively elsewhere in this textbook.

MDCT: Are there Disadvantages to the Technology?

Used appropriately, most state-of-the-art MDCT scanners can help reduce overall radiation dose compared with the prior single-slice or conventional CT scanners. Although each technological breakthrough in MDCT has contributed to improved resolution and coverage with expansion of its clinical applications, recent trends in radiation dose contribution from MDCT scanners are alarming. CT scanning contributes the most radiation dose among all medical radiation-based imaging procedures. Several experts have raised concerns over potential overuse and inappropriate use of MDCT scanners. Several vendors have introduced sophisticated techniques, such as automatic exposure control, detectors with better dose efficiency, improved reconstruction kernels, and noise-reduction filters, but much remains to be accomplished for optimization of radiation dose. Most importantly, the definition of "optimum image quality at lowest possible dose" for different-sized patients in different body regions for different clinical indications remains elusive. In the absence of these guidelines, users must employ strategies for dose reduction, when indicated.

Summary

In summary, understanding the fundamentals of MDCT helps adequate planning of scanning protocols.

References

1. Kalra MK, Maher MM, D'Souza R, Saini S (2004) Multidetector computed tomography technology: current status and emerging developments. J Comput Assist Tomogr 28 [Suppl 1]:S2–6
2. Kalra MK, Maher MM, Toth TL et al (2004) Strategies for CT radiation dose optimization. Radiology 230(3):619–628
3. Kalra MK, Schmidt B, Flohr TG et al (2005) Can dual-source MDCT technology provide 83 millisecond temporal resolution for single segment reconstruction of coronary CT angiography? 91st Annual Meeting and Scientific Assembly of Radiological Society of North America, November 27–December 2, 2005
4. Kalra MK, Schmidt B, Flohr TG (2005) Coronary stent imaging with dual source MDCT Scanner: an in vivo study with an ECG synchronized moving heart phantom. 91st Annual Meeting and Scientific Assembly of Radiological Society of North America, November 27–December 2, 2005
5. Saini S (2004) Multi-detector row CT: principles and practice for abdominal applications. Radiology 233(2):323–327

6. Campbell J, Kalra MK, Rizzo S (2005) Scanning beyond anatomic limits of the thorax in chest CT: findings, radiation dose, and automatic tube current modulation. AJR Am J Roentgenol 185(6):1525–1530

7. Jhaveri KS, Saini S, Levine LA et al (2001) Effect of multislice CT technology on scanner productivity. AJR Am J Roentgenol 177(4):769–772

8. Kalra MK, Maher MM, Toth TL et al (2004) Radiation from "extra" images acquired with abdominal and/or pelvic CT: effect of automatic tube current modulation. Radiology 232(2):409–414

9. Kalra MK, Maher MM, Toth TL et al (2004) Techniques and applications of automatic tube current modulation for CT. Radiology 233(3):649–657

10. Kalra MK, Maher MM, Kamath RS et al (2004) Sixteen-detector row CT of abdomen and pelvis: study for optimization of Z-axis modulation technique performed in 153 patients. Radiology 233(1):241–249

11. Abdelmoumene A, Chevallier P, Chalaron M et al (2005) Detection of liver metastases under 2 cm: comparison of different acquisition protocols in four row multidetector-CT (MDCT). Eur Radiol 15(9):1881–1887

12. Kalra MK, Prasad S, Saini S et al (2002) Clinical comparison of standard-dose and 50% reduced-dose abdominal CT: effect on image quality. AJR Am J Roentgenol 179(5):1101–1106. Erratum in: AJR Am J Roentgenol 179(6):1645

13. Kalra MK, Rizzo S, Maher MM et al (2005) Chest CT performed with z-axis modulation: scanning protocol and radiation dose. Radiology 237(1):303–308

I.2

Principles of Contrast Medium Delivery and Scan Timing in MDCT

Kyongtae T. Bae

Introduction

The advent of multidetector-row computed tomography (MDCT) technology has brought substantial advantages over single-detector-row CT (SDCT) in terms of image quality and clinical practice. The dramatically improved spatial and temporal resolution achievable on MDCT permits previously highly technically demanding clinical applications such as CT angiography and cardiac CT to be practiced routinely.

Another major advantage of MDCT over SDCT is that contrast medium can be used more efficiently and flexibly. However, in order to fully appreciate the benefits of MDCT, certain technical challenges involving scan timing and optimization of contrast enhancement need to be overcome. This chapter aims to review the numerous factors associated with contrast medium delivery and scan timing. Moreover, modifications to protocol design that are necessary for optimized contrast enhancement in MDCT are discussed, along with clinical considerations for CT angiography (CTA) and hepatic imaging.

Scan Timing and Factors Affecting Contrast Medium Delivery

The principal factors affecting contrast medium enhancement in CT imaging can be grouped into three broad categories: the patient, the injection of contrast medium, and the CT scan. Whereas factors associated with the former two categories determine the contrast enhancement process itself (independently of the CT scan), factors associated with the latter category (i.e., image acquisition parameters) play a critical role in permitting optimal visualization of the resulting contrast enhancement at specific time points. Whereas patient and injection factors involved in contrast enhancement are highly interrelated, some factors more closely affect the magnitude of contrast enhancement while others more closely affect the timing of contrast enhancement.

Patient Factors

The principal patient-related factors that influence contrast enhancement are body weight and cardiac output (cardiovascular circulation time). Other factors that can be considered of less significance include height, gender, age, venous access, renal function, and various pathological conditions.

Body Weight

The most important patient-related factor affecting the magnitude of vascular and parenchymal contrast enhancement is body weight [1–4]. Since large patients have larger blood volumes than small patients, contrast medium administered into the blood compartment of a large patient is diluted more than that administered to a small patient. The result is a reduced magnitude of contrast enhancement. Patient weight and the magnitude of enhancement are inversely related in a nearly one-to-one linear fashion. For a given administered dose of contrast medium, the magnitude of contrast enhancement is reduced proportionally to patient weight (Fig. 1). However, whereas the magnitude of contrast enhancement is strongly affected by patient weight, the timing of enhancement is largely unaffected by this parameter due to the concomitant proportional increase in both blood volume and cardiac output [3, 5, 6]. The result is a largely unaltered contrast medium circulation time that is independent of patient weight.

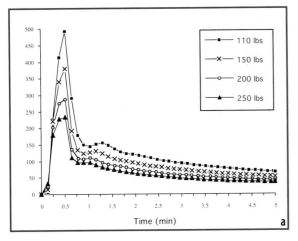

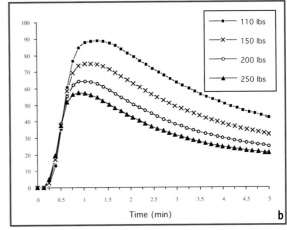

Fig. 1a, b. Simulated contrast enhancement curves with four different body weights. Simulated enhancement curves of the **a** aorta and **b** liver based on a hypothetical adult male with a fixed height (5'8" or 173 cm) and varying body weight (110, 160, 200, and 260 lbs, or 49.8, 72.5, 90.7, and 117.9 kg), subjected to injection of 125 ml of contrast medium at 5 ml/s (14). The magnitude of contrast enhancement is inversely proportional to body weight. (Reprinted from [53])

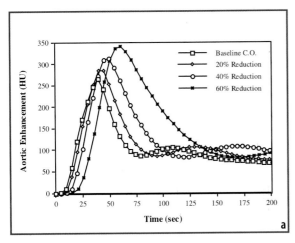

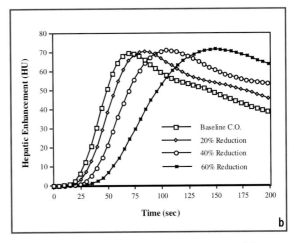

Fig. 2a, b. Simulated contrast enhancement curves at baseline and reduced cardiac outputs. Simulated enhancement curves of the **a** aorta and **b** liver based on a hypothetical adult male with a fixed height (5'8", or 173 cm) and body weight (150 lbs, or 68 kg), subjected to injection of 120 ml of contrast agent at 4 ml/s. A set of aortic and hepatic contrast enhancement curves was generated by reducing the baseline cardiac output, i.e., 6,500 ml/min, by 20%, 40%, and 60%. (Reprinted from [53])

Practical Tips

1. To maintain a constant degree of contrast enhancement in larger patients, one should consider increasing the overall iodine dose by increasing contrast medium volume and/or concentration. Increasing injection rate also increases the magnitude of vascular contrast enhancement (and hepatic enhancement in limited circumstances).
2. The timing of enhancement is largely unaffected by patient weight.

Cardiac Output

The most important patient-related factor affecting the timing of contrast enhancement is cardiac output (or cardiovascular circulation time) [7]. As cardiac output is reduced, the circulation of contrast

medium slows, resulting in delayed contrast bolus arrival and delayed peak arterial and parenchymal enhancement (Fig. 2). The time delay between injection of the contrast medium bolus and the arrival of peak enhancement in the aorta and liver is highly correlated with, and linearly proportional to, cardiac output. Thus, in patients with reduced cardiac output, once the contrast bolus arrives in the central blood compartment, it is cleared more slowly, resulting in a higher, prolonged enhancement.

A consequence of the slower contrast bolus clearance in patients with reduced cardiac output is an increased magnitude of peak aortic and parenchymal enhancement. The rate of increase, however, is different in the aorta and liver. Whereas the magnitude of peak aortic enhancement increases substantially in patients with reduced cardiac output, the magnitude of peak hepatic enhancement increases only slightly.

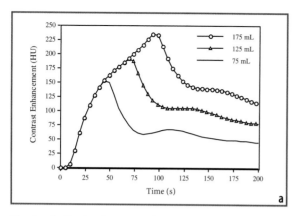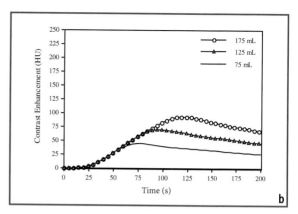

Fig. 3a, b. Simulated contrast enhancement curves with three different contrast medium volumes. Simulated enhancement curves of the **a** aorta and **b** liver based on a hypothetical adult male with a fixed height (5′8″, or 173 cm) and body weight (150 lbs, or 68 kg), subjected to injection of 75, 125, and 175 ml of contrast medium at 2 ml/s. Time-to-peak and magnitude of enhancement peak increases with contrast medium volume. (Reprinted from [53])

Practical Tips

1. When scan timing is critical, it is important to individualize the scan delay to account for variations in cardiac output among patients. Scan delay can be individualized by using a test bolus or a bolus tracking technique.

Contrast Injection Factors

Key factors related to the injection of contrast medium include injection duration, injection rate, contrast medium volume (injection duration × rate), concentration, and use of a saline flush.

Injection Duration

Injection duration, which is determined by the volume of contrast medium and the rate at which it is administered (injection duration = contrast volume ÷ injection rate), critically affects both magnitude and timing of contrast enhancement [8–13]. Increased injection duration at a fixed rate of injection leads to greater deposition of iodine mass. This results in increased magnitude of vascular and parenchymal enhancement, which is proportional to injection duration (Fig. 3).

The appropriate injection duration is determined by scanning conditions and the clinical objectives of the examination. Injection duration should be prolonged for a long CT scan to maintain good enhancement throughout image acquisition. An injection duration that is too short leads to insufficient contrast enhancement. On the other hand, too long an injection duration results in a waste of contrast medium and the generation of undesirable tissue and venous contrast enhancement. Pertinent clinical factors to be considered in determining injection duration include body size,

the vessel or organ of interest, and the desired level of enhancement [14].

A sufficiently long injection is particularly crucial in portal-venous phase imaging of the liver because the principal determinant of hepatic enhancement is total iodine dose administered [9–11, 13, 15–21]. Thus, for a fixed injection rate, the injection duration for a large patient should be longer than that for a small patient. On the other hand, for a fixed injection duration and contrast medium concentration, the injection rate should be adjusted according to the patient's body size to deliver the appropriate amount of iodine mass. In this case, larger patients require faster injections.

The duration of contrast medium injection is the most important technical factor that affects scan timing. In patients with normal cardiac output, peak arterial contrast enhancement is achieved shortly after termination of a contrast medium injection [20]. As the volume of contrast medium increases, so too does the time required to reach the peak of arterial or parenchymal contrast enhancement (Fig. 3). Conversely, a shorter time-to-peak enhancement is noted for a fixed volume of contrast medium injected at a faster injection rate (Fig. 4).

Practical Tips

1. The use of a higher contrast medium concentration or a faster injection rate facilitates faster delivery of the total iodine load, allowing use of a shorter injection to achieve the desired degree of contrast enhancement.
2. A rapid contrast delivery rate and short injection duration are desirable for arterial enhancement with MDCT but are much less important for parenchymal or venous enhancement.
3. A short injection duration (i.e., low volume and/or high injection rate) results in earlier

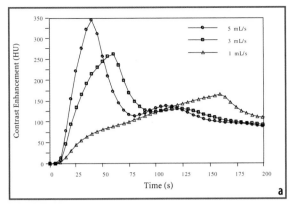 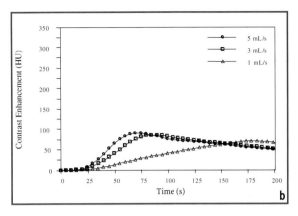

Fig. 4a, b. Simulated contrast enhancement curves with three different contrast medium injection rates. Simulated enhancement curves of the **a** aorta and **b** liver based on a hypothetical adult male with a fixed height (5'8", or 173 cm) and body weight (150 lbs, or 68 kg) subjected to 150 ml of contrast medium injected at 1, 3, and 5 ml/s. The curves show that for a fixed volume of contrast medium, as the rate of injection increases, the magnitude of contrast enhancement increases and the duration of high-magnitude contrast enhancement decreases. (Reprinted with permission from Bae KT (2005) Technical aspects of contrast delivery in advanced CT. Applied Radiology 32 [Suppl]: 12-19)

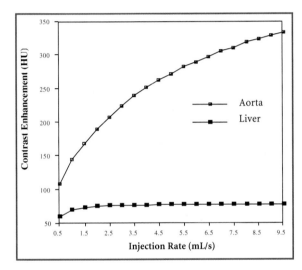

Fig. 5. Effect of contrast medium injection rate on the magnitude of peak contrast enhancement. Simulation of peak aortic and hepatic contrast enhancement at different injection rates based on a hypothetical adult male with a fixed height (5'8", or 173 cm) and body weight (150 lbs, or 68 kg) subjected to injection of 120 ml of contrast medium. (Reprinted with permission from Bae KT, Heiken JP, Brink JA (1998) Aortic and hepatic peak enhancement at CT: effect of contrast medium injection rate-pharmacokinetic analysis and experimental porcine model. Radiology 206:455-464)

peak arterial and parenchymal enhancement and requires a short scan delay. A long injection duration (i.e., high volume and/or low injection rate) results in later peak enhancement, and thus a longer scan delay is preferable.

Injection Rate

Both rate of delivery and total delivered mass of iodine are increased when the injection rate is increased at a fixed duration of injection. The magnitude of peak vascular and parenchymal enhancement increases with a wider temporal window of desired contrast enhancement. On the other hand, when the injection rate is increased at a fixed volume of contrast medium, the peaks of enhancement increase in magnitude and occur earlier and the duration of high-magnitude enhancement decreases (Fig. 4). However, for a given increase in injection rate, the rate of increase in the magnitude of aortic contrast enhancement is substantially greater than that of the liver (Fig. 5) [22–24].

To obtain a fast arterial CT scan (e.g., for MDCT angiography applications), an increased injection rate resulting in a shortened but elevated magnitude of arterial enhancement is beneficial. On the other hand, a longer injection duration resulting in more prolonged vascular enhancement is preferable for slower CT scans. Faster injection rate and shorter injection duration result in a longer interval between peak arterial enhancement and hepatic parenchymal equilibrium enhancement. Thus, a faster injection results not only in a higher magnitude of arterial enhancement but also in a greater temporal separation between the arterial and venous phases of hepatic enhancement (Fig. 6).

Practical Tips

1. The magnitude of peak aortic enhancement increases almost linearly with increases of injection rate (up to 8–10 ml/s) while peak hepatic enhancement increases much more gradually and is apparent only at relatively low injection rates (<3 ml/s).
2. A fast injection improves the separation of contrast-enhancement phases and thus is beneficial for multiphase examinations of the liver, pancreas, and kidneys, as optimized enhancement during each contrast enhancement phase may improve lesion detection and characterization.

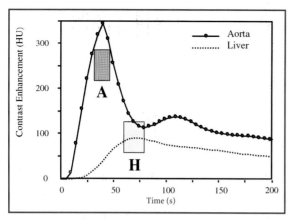

Fig. 6. Simulated aortic and hepatic contrast enhancement curves with a high contrast injection rate. Aortic (*solid line*) and hepatic (*dashed line*) contrast enhancement curves are simulated using a physiologically based compartment model (body weight 150 lbs, or 68 kg, and height 5'8", or 173 cm) subjected to a high injection rate protocol (150 ml of contrast medium injected at 5 ml/s) (14). A high injection rate not only increases the magnitude of arterial enhancement, but it also provides greater temporal separation between the arterial (*A*) and venous (*H*) phases of enhancement. This distinct phase separation is beneficial for multiphase scanning of the liver, pancreas, and kidneys. (Reprinted from [94])

Concentration

The availability of contrast media with high iodine concentrations (350 mgI/ml and above) has attracted a great deal of interest recently for MDCT applications [21, 25–39]. For injections of fixed duration, rate, and volume, a contrast medium with a high iodine concentration will deliver a larger total iodine load more rapidly. The resulting magnitude of peak contrast enhancement is increased, and the temporal window at a given level of enhance-

ment is wider. Conversely, time-to-peak enhancement is unaffected because duration and rate of injection remain constant.

On the other hand, when the need is to maintain a constant total iodine mass and injection rate, injection volume and duration vary with contrast medium concentration. Under these conditions, the injected volume of a contrast medium with high iodine concentration is smaller than that of a contrast medium with low iodine concentration. The duration of enhancement is shorter with the higher concentration agent because of reduced contrast medium volume. Nevertheless, contrast medium with a higher iodine concentration delivers more iodine mass per unit time and thus results in earlier and greater peak aortic enhancement (Fig. 7). The effect is the same as that seen with the use of a high injection rate.

Practical Tips

1. For a fast MDCT scan, a high iodine delivery rate is desirable to maximize arterial enhancement for CTA and to depict hypervascular tumors.
2. Use of a contrast medium with high iodine concentration is an alternative approach to using an increased injection rate to increase iodine delivery rate.

Saline Flush

A saline flush "pushes" the tail of the injected contrast medium bolus into the central blood volume and thus makes use of contrast medium that would otherwise remain unused in the injection

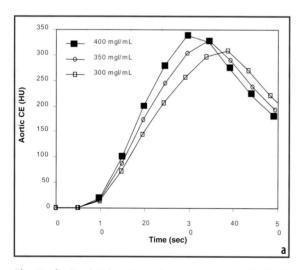

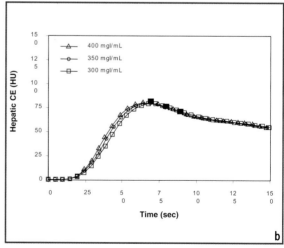

Fig. 7a, b. Simulated contrast enhancement curves with a fixed amount of iodine mass but three different contrast medium concentrations injected at a constant rate. Simulated enhancement curves of the **a** aorta and **b** liver based on a hypothetical adult male with a fixed height (5,8", or 173 cm) and body weight (150 lbs, or 68 kg) subjected to 5 ml/s injection of the same amount of iodine mass but at three different concentrations and volumes: 300 mgI/ml, 140 ml; 350 mgI/ml, 120 ml; and 400 mgI/ml, 105 ml. The aortic time-enhancement curves demonstrate that the use of high-concentration contrast material is associated with earlier and greater peak aortic enhancement. The effect of high iodine concentration contrast material on liver enhancement is minimal if iodine mass is unchanged. (Reprinted with permission from Bae KT (2003) Technical aspects of contrast delivery in advanced CT. Applied Radiology 32 [Suppl]:12-19)

tubing and peripheral veins. A saline flush therefore increases both the level of contrast enhancement and the efficiency of contrast medium utilization [40–47]. Additional advantages of a saline flush include improved bolus geometry due to reduced intravascular contrast medium dispersion and, on thoracic CT studies, reduced streak artifact from dense contrast material in the brachiocephalic vein and superior vena cava. A saline flush is particularly beneficial when a small volume of contrast medium is used. For this reason, a saline flush is commonly used for gadolinium-enhanced magnetic resonance imaging (MRI) but has not been widely used in CT, in part because a double-barrel CT contrast injector has not been commercially available until recently. With the increasing use of MDCT and the increasing clinical application of CTA, use of a saline flush is rapidly becoming accepted in clinical practice to compensate for the use of smaller contrast medium volumes.

The volume of contrast medium that can be substituted by saline flush without affecting the degree of contrast enhancement depends on the "dead space" volume of the injection tubing and the peripheral venous blood volume between the brachial vein and the superior vena cava. The peripheral venous blood volume is in turn related to patient size or weight. In a typical clinical setting, the amount of contrast medium saving may be anything between 12 ml and 20 ml.

Practical Tips

1. A saline flush improves contrast enhancement, the efficiency of contrast medium use and reduces artifacts; this is particularly beneficial when a small total amount of contrast medium is used.
2. Twenty to thirty milliliters of saline flush may be sufficient, and injection of a larger quantity might not further improve contrast enhancement.

Arterial CT Angiography

MDCT readily permits acquisition of images with high spatial and temporal resolution. The benefits of MDCT angiography are such that most conventional catheter-based diagnostic angiography examinations have been replaced by this technique.

For example, pulmonary CTA is now the most commonly practiced CTA application in the routine clinical setting. Improved spatial resolution on MDCT permits excellent delineation of peripheral pulmonary arteries and detection of small emboli. Improved temporal resolution deriving from increased scan speeds on the more recent 16- and 64-slice MDCT scanners permits a pulmonary CTA

examination to be performed within a few seconds. Moreover, better temporal resolution results in reduced motion artifacts, with improved contrast enhancement and image quality. Advances in MDCT and electrocardiogram (ECG)-gating technology enable acquisition of high-resolution, motion-free images of the heart and coronary CTA within a single short breath hold. Aortic CTA and peripheral run-off CTA are additional routine applications with MDCT.

Contrast Enhancement Magnitude

As discussed above, the magnitude of arterial contrast enhancement for CTA depends on a number of patient-related and injection-related factors, including body weight and cardiac output, contrast medium volume and concentration, injection rate, type of contrast medium, and saline flush. The magnitude of arterial enhancement increases in direct proportion to the rate of iodine delivery, which is dependent on injection rate and contrast medium concentration (Figs. 4 and 7). In addition, when contrast medium is injected at a constant rate, enhancement increases continuously over time, with increasing injection duration due to the cumulative effects of new incoming contrast medium and recirculated contrast medium. Without recirculation, contrast enhancement reaches a steady-state plateau. The use of a contrast medium with a higher iodine concentration results in a greater magnitude of aortic contrast enhancement, even if the total iodine dose and injection rate are unchanged. This is due to the increased rate of iodine delivery into the vascular system.

The amount of contrast medium required for CTA is determined by the desired level of enhancement, vessels of interest, and scan duration. Although the magnitude of hepatic enhancement needed to detect focal lesions has been investigated extensively, to date, only a few studies have addressed the minimum degree of enhancement needed for CTA. Becker et al. [26] considered an attenuation of 250–300 HU to be optimal for coronary CTA since this attenuation permitted adequate differentiation of low-density coronary artery atherosclerotic lesions (which typically have a density of approximately 40 HU), intermediate fibrous plaques (approximately 90 HU), and calcified plaques (>350 HU) without obscuring coronary calcifications. However, when imaging is performed to identify significant stenoses, visualization of the lumen is more important, and higher vascular attenuation (>300 HU) may improve visualization of small coronary vessels [39]. In our opinion, for most CTA applications, contrast enhancement of 250–300 HU (i.e., attenuation of

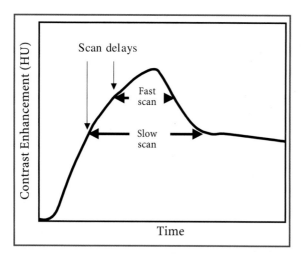

Fig. 8. Simulated aortic contrast enhancement curve with two different scan delays designated for the fast and the slow scans. For given duration of contrast enhancement or injection, the shorter the scan duration, the longer the additional delay needed to ensure that imaging takes place during the peak of aortic enhancement

300–350 HU) is adequate for the diagnosis of a wide range of vascular pathology.

In a coronary CTA study performed on a 4-row MDCT scanner, Becker et al. [26] reported that 40 g iodine (gI) (equivalent to 114 ml of a 350 mgI/ml concentration) injected at a flow rate of 1 gI/s (equivalent to 3.3 ml/s of a 350 mgI/ml concentration) resulted in an attenuation of 250–300 HU although no information was given about patient weight. In a similar but more elaborate comparative coronary CTA study with 16-row MDCT, Cademartiri et al. [39] reported that 42–49 gI at an injection rate of 1.2–1.4 gI/s generated a mean coronary artery attenuation of 273–333 HU (average patient weight 72–74 kg). In our experience, with a 64-row MDCT scanner, a volume of approximately 1.2 ml/kg of 350 mgI/ml contrast medium injected at a rate of 4 ml/s (i.e., 0.4 gI/kg of contrast medium injected at 1.4 gI/s) yields a contrast enhancement of approximately 250 HU in the pulmonary artery. Based on these observations, we thus estimate that diagnostically adequate coronary artery enhancement may be obtained for a 70-kg patient with (1) 45 gI injected at 1.2 gI/s (e.g., 128 ml of 350 mgI/ml concentration @ 3.3 ml/s) over 40 s for 4-row MDCT, (2) 42 gI injected at 1.4 gI/s (e.g., 120 ml of 350 mgI/ml concentration @ 4 ml/s) over 30 s for 16-row MDCT, and (3) 35 gI injected at 1.4 gI/s (e.g., 100 ml of 350 mgI/ml concentration @ 4 ml/s) over 25 s for 64-row MDCT. With these contrast medium administration schemes, a mean coronary artery attenuation of 300–350 HU can be expected for a 70-kg patient. A saline flush may further reduce the contrast medium requirement by 15–25 ml as well as helping to reduce the level of artifact in the superior vena cava and right heart. In order to maintain an equivalent degree of

contrast enhancement, larger patients require a larger iodine dose while smaller patients require a smaller iodine dose.

For peripheral run-off CTA, the amount of contrast medium required for adequate enhancement of the abdominal aorta and peripheral arteries depends on patient weight and scan duration. For a patient with a body weight of 60–80 kg, an injection rate of 1.4 gI/s (4 ml/s of a 350 mgI/ml concentration) is probably sufficient. This is similar to the scheme for pulmonary and coronary CTA described above. The rate can be increased or decreased depending on the patient's body weight and the concentration of contrast medium used.

A common approach to selecting the injection duration for a CTA examination with a long scan time (>25 s) is to keep injection duration identical to scan duration. This approach, however, does not work with a short scan time (<15 s). If scan time and injection duration are equally short, then the result will be poor overall enhancement. Although enhancement can be improved by using a faster injection rate or a higher iodine concentration, there are clear practical restrictions on the extent to which these parameters can be increased to compensate for a short injection duration or low contrast volume.

Practical Tips

1. When contrast medium volume is reduced for CT angiography with MDCT, an increased injection rate and high contrast medium concentration can compensate for the somewhat decreased magnitude of aortic enhancement achieved with the smaller contrast medium volume.

2. One approach to estimating the injection duration for a short scan may be to add a constant factor to the scan duration. For a patient with body weight of 60–80 kg who receives contrast medium injected at 1.4 gI/s (e.g., 4 ml/s of 350 mgI/ml concentration), our proposed injection duration is "15 s + $\frac{1}{2}$ scan duration" with a saline flush or "20 s + $\frac{1}{2}$ scan duration" without a saline flush. The injection rate can be increased or decreased depending on body weight and the concentration of contrast medium used.

Scan Timing

Three factors should be considered for determination of scan delays for CTA or parenchymal imaging: (1) contrast medium injection duration, (2) contrast arrival time (*Tarr*), and (3) scan duration. In patients with normal cardiac output, peak arterial contrast enhancement is achieved shortly after termination of the contrast medium injection [20,

23]. Thus, in general, an injection of short duration (i.e., low volume and/or high injection rate) results in earlier peak arterial and parenchymal enhancement. In such cases, a short scan delay is required for CTA. On the other hand, an injection of long duration (i.e., high volume and/or low injection rate) results in later peak enhancement, and thus a longer scan delay is needed for CTA (Figs. 3 and 4).

In addition to injection duration, variation among patients in cardiac output (cardiovascular circulation time) should be taken into account when individualizing the scan delay for CTA studies. *Tarr* is related to the patient's cardiac output and can be measured using a test-bolus or bolus-tracking method. In our experience, the bolus-tracking method is a more efficient and practical approach although some radiologists prefer the test-bolus method because it provides an additional opportunity to "test" the integrity of the venous access prior to injecting the full bolus of contrast medium. With both techniques, a region of interest (ROI) is usually placed just proximal to the organ of interest, e.g., on the main pulmonary artery or right ventricle for pulmonary CTA or on the ascending aorta or left ventricle for coronary CTA.

Traditionally, for slow CTA studies (single-row and 4-detector-row scanners), the scan delay was chosen to equal a patient's *Tarr*. However, this approach does not provide precise scan timing when faster MDCT scanners and shorter injection durations are utilized. This is because *Tarr* merely represents time of contrast arrival rather than optimal scan delay. For fast (i.e., 16- and 64-row) MDCT scanners, an "additional or diagnostic delay" must be included to determine the appropriate scan delay [20, 28]. The significance of the additional delay for optimal enhancement has been demonstrated both empirically [48] and theoretically [49]. Determination of the appropriate additional delay, which is related to scan speed and injection duration, is critical for fast MDCT. The shorter the scan duration, the longer the additional delay needed to ensure that imaging takes place during the peak of aortic enhancement (Fig. 8), unless the injection duration is shortened to match the reduced scan duration.

For the majority of pulmonary CTA studies, well-designed fixed scan delays (typically 15 s) are usually adequate because contrast enhancement in the pulmonary arteries increases rapidly with fast injections of contrast medium. However, precise timing in pulmonary CTA is crucial when a "tight" contrast bolus is used with fast MDCT because pulmonary artery enhancement can be delayed considerably in patients with cardiac dysfunction, pulmonary artery hypertension, or compromised central or peripheral venous flow [50, 51]. The need to individualize the scan delay for cardiac and coronary artery CTA is well recognized. For peripheral run-off CTA, it is crucial that the scan delay is long enough that the scan does not outpace the contrast bolus but is completed when the bolus reaches the pedal arteries. One approach is to reduce scan speed and to use a longer injection to match scan duration; this may be particularly appropriate for imaging diseased peripheral vessels [52].

Our proposed approach to determining a scan delay involves: (1) estimating time-to-peak contrast enhancement from injection duration and *Tarr*, and (2) calculating scan delay by subtracting one-half of the scan duration from the estimated peak enhancement time (Table 1, Fig. 9). Time-to-peak enhancement may be estimated using either a "variable" approach, in which *Tarr* is estimated assuming normal circulation, or a "circulation-adjusted" approach, in which *Tarr* is measured using a test-bolus or bolus-tracking technique.

For the variable scan delay approach, time-to-peak aortic enhancement is determined as "injection duration + (x s)," in which "x" is larger for shorter injection durations but is typically a number between 0 and 10 [23]. For example, for a 30-s injection, the peak aortic enhancement would occur at "30+5=35" s (a 5-s additional delay is used in this example because a 30-s injection is considered to be of intermediate duration). Using this estimated peak time, scan delay for the arterial phase for a 20-s scan would be calculated as "35 – 20/2=25" s. Likewise, the scan delay for a 10-s scan would be "35 – 10/2=30" s.

For the circulation-adjusted delay approach, either a test-bolus or a bolus-tracking technique is used to measure *Tarr*. If 15 s is taken as the normal default value for *Tarr* (i.e., a typical value in a patient with normal circulation), time-to-peak aortic enhancement corresponds to "injection duration + (*Tarr* – 15)+(0 to 10 s)" or " injection duration + *Tarr* – (5 to 15 s)." Thus, at *Tarr* = 15, the circulation-adjusted and variable delay approaches are equivalent. The scan delay can be computed from this equation using the same steps as for the variable delay approach: for example, for a 10-s scan with a 30-s injection, the scan delay would be "30 + (*Tarr* – 15)+(5) – (10/2)" or "*Tarr* +15." Thus, when a test-bolus method is used, the scan delay is determined by adding 15 s to the measured *Tarr*. On the other hand, when a bolus-tracking method is used, *Tarr* is not estimated prior to the injection of a full bolus of contrast medium. In this case, the scan will start at "*Tarr* + 15": i.e., after 15 s of additional "diagnostic delay" once the 50-HU enhancement threshold is reached [53].

Practical Tips

1. Three factors should be considered when determining a scan delay for CTA: (1) contrast

Table 1. Contrast enhancement times and proposed scan delays in different applications

	Pulmonary CTA	Coronary thoracic aorta CTA	Abdominal aorta/peripheral runoff	Hepatic parenchyma/portal vein
Contrast arrival time (s)[a]	$Tarr = 7–10$	$Tarr = 12–15$	$Tarr = 15–18$	30–40 ($Tarr = 15–18$)
Peak time (s)[a]	From 15 to ID (peak reaches a plateau rapidly)	ID + (0 to 5)[b]	ID + (5 to 10)[b]	ID + (25 to 40)[b]
Fixed scan delay (s)	15 (20 for slow injection)	20	30 (20-25 for slow scan)	60–70
Variable scan delay (s)	15 (20 for slow injection)	ID + 5 – SD/2	ID + 5 – SD/2	ID + 35 – SD/2
Circulation-adjusted delay	$Tarr + 5$	ID + ($Tarr – 10$) – SD/2	ID + ($Tarr – 10$) – SD/2	ID + ($Tarr \times 2+5$) – SD/2

CTA computed tomography angiography, *Tarr* contrast arrival time, *ID* injection duration (s), *SD* scan duration (s)
For CTA, ID = "15 s + $^{1}/_{2}$ SD" (with saline flush) or "20 s + $^{1}/_{2}$ SD" (without saline flush) is suggested with the injection rate of 4 ml/s
For the liver, ID is determined by considering the total iodine load of 0.5 gI/kg
Peak time increases by 3–5 s with the use of saline flush
Tarr. **a** for pulmonary CTA, 100 HU threshold over the pulmonary artery with the first scan at 10 s after the start of the injection; **b** for aorta and hepatic phases, 50 HU threshold over the aorta with the first scan at 10 s after the start of the injection
[a] Assuming normal cardiac circulation, body weight of 60–80 kg, and the injection rate of 3–5 ml/s via the antecubital vein
[b] A larger number is used for a shorter injection duration

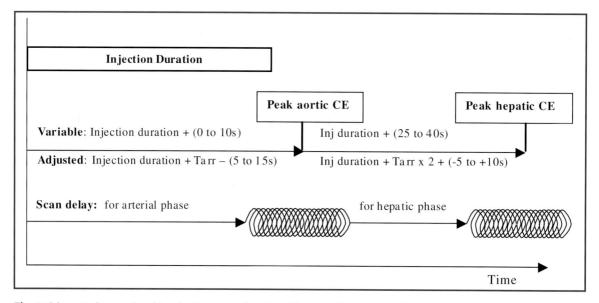

Fig. 9. Schematic diagram describing the times-to-peak aortic and hepatic enhancement and associated scan delays for a given injection duration. Times-to-peak enhancement of the arterial and hepatic phases are estimated from injection durations and contrast arrival times. We propose two approaches of estimating time-to-peak enhancement: variable (contrast arrival time is empirically estimated assuming normal circulation) and circulation-adjusted (contrast arrival time is measured using a test-bolus or bolus-tracking technique). From estimated peak time, scan delay can be calculated by subtracting one-half of the scan duration

medium injection duration, (2) *Tarr*, and (3) scan duration.

2. Traditionally, for slow CTA studies, the scan delay was chosen to equal a patient's *Tarr*. Because this approach does not provide precise scan timing with faster MDCT scanners and shorter injection durations, an additional diag-

nostic delay must be included to determine the appropriate scan delay.

3. The shorter the scan duration, the longer the additional delay needed to ensure that imaging takes place during the peak of aortic enhancement.

4. The scan delay can be calculated by subtracting

one-half of the scan duration from time-to-peak enhancement time. The time-to-peak enhancement in turn is estimated from the injection duration and *Tarr* using either a variable approach or a circulation-adjusted approach.

Hepatic Imaging

Among the many clinical applications for MDCT in hepatic imaging are: detection and characterization of primary or metastatic hepatic lesions, diagnosis of diffuse liver diseases, assessment of vascular and biliary patency or obstruction, tumor staging, monitoring treatment response, and preoperative evaluation for surgical resection. The high temporal resolution of MDCT permits the liver to be imaged during multiple precisely defined phases of contrast enhancement.

Multiphasic Hepatic Imaging

Approximately 20% of the blood supply to the liver derives from the hepatic artery while the remaining 80% derives from the portal vein. Injected contrast medium initially reaches the liver via the hepatic artery; in patients with normal circulation, the typical hepatic artery arrival time is approximately 15 s after the start of the injection. During the next 10–20 s, contrast medium from the splanchnic venous return enters the portal vein and hepatic parenchyma. However, whereas contrast medium from the splenic and pancreatic circulation arrives in the portal vein earlier than that from the intestinal circulation, the contribution of the portal vein to hepatic enhancement is usually very small within the first 30 s after initiation of the contrast injection [54, 55].

For routine abdominal CT or as part of a thoraco-abdominal and pelvic imaging survey, the liver is scanned once during the hepatic phase, i.e., during the phase of maximal liver parenchyma enhancement. However, to detect hypervascular liver lesions or to evaluate the hepatic vascular anatomy, it is highly desirable to scan during at least one phase prior to the hepatic phase. When optimizing multiphasic hepatic imaging, the goal is to scan during maximal enhancement for each phase and to minimize the influence of other enhancement phases.

For dedicated hepatic CT imaging, the three contrast-enhancement phases of interest are early arterial phase, late arterial/portal vein inflow phase, and hepatic parenchymal phase [56]. The early arterial phase begins with the arrival of contrast medium in the hepatic artery and ends prior to portal vein enhancement. The diagnostically useful early arterial phase begins about 10 s after contrast arrival and lasts for approximately 10 s (20–30 s from the start of contrast medium injection with a typical injection protocol and normal circulation). Prior to this, at the time of earliest contrast arrival in the hepatic artery, enhancement is too weak for adequate early arterial phase imaging. The late arterial/portal vein inflow phase (referred to simply as the late arterial phase in this chapter) corresponds to the time of maximum aortic enhancement. This occurs shortly (typically 0–10 s) after completion of injection, with the optimal temporal window lasting approximately 10 s. The hepatic parenchymal phase occurs when the peak contrast bolus has traveled through the splanchnic circulation and has returned to the portal venous system. This occurs typically at 25–40 s after completion of the injection and corresponds to the phase of maximum hepatic parenchyma enhancement.

The early arterial phase of enhancement is useful primarily for acquisition of a pure arterial data set for CTA and has only a limited role in imaging the liver. For detection of hypervascular primary or metastatic neoplasms, the late arterial phase is the preferred imaging phase [25, 57–67]. During this phase, hypervascular hepatic lesions enhance maximally while the hepatic parenchyma remains relatively unenhanced, commensurate with the relatively small contribution of the hepatic artery to the total hepatic blood supply. The hepatic parenchymal phase, the period of peak hepatic enhancement, is the phase used for routine abdominal CT imaging. Most hepatic lesions, including most metastases, are hypovascular and are therefore best depicted against the maximally enhanced hepatic parenchyma during this phase. The delayed imaging phase (>3 min after the start of contrast injection) is useful for detecting and characterizing some hepatocellular carcinomas [68] and for characterizing cholangiocarcinomas [69]. During this phase, hepatocellular carcinomas typically appear hypoattenuating whereas cholangiocarcinomas often demonstrate delayed contrast enhancement relative to the background hepatic parenchyma.

Contrast Enhancement Magnitude

The magnitude of hepatic enhancement is affected by numerous factors, such as contrast medium volume and concentration, rate and type of injection, scan delay time, and body weight [2, 7–10, 13–15, 22, 23, 25, 32, 33, 70–78]. The magnitude of hepatic parenchymal enhancement is directly and almost linearly related to the amount of total iodine mass administered (i.e., total contrast medium volume $\times$ concentration) [2, 8, 10, 15, 22, 23, 70–73, 75, 77, 78] (Fig. 3b). The most important patient-related factor affecting the magnitude of hepatic enhancement is body weight, which demonstrates a linear inverse relationship with the magnitude of enhancement: as body weight increases, the magnitude of hepatic parenchymal enhancement decreases [1, 2, 73] (Fig. 1b). As a consequence, the total iodine load should be increased when imaging large patients in order to achieve a constant degree of hepatic enhancement. The iodine load can be increased by increasing contrast medium concentration, volume injected, or injection rate [13, 23, 78].

Insufficient hepatic parenchymal enhancement results in diminished lesion conspicuity [16, 17, 73]. The minimum level of hepatic enhancement acceptable for adequate liver imaging has variously been reported to be 30 HU [79], 40 HU [80–82], or 50 HU [9, 33, 74, 77, 83, 84]. In a multicenter study, Megibow et al. [19] found that 30 HU was the lowest limit of acceptable hepatic enhancement and that no definite clinical gain was achieved with hepatic enhancement greater than 50 HU. The iodine mass required to achieve this enhancement can be estimated on the basis of patient weight [2, 77]. In this regard, Heiken et al. [2] found that the maximum hepatic enhancement calculated as a function of patient weight was 96±19 HU per gram of iodine per kilogram of body weight. Thus, approximately 0.5 gI/kg is needed to achieve the maximum hepatic enhancement of 50 HU; i.e., 35 gI for a 70-kg patient. A similar weight-adjusted dose conversion ratio was reported in later studies [37, 67, 73, 78, 85].

Hepatic parenchymal enhancement increases mildly with an increase in injection rate although this is apparent only at relatively low injection rates (<3 ml/s) [22, 23, 74] (Figs. 4 and 5). Although the magnitude of hepatic parenchymal enhancement may not increase substantially at high injection rates (e.g., 4– 6 ml/s) compared with intermediate injection rates (e.g., 2–3 ml/s), a fast injection rate increases the magnitude of hepatic arterial enhancement and thus better separates the peaks of hepatic arterial and hepatic parenchymal enhancement [23, 62, 86]. As a result, fast injection rates are desirable in multiphase hepatic imaging and for detection of hypervascular liver masses [62, 73–75, 86, 87] (Fig. 6). Likewise, recent studies [25, 33, 35, 37, 38] that compared contrast media with different iodine concentrations for dual-phase MDCT liver imaging found that high-concentration contrast medium increases detection of hypervascular lesions by increasing the iodine delivery rate (Fig. 7a).

Practical Tips

1. The magnitude of hepatic parenchymal enhancement is directly and almost linearly related to the total administered iodine mass per body weight. When imaging large patients, the total iodine load should be increased to achieve a constant degree of hepatic enhancement.
2. Approximately 0.5 gI/kg is needed to achieve the maximum hepatic enhancement of 50 HU; i.e., 35 gI for a 70-kg patient.
3. Although increasing the delivery rate of iodine (i.e., use of high injection rate or high concentration contrast medium) may not substantially increase the magnitude of hepatic parenchymal enhancement, it is desirable in multiphase hepatic imaging and for detection of hypervascular liver masses because it increases the magnitude of hepatic arterial enhancement and better separates the peaks of hepatic arterial and hepatic parenchymal enhancement.

Scan Timing

Fixed scan delays from the initiation of contrast medium injection are commonly used for hepatic imaging. The typical scan delay for arterial phase imaging for a 30-s contrast medium injection is 20–30 s for SDCT [58] and 30–35 s for MDCT. For both SDCT and MDCT, the scan delay for hepatic parenchymal phase imaging is approximately 55–70 s. Note that the scan delay required for arterial phase imaging on MDCT is longer than that on SDCT because the shorter image acquisition time of MDCT permits scanning to be performed more closely to the peak of aortic enhancement.

Whereas the hepatic enhancement phase lasts 20–30 s, with gradual changes in enhancement, the arterial phase lasts for only 10-15 s, with abrupt changes in enhancement [88]. Thus, it is more critical to accurately determine the scan delay for the arterial phase. The time to aortic contrast arrival varies widely, from 10–36 s [64, 66, 86, 89], due to interindividual variations in circulation time. It is therefore necessary to use a test-bolus or bolus-tracking technique to acquire images during individualized enhancement phases.

Both test-bolus [13, 25, 37, 64, 66, 78] and bolus-tracking methods [11, 32, 34, 86, 89–92] have been used to determine the arterial phase scan delay for dual-phase hepatic imaging studies. Typically, an ROI is placed over the descending thoracic aorta just above the diaphragmatic dome at the same level as the start of the diagnostic scan. *Tarr* in the aorta is measured from the peak timing of a test bolus (15–20 ml of contrast) or, when using a bolus-tracking program, from the time to reach a contrast enhancement threshold of 50–100 HU above baseline attenuation. In order to avoid the early arterial phase and to scan during the late arterial phase, a further 5- to 15-s delay is added to determine scan delay. As discussed above, the magnitude of this additional delay depends on injection duration and scan speed.

Scan delays for both the arterial and hepatic phases can be determined by considering injection duration, *Tarr*, and scan duration. The time-to-peak enhancement of the arterial and hepatic phases can be estimated from injection duration and arterial *Tarr* (Table 1, Fig. 9). The scan delay can be calculated from the estimated peak enhancement time by subtracting one-half of the scan duration. Again, both variable and circulation-adjusted approaches can be used.

Time-to-peak aortic enhancement is estimated as described previously in the section on CTA. For the variable scan delay approach, using an estimated peak time derived as "injection duration + (0 to 10 s)" [23], the scan delay for the arterial phase for a 20-s scan with a 30-s injection would be "30+5 – 20/2=25" s, while that for a 10-s scan would be "30+5 – 10/2=30" s. For the circulation-adjusted scan delay approach, the time-to-peak aortic enhancement corresponds to "injection duration + (*Tarr* – 15)+(0 to 10 s)" or "injection duration + *Tarr* – (5 to 15 s)." For a 10-s scan with a 30-s injection, the scan delay would be "30 + (*Tarr* – 15)+(5) – (10/2)" or "*Tarr* +15." When a bolus-tracking method is used, the scan will start at "*Tarr* + 15," i.e., after 15 s of additional diagnostic delay once the 50 HU enhancement threshold is reached [53].

Time-to-peak hepatic enhancement for the variable scan delay approach is estimated as "injection duration + (25 to 40 s)" [23, 73, 93]. Again, a longer additional delay is added for injections of shorter duration. For example, for a 30-s injection, peak hepatic enhancement would occur at "30 + 35 = 65" s. The scan delay for the hepatic phase for a 20-s scan would then be "65 – 20/2=55" s, while that for a 10-s scan would be "65 – 10/2=60" s. Using arterial *Tarr* measured over the abdominal aorta, for the circulation-adjusted scan delay approach, time-to-peak hepatic enhancement can be estimated as "injection duration + *Tarr*×2+(–5 to +10 s)." When *Tarr* is 15 s, this equation is again identical to that of a delay determined using the variable approach. For a 10-s scan with 30-s injection, the scan delay would be "30 + *Tarr*×2+(5) – (10/2)" s, or "*Tarr*×2+30" s. At a *Tarr* of 15 s, the scan delay for the hepatic phase would be 60 s.

Practical Tips

1. Three factors should be considered when determining scan delays for hepatic imaging: (1) contrast medium injection duration, (2) *Tarr*, and (3) scan duration.
2. For multiphase hepatic imaging, it is more critical to accurately determine the scan delay for the arterial phase than for the hepatic phase. A test-bolus or bolus-tracking technique is used to acquire images during individualized enhancement phases.

3. Time-to-peak enhancement of the arterial and hepatic phases can be estimated from injection duration and arterial *Tarr*. From the estimated peak enhancement time, the scan delay can be calculated by subtracting one-half of the scan duration. Just as with CTA, both the variable and circulation-adjusted approaches to estimating the times-to-peak enhancement are possible for hepatic imaging.

Summary

A variety of patient-related and injection-related factors can affect the magnitude and timing of intravenous contrast medium enhancement. Although these factors are interrelated, some (body size, contrast volume and iodine concentration, saline flush) have more of an effect on enhancement magnitude while others (cardiac output, contrast injection duration, contrast injection rate) have more of an effect on the temporal pattern of contrast enhancement.

MDCT, with its dramatically shorter image acquisition times, permits images with high spatial resolution to be acquired at multiple, precisely defined phases of contrast enhancement. However, to make full use of the benefits that MDCT provides, protocols for contrast administration and scan timing must be modified to take into account the specific objectives of each clinical imaging application and the different MDCT scanners available. For example, a faster injection rate or a contrast medium with high iodine concentration may be desirable for many MDCT applications to improve arterial enhancement and tumor-to-parenchyma attenuation difference during the hepatic arterial phase. Injection duration should be considered for determinations of scan delay because it critically affects time-to-peak enhancement. Individualized scan delay is more critical with MDCT than with SDCT. The contrast arrival time (*Tarr*) measured using test-bolus or bolus-tracking techniques can be integrated with injection duration to predict peak enhancement time. The scan delay is then estimated such that the center of the scan is timed to the peak of contrast enhancement.

References

1. Kormano M, Partanen K, Soimakallio S, Kivimaki T (1983) Dynamic contrast enhancement of the upper abdomen: effect of contrast medium and body weight. Invest Radiol 18:364–367
2. Heiken JP, Brink JA, McClennan BL et al (1995) Dynamic incremental CT: effect of volume and concentration of contrast material and patient weight on hepatic enhancement. Radiology 195:353–357
3. Platt JF, Reige KA, Ellis JH (1999) Aortic enhance-

ment during abdominal CT angiography: correlation with test injections, flow rates, and patient demographics. AJR Am J Roentgenol 172:53–56

4. Bae KT (2003) Technical aspects of contrast delivery in advanced CT. Applied Radiology 32 [Suppl]:12–19

5. van Hoe L, Marchal G, Baert AL et al (1995) Determination of scan delay time in spiral CT-angiography: utility of a test bolus injection. J Comput Assist Tomogr 19:216–220

6. Kirchner J, Kickuth R, Laufer U (2000) Optimized enhancement in helical CT: experiences with a real-time bolus tracking system in 628 patients. Clin Radiol 55:368–373

7. Bae KT, Heiken JP, Brink JA (1998) Aortic and hepatic contrast medium enhancement at CT. Part II. Effect of reduced cardiac output in a porcine model. Radiology 207:657–662

8. Dean PB, Violante MR, Mahoney JA (1980) Hepatic CT contrast enhancement: effect of dose, duration of infusion, and time elapsed following infusion. Invest Radiol 15:158–161

9. Heiken JP, Brink JA, McClennan BL et al (1993) Dynamic contrast-enhanced CT of the liver: comparison of contrast medium injection rates and uniphasic and biphasic injection protocols. Radiology 187:327–331

10. Chambers TP, Baron RL, Lush RM (1994) Hepatic CT enhancement. Part I. Alterations in the volume of contrast material within the same patients. Radiology 193:513–517

11. Kopka L, Rodenwaldt J, Fischer U et al (1996) Dual-phase helical CT of the liver: effects of bolus tracking and different volumes of contrast material. Radiology 201:321–326

12. Han JK, Kim AY, Lee KY et al (2000) Factors influencing vascular and hepatic enhancement at CT: experimental study on injection protocol using a canine model. J Comput Assist Tomogr 24:400–406

13. Awai K, Hiraishi K, Hori S (2004) Effect of contrast material injection duration and rate on aortic peak time and peak enhancement at dynamic CT involving injection protocol with dose tailored to patient weight. Radiology 230:142–150

14. Bae KT, Heiken JP, Brink JA (1998) Aortic and hepatic contrast medium enhancement at CT. Part I. Prediction with a computer model. Radiology 207:647–655

15. Berland LL, Lee JY (1988) Comparison of contrast media injection rates and volumes for hepatic dynamic incremented computed tomography. Investigative Radiology 23:918–922

16. Small WC, Nelson RC, Bernardino ME, Brummer LT (1994) Contrast-enhanced spiral CT of the liver: effect of different amounts and injection rates of contrast material on early contrast enhancement. AJR Am J Roentgenol 163:87–92

17. Freeny PC, Gardner JC, von Ingersleben G et al (1995) Hepatic helical CT: effect of reduction of iodine dose of intravenous contrast material on hepatic contrast enhancement. Radiology 197:89–93

18. Han JK, Choi BI, Kim AY, Kim SJ (2001) Contrast media in abdominal computed tomography: optimization of delivery methods. Korean J Radiol 2:28–36

19. Megibow AJ, Jacob G, Heiken JP et al (2001) Quantitative and qualitative evaluation of volume of low osmolality contrast medium needed for routine helical abdominal CT. AJR Am J Roentgenol 176:583–589

20. Bae KT (2003) Peak contrast enhancement in CT and MR angiography: When does it occur and why? Pharmacokinetic study in a porcine model. Radiology 2003; 227:809–816

21. Roos JE, Desbiolles LM, Weishaupt D et al (2004) Multi-detector row CT: effect of iodine dose reduction on hepatic and vascular enhancement. Rofo 176:556–563

22. Garcia PA, Bonaldi VM, Bret PM et al (1996) Effect of rate of contrast medium injection on hepatic enhancement at CT. Radiology 199:185–189

23. Bae KT, Heiken JP, Brink JA (1998) Aortic and hepatic peak enhancement at CT: effect of contrast medium injection rate – pharmacokinetic analysis and experimental porcine model. Radiology 206:455–464

24. Garcia P, Genin G, Bret PM et al (1999) Hepatic CT enhancement: effect of the rate and volume of contrast medium injection in an animal model. Abdom Imaging 24:597–603

25. Awai K, Takada K, Onishi H, Hori S (2002) Aortic and hepatic enhancement and tumor-to-liver contrast: analysis of the effect of different concentrations of contrast material at multi-detector row helical CT. Radiology 224:757–763

26. Becker CR, Hong C, Knez A et al (2003) Optimal contrast application for cardiac 4-detector-row computed tomography. Invest Radiol 38:690–694

27. Brink JA (2003) Use of high concentration contrast media (HCCM): principles and rationale-body CT. Eur J Radiol 45 [Suppl 1]:S53–58

28. Fleischmann D (2003) High-concentration contrast media in MDCT angiography: principles and rationale. Eur Radiol 13 [Suppl 3]:N39–43

29. Fleischmann D (2003) Use of high-concentration contrast media in multiple-detector-row CT: principles and rationale. Eur Radiol 13 [Suppl 5]:M14–20

30. Fleischmann D (2003) Use of high concentration contrast media: principles and rationale-vascular district. Eur J Radiol 45 [Suppl 1]:S88–93

31. Shinagawa M, Uchida M, Ishibashi M et al (2003) Assessment of pancreatic CT enhancement using a high concentration of contrast material. Radiat Med 21:74–79

32. Awai K, Inoue M, Yagyu Y et al (2004) Moderate versus high concentration of contrast material for aortic and hepatic enhancement and tumor-to-liver contrast at multi-detector row CT. Radiology 233:682–688

33. Furuta A, Ito K, Fujita T et al (2004) Hepatic enhancement in multiphasic contrast-enhanced MDCT: comparison of high- and low-iodine-concentration contrast medium in same patients with chronic liver disease. AJR Am J Roentgenol 183:157–162

34. Suzuki H, Oshima H, Shiraki N et al (2004) Comparison of two contrast materials with different iodine concentrations in enhancing the density of the the aorta, portal vein and liver at multi-detector row CT: a randomized study. Eur Radiol 14:2099–2104

35. Yagyu Y, Awai K, Inoue M et al (2005) MDCT of hypervascular hepatocellular carcinomas: a prospective study using contrast materials with different iodine concentrations. AJR Am J Roentgenol 184:1535–1540

36. Schoellnast H, Deutschmann HA, Fritz GA et al (2005) MDCT angiography of the pulmonary arteries: influence of iodine flow concentration on vessel attenuation and visualization. AJR Am J Roentgenol 184:1935–1939

37. Marchiano A, Spreafico C, Lanocita R et al (2005) Does iodine concentration affect the diagnostic efficacy of biphasic spiral CT in patients with hepatocellular carcinoma? Abdom Imaging 30:274–280

38. Itoh S, Ikeda M, Achiwa M (2005) Multiphase con-

trast-enhanced CT of the liver with a multislice CT scanner: effects of iodine concentration and delivery rate. Radiat Med 23:61–69

39. Cademartiri F, Mollet NR, van der Lugt A et al (2005) Intravenous contrast material administration at helical 16-detector row CT coronary angiography: effect of iodine concentration on vascular attenuation. Radiology 236:661–665

40. Hopper KD, Mosher TJ, Kasales CJ et al (1997) Thoracic spiral CT: delivery of contrast material pushed with injectable saline solution in a power injector. Radiology 205:269–271

41. Dorio PJ, Lee FT Jr, Henseler KP et al (2003) Using a saline chaser to decrease contrast media in abdominal CT. AJR Am J Roentgenol 180:929–934

42. Haage P, Schmitz-Rode T, Hubner D et al (2000) Reduction of contrast material dose and artifacts by a saline flush using a double power injector in helical CT of the thorax. AJR Am J Roentgenol 174:1049–1053

43. Irie T, Kajitani M, Yamaguchi M, Itai Y (2002) Contrast-enhanced CT with saline flush technique using two automated injectors: how much contrast medium does it save? J Comput Assist Tomogr 26:287–291

44. Schoellnast H, Tillich M, Deutschmann HA et al (2003) Abdominal multidetector row computed tomography: reduction of cost and contrast material dose using saline flush. J Comput Assist Tomogr 27:847–853

45. Cademartiri F, Mollet N, van der Lugt A et al (2004) Non-invasive 16-row multislice CT coronary angiography: usefulness of saline chaser. Eur Radiol 14:178–183

46. Schoellnast H, Tillich M, Deutschmann MJ et al (2004) Aortoiliac enhancement during computed tomography angiography with reduced contrast material dose and saline solution flush: influence on magnitude and uniformity of the contrast column. Invest Radiol 39:20–26

47. Schoellnast H, Tillich M, Deutschmann HA et al (2004) Improvement of parenchymal and vascular enhancement using saline flush and power injection for multiple-detector-row abdominal CT. Eur Radiol 14:659–664

48. Cademartiri F, Nieman K, van der Lugt A et al (2004) Intravenous contrast material administration at 16-detector row helical CT coronary angiography: test bolus versus bolus-tracking technique. Radiology 233:817–823

49. Bae KT (2005) Test-bolus versus bolus-tracking techniques for CT angiographic timing. Radiology 236:369–370 (Author reply 370)

50. Yankelevitz DF, Shaham D, Shah A et al (1998) Optimization of contrast delivery for pulmonary CT angiography. Clin Imaging 22:398–403

51. Washington L, Gulsun M (2003) CT for thromboembolic disease. Curr Probl Diagn Radiol 32:105–126

52. Fleischmann D, Rubin GD (2005) Quantification of intravenously administered contrast medium transit through the peripheral arteries: implications for CT angiography. Radiology 236:1076–1082

53. Bae KT, Heiken JP (2000) Computer modeling approach to contrast medium administration and scan timing for multislice CT. In: Marincek B, Ros PR, Reiser M, Baker ME, eds. Multislice CT: a practical guide: Springer, Berlin, Heidelberg, New York, pp 28–36

54. Leggett RW, Williams LR (1995) A proposed blood circulation model for Reference Man. Health Phys 69:187–201

55. Frederick MG, McElaney BL, Singer A et al (1996) Timing of parenchymal enhancement on dual-phase dynamic helical CT of the liver: how long does the hepatic arterial phase predominate? AJR Am J Roentgenol 166:1305–1310

56. Foley WD, Kerimoglu U (2004) Abdominal MDCT: liver, pancreas, and biliary tract. Semin Ultrasound CT MR 25:122–144

57. Hollett MD, Jeffrey RB Jr, Nino-Murcia M et al (1995) Dual-phase helical CT of the liver: value of arterial phase scans in the detection of small (< or = 1.5 cm) malignant hepatic neoplasms. AJR Am J Roentgenol 164:879–884

58. Oliver JH 3rd, Baron RL (1996) Helical biphasic contrast-enhanced CT of the liver: technique, indications, interpretation, and pitfalls. Radiology 201:1–14

59. Oliver JH 3rd, Baron RL, Federle MP et al (1997) Hypervascular liver metastases: do unenhanced and hepatic arterial phase CT images affect tumor detection? Radiology 205:709–715

60. Oliver JH 3rd, Baron RL, Federle MP, Rockette HE Jr (1996) Detecting hepatocellular carcinoma: value of unenhanced or arterial phase CT imaging or both used in conjunction with conventional portal venous phase contrast-enhanced CT imaging. AJR Am J Roentgenol 167:71–77

61. Paulson EK, McDermott VG, Keogan MT et al (1998) Carcinoid metastases to the liver: role of triple-phase helical CT. Radiology 206:143–150

62. Mitsuzaki K, Yamashita Y, Ogata I et al (1996) Multiple-phase helical CT of the liver for detecting small hepatomas in patients with liver cirrhosis: contrast-injection protocol and optimal timing. AJR Am J Roentgenol 167:753–757

63. Baron RL, Oliver JH 3rd, Dodd GD 3rd et al (1996) Hepatocellular carcinoma: evaluation with biphasic, contrast-enhanced, helical CT. Radiology 199:505–511

64. Foley WD, Mallisee TA, Hohenwalter MD et al (2000) Multiphase hepatic CT with a multirow detector CT scanner. AJR Am J Roentgenol 175:679–685

65. Lee KH, Choi BI, Han JK et al (2000) Nodular hepatocellular carcinoma: variation of tumor conspicuity on single-level dynamic scan and optimization of fixed delay times for two-phase helical CT. J Comput Assist Tomogr 24:212–218

66. Murakami T, Kim T, Takamura M et al (2001). Hypervascular hepatocellular carcinoma: detection with double arterial phase multi-detector row helical CT. Radiology 218:763–767

67. Kanematsu M, Goshima S, Kondo H et al (2005) Optimizing scan delays of fixed duration contrast injection in contrast-enhanced biphasic multidetector-row CT for the liver and the detection of hypervascular hepatocellular carcinoma. J Comput Assist Tomogr 29:195–201

68. Lim JH, Choi D, Kim SH et al (2002) Detection of hepatocellular carcinoma: value of adding delayed phase imaging to dual-phase helical CT. AJR Am J Roentgenol 179:67–73

69. Lacomis JM, Baron RL, Oliver JH 3rd et al (1997) Cholangiocarcinoma: delayed CT contrast enhancement patterns. Radiology; 203:98–104

70. Claussen CD, Banzer D, Pfretzschner C et al (1984) Bolus geometry and dynamics after intravenous contrast medium injection. Radiology 153:365–368

71. Harmon BH, Berland LL, Lee JY (1992) Effect of varying rates of low-osmolarity contrast media injection for hepatic CT: correlation with indocyanine green transit time. Radiology 184:379–382

72. Chambers TP, Baron RL, Lush RM (1994) Hepatic CT enhancement. Part II. Alterations in contrast material volume and rate of injection within the same patients. Radiology 193:518–522

73. Tello R, Seltzer SE, Polger M et al (1997) A contrast agent delivery nomogram for hepatic spiral CT. J Comput Assist Tomogr 21:236–245

74. Kim T, Murakami T, Takahashi S et al (1998) Effects of injection rates of contrast material on arterial phase hepatic CT. AJR Am J Roentgenol 171:429–432

75. Tublin ME, Tessler FN, Cheng SL et al (1999) Effect of injection rate of contrast medium on pancreatic and hepatic helical CT. Radiology 210:97–101

76. Hanninen EL, Vogl TJ, Felfe R et al (2000) Detection of focal liver lesions at biphasic spiral CT: randomized double-blind study of the effect of iodine concentration in contrast materials. Radiology 216:403–409

77. Yamashita Y, Komohara Y, Takahashi M et al (2000) Abdominal helical CT: evaluation of optimal doses of intravenous contrast material – a prospective randomized study. Radiology 216:718–723

78. Awai K, Hori S (2003) Effect of contrast injection protocol with dose tailored to patient weight and fixed injection duration on aortic and hepatic enhancement at multidetector-row helical CT. Eur Radiol 13:2155–2160

79. Bluemke DA, Fishman EK, Anderson JH (1994) Dose requirements for a nonionic contrast agent for spiral computed tomography of the liver in rabbits. Invest Radiol 29:195–200

80. Baker ME, Beam C, Leder R et al (1993) Contrast material for combined abdominal and pelvic CT: can cost be reduced by increasing the concentration and decreasing the volume? AJR Am J Roentgenol 160:637–641

81. Herts BR, Paushter DM, Einstein DM et al (1995) Use of contrast material for spiral CT of the abdomen: comparison of hepatic enhancement and vascular attenuation for three different contrast media at two different delay times. AJR Am J Roentgenol 164:327–331

82. Herts BR, O'Malley CM, Wirth SL et al (2001) Power injection of contrast media using central venous catheters: feasibility, safety, and efficacy. AJR Am J Roentgenol 176:447–453

83. Walkey MM (1991) Dynamic hepatic CT: how many years will it take 'til we learn? Radiology 181:17–18

84. Brink JA, Heiken JP, Forman HP et al (1995) Hepatic spiral CT: reduction of dose of intravenous contrast material. Radiology 197:83–88

85. Takeshita K (2001) Prediction of maximum hepatic enhancement on computed tomography from dose of contrast material and patient weight: proposal of a new formula and evaluation of its accuracy. Radiat Med 19:75–79

86. Shimizu T, Misaki T, Yamamoto K et al (2000) Helical CT of the liver with computer-assisted bolus-tracking technology: scan delay of arterial phase scanning and effect of flow rates. J Comput Assist Tomogr 24:219–223

87. Schoellnast H, Brader P, Oberdabernig B et al (2005) High-concentration contrast media in multiphasic abdominal multidetector-row computed tomography: effect of increased iodine flow rate on parenchymal and vascular enhancement. J Comput Assist Tomogr 29:582–587

88. Bader TR, Prokesch RW, Grabenwoger F (2000) Timing of the hepatic arterial phase during contrast-enhanced computed tomography of the liver: assessment of normal values in 25 volunteers. Invest Radiol 35:486–492

89. Kim T, Murakami T, Hori M et al (2002) Small hypervascular hepatocellular carcinoma revealed by double arterial phase CT performed with single breath-hold scanning and automatic bolus tracking. AJR Am J Roentgenol 178:899–904

90. Mehnert F, Pereira PL, Trubenbach J et al (2001) Biphasic spiral CT of the liver: automatic bolus tracking or time delay? Eur Radiol 11:427–431

91. Sandstede JJ, Tschammler A, Beer M et al (2001) Optimization of automatic bolus tracking for timing of the arterial phase of helical liver CT. Eur Radiol 11:1396–1400

92. Itoh S, Ikeda M, Achiwa M et al (2004) Late-arterial and portal-venous phase imaging of the liver with a multislice CT scanner in patients without circulatory disturbances: automatic bolus tracking or empirical scan delay? Eur Radiol 14:1665–1673

93. Irie T, Kusano S (1996) Contrast-enhanced spiral CT of the liver: effect of injection time on time to peak hepatic enhancement. J Comput Assist Tomogr 20:633–637

94. Bae KT (2004) Contrast injection techniques and CT scan timing. In: Claussen CD, Fishman EK, Marincek B, Reiser M (eds.) Multislice CT: a practical guide. Springer, Berlin, Heidelberg, New York, pp 121–128

I.3

Contrast-Induced Nephropathy: Managing At-Risk Patients

Richard Solomon

Introduction

The administration of iodinated contrast media (CM) is a standard component of many computed tomography (CT) examinations. The large number of procedures performed each year and the infrequency of adverse events attests to the safety of CM. However, a small number of patients experience adverse events that are directly related to the CM or the procedure being performed. In this chapter, we examine the issue of renal toxicity. Objectives of this review include recognizing the patients at risk for renal complications following CM administration and understanding strategies to minimize the risk in those who will receive CM.

Who is At-Risk?

Risk factors for the development of contrast-induced nephropathy (CIN) are well characterized. These risk factors include: (1) a baseline decrease in glomerular filtration rate (GFR <60 ml/min), (2) increasing age, (3) female gender, (4) intravascular volume depletion, such as might occur with chronic use of diuretics, (5) diabetes, congestive heart failure, or cirrhosis, and (6) the concomitant administration of drugs that diminish renal function, such as NSAIDs, cyclosporin, and cisplatin [1].

Appropriate screening before contrast administration is necessary to identify these high-risk patients. The most important risk factor, a low GFR, is most easily identified using a serum creatinine measurement and applying a formula to convert creatinine to GFR [2]. The most widely used formula, called the Modification of Diet in Renal disease (MDRD) or Levey formula (Fig. 1), can be found online at a number of sites (Table 1) or put on a personal digital assistant (PDA) for easy use in a screening protocol. A protocol to identify and manage high-risk patients is presented in Figure 2 [3]. Modification of this protocol to reflect the realities of the practice environment is appropriate, but the basic intent should not be lost. High-risk patients should be identified *before* contrast administration, and steps to minimize CIN need to be taken.

Estimated GFR/1.73 m^2 = 186 x Serum [creatinine]-1.154 x Age -0.203

x 0.74 if female x 1.21 if African American

Formula was empirically determined in a cohort of individuals (1628) (mostly white) with chronic kidney disease (determined by iothalamate clearance <55 mL/min/1.73 m^2).

Evidence from other studies suggests that it underestimates GFR by 25-30% in subjects with "normal" renal function.

Fig. 1. MDRD or Levey Formula

Table 1. Websites for Glomerular Filtration Calculators

Website	Calculation formula used
http://www.nkdep.nih.gov/ go to Health Professionals /Tools	MDRD
http://www.kidney.org/ go to professionals/Clinical tools/gfr calculator	MDRD
http://www.nephron.com/	MDRD
http://www.hdcn.com/calc.gfr.htm	MDRD

MDRD Modification of Diet in Renal Disease

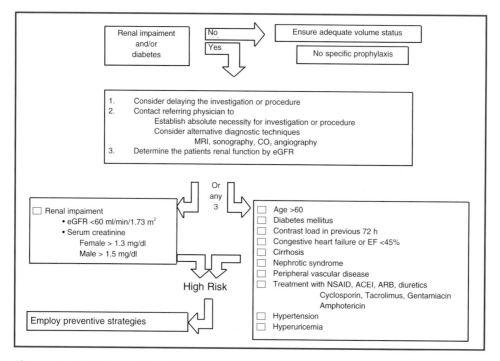

Fig. 2. Protocol (modified from [3])

Characteristics of the Contrast-Enhanced Examination That Enhance the Risk of CIN

In addition to these patient-specific risk factors, there are independent risk factors related to the procedure, including: (1) the volume of CM administered, (2) the route of administration, e.g., intraarterial versus intravenous, (3) a second CM study within 72 h, and (4) the specific CM used.

Since these are potentially modifiable factors, it is important to consider each factor when a high-risk patient has been identified. The risk of CIN is proportional to the volume of contrast administered, with no clear threshold dose [4]. There

is an interaction with the patient's level of renal function. A smaller volume of contrast can cause CIN as the level of renal function (GFR) falls. This has led to the development of a recommended maximum volume of contrast based upon serum creatinine although this has not been extensively validated [5]. Multidetector CT (MDCT) technology offers the opportunity to decrease the volume of contrast needed for a number of applications. Contrast volume can be decreased by a higher initial injection rate with subsequent variable flow rates, saline flushing, and appropriate timing of the acquisition of images after contrast administration. Use of the contrast agent with the highest amount of iodine per unit volume will also reduce overall contrast volume. Strategies for protocol

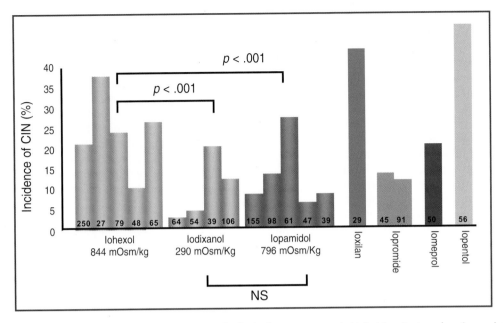

Fig. 3. Review of 17 prospective randomized trials of a single contrast agent in high-risk patients undergoing angiographic studies or interventions [9]. The studies included head-to-head comparisons and placebo arms of trials investigating prophylactic therapies such as theophylline, fenoldopam, and N-acetylcysteine. Number of patients studied is indicated on each bar. CIN = contrast-induced nephropathy, NS = not significant

building are beyond the scope of this chapter but are covered in other chapters in this volume.

At this time, CM use in CT is exclusively intravenous. Although the risk of CIN may be less with intravenous injection than with intra-arterial injection, this is not a reason to reduce one's efforts to prevent nephropathy. A second contrast exposure within 72 h increases the risk of nephropathy significantly. Often, the first indication that a patient was recently given contrast and is at risk for nephropathy is to see delayed retention of contrast in the cortex of the kidneys when performing the initial noncontrast scout images [6]. A second exposure to contrast should be delayed whenever possible in such a circumstance, and contrast should not be administered twice within 72 h unless it is urgently needed for patient management.

The type of contrast used also impacts on the development of nephropathy. Osmolality of the CM is one potential mediator of this toxic effect. Support for the role of osmolality comes from experimental animal data as well as clinical trial data. A meta-analysis of prospective randomized trials comparing high osmolality (>1,500 mOsm/kg) to low osmolality CM (700–800 mOsm/kg) found a reduction in the incidence of CIN with the use of low-osmolality CM. However, the risk reduction was statistically significant only in patients with a GFR <55 ml/min [relative risk (RR 0.50)] [7]. The recent availability of iso-osmolality CM (290 mOsm/kg) has raised the question of whether these agents would be less nephrotoxic than low-osmolality

agents. One comparative trial of iso-osmolality (iodixanol) versus low-osmolality (iohexol) CM in patients with both diabetes and renal insufficiency showed a lower incidence of CIN with the use of the iso-osmolality CM [8]. However, a systematic review of available data in high-risk patients from prospective trials involving low- and iso-osmolality CM does not support a benefit of iso-osmolality CM over all other low-osmolality CM [9]. In particular, the data show comparable rates of CIN with the use of iodixanol and iopamidol, another non-ionic monomer contrast agent. Indeed, it appears that the benefit observed in the study comparing iodixanol and iohexol may be related to the choice of that particular low-osmolality CM rather than a benefit attributable to the use of the iso-osmolality CM (Fig. 3). Randomized trials comparing the renal effects of iopamidol and iodixanol in high-risk patients may help answer this question more definitively.

Other Strategies to Minimize Contrast-Induced Nephropathy

A number of other strategies have been studied to minimize risk, particularly in high-risk patients. These include use of saline volume expansion and pharmacologic agents to produce renal vasodilation or interfere with generation of free oxygen radicals.

Contrast-induced toxicity to the kidneys is reduced by enhancing renal blood flow and urine flow. In practical terms, this means that patients should drink liberally the night before a contrast study or receive intravenous fluids starting the night before if they are high risk. The ideal combination of water and electrolytes is not known and may be patient specific. Correcting known extracellular volume depletion with saline, holding diuretics for 12 h, and encouraging oral water intake will suffice for most patients [1]. In situations that do not permit corrective measures beginning the evening before contrast exposure, a single-center trial found that an isotonic sodium bicarbonate solution (three ampules of $NaHCO_3$ in 1,000 ml D5W) significantly reduced the incidence of CIN in high-risk patients receiving intra-arterial CM. The isotonic sodium bicarbonate solution was given at 3 mL/kg/hr for 1 h before CM exposure and at 1 mL/kg/hr for 6 h postexposure [10].

Attempts to enhance renal blood flow with systemic vasodilator therapy have not been particularly successful. These agents – dopamine, fenoldopam, theophylline, atrial natriuretic peptide, endothelin antagonists, and calcium-channel blockers – have systemic effects that limit the degree of renal vasodilation. Strategies to find more specific renal vasodilators or to deliver these agents directly into the kidney are being evaluated.

Inhibition of the generation of reactive oxygen species may be protective in some patients. The initial trial of N-acetylcysteine (NAC) was performed in patients with renal insufficiency receiving contrast as part of abdominal CT procedures. A significant reduction in the incidence of CIN was found when NAC was administered orally at 600 mg twice daily on the day before and day of contrast exposure [11]. Subsequent prospective randomized trials conducted primarily in high-risk patients undergoing cardiac catheterization and percutaneous coronary intervention (PCI) found equivocal results [12]. Different patient populations and dosing schedules may account for some of these contradictory results. However, when taking into account the failure of many negative trials to get published (presented in abstracts at meeting), it seems our current enthusiasm for using NAC routinely in all high-risk patients needs to be tempered. Administration of NAC, however, is inexpensive and associated with little or no side effects. While this favors use of NAC, it does not obviate the necessity of the other protective strategies described above. Additional trials with other NAC dosing strategies – acute intravenous administration [13], double-dose oral administration [14] – have suggested an enhanced effect, but these strategies need further validation.

Conclusion

As the number of contrast-enhanced CT procedures increase and the target patient population has an increasing prevalence of comorbidities, the number of adverse renal effects will likely increase. However, appropriate screening for those patients at high risk and the employment of preventative strategies should minimize the percentage of patients who suffer from this adverse event.

For the CT service, a screening protocol (Fig. 2) can be employed to identify high-risk patients by using simple demographic, historical, and laboratory data. MDCT protocols to minimize the volume of CM used and the choice of an appropriate nonionic contrast agent may also reduce risk (Fig. 3). Collaboration with local nephrologists to develop practical pharmacologic interventions and volume expansion strategies is highly recommended.

References

1. Solomon R (1998) Contrast-medium-induced acute renal failure. Kidney Int 53:230–242
2. Levey A, Bosch JP, Lewis JB et al (1999) A more accurate method to estimate glomerular filtration rate from serum creatinine: A new prediction equation. Ann Intern Med 130:461–470
3. Gleeson T, Bulugahapitiya S (2004) Contrast-induced nephropathy. AJR Am J Roentgenol 183:1673–1689
4. McCullough P, Sandberg KA (2003) Epidemiology of contrast-induced nephropathy. Rev Cardiovasc Med 4 [Suppl 5]:S3–S9
5. Cigarroa R, Lange RA, Williams RH, Hillis LD (1989) Dosing of contrast material to prevent contrast nephropathy in patients with renal disease. Am J Med 86:649–652
6. Love L, Lind JA Jr, Olson MC (1989) Persistent CT nephrogram: significance in the diagnosis of contrast nephropathy. Radiology 172:125–129
7. Barrett B, Carlisle EJ (1993) Meta-analysis of the relative nephrotoxicity of high- and low-osmolality iodinated contrast media. Radiology 188:171–178
8. Aspelin P, Aubry P, Fransson S et al (2003) Nephrotoxic effects in high-risk patients undergoing angiography. N Engl J Med 348:491–499
9. Solomon R (2005) The role of osmolality in the incidence of contrast induced nephropathy: a systematic review of angiographic contrast media in high risk patients. Kidney Int 68(5):2256–2263
10. Merten G, Burgess WP, Gray LV et al (2004) Prevention of contrast-induced nephropathy with sodium bicarbonate: a randomized controlled trial. JAMA 291:2328–2334
11. Tepel M, Van Der Giet M, Schwarzfeld C et al (2000) Prevention of radiographic-contrast-agent-induced reductions in renal function by acetylcysteine. N Engl J Med 343:180–184
12. Kshirsagar A, Poole C, Mottl A et al (2004) N-acetylcysteine for the prevention of radiocontrast induced nephropathy: a meta-analysis of prospective con-

trolled trials. J Am Soc Nephrol 15:761–769

13. Baker C, Wragg A, Kumar S et al (2003) A rapid protocol for the prevention of contrast-induced renal dysfunction: the RAPPID study. J Am Coll Cardiol 41:2114–2118

14. Briguori C, Columbo A, Violante A et al (2004) Standard vs double dose of N-acetylcysteine to prevent contrast agent associated nephrotoxicity. Eur Heart J 25:206–211

I.4

MDCT Radiation Dose

Mannudeep K. Kalra

Introduction

Emergence of multidetector computed tomography (MDCT) scanners in radiology practice has increased the number of CT studies being performed for different clinical applications. This has raised concerns about risk of radiation-induced cancer with low-dose exposure associated with CT scanning. This chapter describes radiation dose quantities, scanning parameters that can be adjusted to optimize CT dose, and strategies for CT dose reduction.

Radiation Dose Quantities

Absorbed dose is the energy deposited in tissue/organs per unit mass measured in Gray (Gy). It is the basic quantity used for assessing the relative radiation risk to the tissue or organ. Effective dose represents a calculated quantity that accounts for the difference in radiosensitivity of different tissues. It compares relative radiation risk from different radiological procedures and is expressed in Sievert (Sv) [1, 2]. However, the principal dosimetric quantities that are displayed on the CT user interface include CT dose index volume (CTDI vol) and dose length product (DLP). These quantities can be applied to sequential or helical scanning for both single-slice or multislice scanners. The CTDI integrates the radiation dose delivered both within and beyond the scan volume. CTDI represents average absorbed dose across the field of view for contiguous CT acquisitions and takes into account regional variations in the absorbed dose. When CT scanning is performed with either gap or overlap between sequential scans (based on pitch values), the CTDI is scaled accordingly and results in the dose descriptor CTDI vol (mGy). While CTDI does not provide the dose given to any specific patient, it is a standardized index of the average dose delivered from the scan series. DLP represents the integrated dose and is equal to the average dose within the scan volume (mGy/cm).

In fact, most scanners provide CTDI vol and DLP values prior to actual patient scanning. These dose quantities can be used to compare radiation dose for different CT examinations, equipments, or imaging centers.

Strategies for Dose Reduction

There are several scanning factors that affect radiation dose associated with MDCT scanning [3]. These factors include those that can be modified by users and those that cannot be adjusted. CT scanning factors that can be adjusted to optimize radiation dose include tube potential, tube current, gantry rotation time, automatic exposure control, detector configuration, pitch, table speed, slice collimation, scan length, scan modes, scan region of interest, scanning phases, postprocessing image-based filters, metal artifact reduction (MAR) software, and shielding devices. In addition, there are several scan features that users cannot change, including scanner geometry, X-ray beam filters, prepatient tracking of X-ray tube focal spot, and projection adaptive reconstruction filters. We will focus on the scanning features that users can adjust to optimize dose.

Although there is an inverse relationship between image noise, an important component of image quality, and radiation dose, several studies have shown that diagnostic information can be achieved with substantial dose reduction [3]. Hence, all efforts to reduce dose must be preceded by evaluation of dose reduction effect on diagnostic requirements for specific indication or region of interest and for specific patient size or age.

Scanner Geometry

There is a considerable difference between geometry of single-slice CT and MDCT scanners that affects the distance between the focal spot of the X-ray tube and isocenter of the scanner. Also, it is not uncommon for large medical centers to have two or more scanner types. If all scanning parameters are kept constant, a scanner with short geometry will produce more interaction of radiation with the patient and lower image noise than a long geometry scanner. Thus, when scanning protocols are prepared for MDCT scanners, it is important to be cautious about the "transfer" of scanning parameters from one scanner type to another. Careful transfer of protocols helps in maintaining image quality with identical or reduced radiation dose depending on scanner geometry and other features (such as reconstruction algorithms) [4].

Tube Current (mA) and Tube Current-Time Product (mAs)

Tube current [milliamperage (mA)] reduction is the most frequently used method of reducing dose. Tube current-time product [milliampere second (mAs)] settings are proportional to the number of photons in the defined exposure time. There is a linear relationship between tube current and radiation dose. Thus, a 50% mAs reduction results in radiation dose reduction by half. However, mAs reduction should be performed carefully, as it leads to increase in image noise that can adversely affect diagnostic image quality.

Reduction in gantry rotation time (scan time) has been a main focus of MDCT developments toward improved temporal resolution. Use of fast scan time on MDCT implies shorter exposure time and lower radiation dose if all other parameters are kept constant. To allow a shorter exposure time, the X-ray tubes are designed to give better radiation output and improved heat capacity and heat dissipation. With development of MDCT scanners, tube cooling issues have been essentially eliminated, thus allowing a substantially higher mA with fast scan time.

Despite improved temporal resolution with MDCT, radiation dose can be higher than single-slice CT due to an increase in overall mAs. Increase in mAs with MDCT may be explained on the basis of increasing applications for thinner slices, which require higher mAs to maintain similar noise. Also, improved temporal resolution of MDCT allows multiphase acquisition protocols with high spatial resolution, which are associated with higher dose. Furthermore, in contradiction to single slice CT, considerably higher mAs values (about 800 mA at half-second rotation) can be used with MDCT

scanners for single- or multiphase CT studies.

Unfortunately, there is no data to limit increasing mAs with decreasing reconstructed slice thickness. Multi-institutional studies are needed to determine the optimum section thickness for various clinical applications and to define maximum possible tolerable image noise for these applications. It is important to remember that MDCT allows volumetric data acquisition, which can be used to retrospectively reconstruct thinner sections, albeit with higher noise. To avoid higher image noise, some institutions acquire thin sections in a prospective manner with smaller pitch and slower table speed. In such circumstances, a relatively higher noise may be acceptable, as thinner sections have higher spatial resolution and less partial volume artifacts. However, in regions with low inherent contrast, such as the abdomen, a small increase in noise can affect conspicuity of small, low-contrast liver lesions.

Several studies have recommended mAs reduction for MDCT scanning [5, 6]. In certain applications and patients, mAs can be reduced due to small patient size (children and small adults), high inherent contrast where diagnostic quality of MDCT is not affected by higher noise (CT colonography, kidney stone CT, routine chest CT, pelvic CT, maxillofacial CT, bony skeleton CT), and applications where lower resolution is acceptable (CT perfusion). Adaptation schemes for adjusting mAs and kilovoltage peak (kVp) to age, weight, or size of children has been evaluated for dose reduction with MDCT scanners [7]. As dose requirements in chest CT are much smaller than for the abdomen because of low X-ray absorption in the lungs, chest CT scanning can be performed at lower tube current than abdominal examinations. For chest MDCT [8], acceptable image quality with 50% reduction in tube current has been reported. Use of reduced tube current (20–80% dose reduction) has also been reported to be as effective as standard-dose scans performed at higher tube current for evaluation of acute lung injury, follow-up of malignant lymphoma and extrapulmonary primary tumors, lung cancer screening, coronary artery calcium screening, pulmonary nodule, benign asbestos-related pleural-based plaques, benign diseases in young patients, and guided lung biopsy [3]. Likewise, tube current reduction (20–80% dose reduction) has also been reported for routine head, paranasal sinuses, neck, abdomen, and pelvis MDCT examinations [3].

Automatic Exposure Control (AEC)

Automatic exposure control (AEC) techniques enable automatic adjustment of tube current to the size and attenuation of the body part being scanned to obtain constant CT examination image quality with lower radiation dose. Available automatic exposure control (AEC) techniques include angular modulation (in the X/Y plane), Z-axis modulation, and combined modulation techniques (both X/Y and z-axis). Several studies have shown 20–70% dose reduction with the use of these AEC techniques, depending on body region and patient size. Dose reduction with AEC has been reported in several MDCT applications, including neck, chest, abdomen, pelvis, and extremities. Furthermore, recent studies have reported substantially higher dose reductions with combined dose modulation techniques compared with angular dose modulation for MDCT of the neck, chest, abdomen, and pelvis [9–12].

Compared with the fixed tube current, AEC techniques can help in homogenizing MDCT scanning protocols for different scanners and applications. This is possible by selection of required or desired image quality (for example, noise index with Auto mA, GE Healthcare, and reference effective mAs with CARE Dose 4D, Siemens Medical Solutions) with AEC techniques instead of fixed-current values. Some vendors allow the user to control the extent of dose reduction to avoid an excessive drop in mA. Users can select desired image quality for AEC based on study indication irrespective of patient size. In fact, initial AEC studies have reported that selection of fixed tube current for scanning was associated with higher dose for small patients and lower dose for large patients [9, 13]. For clinical applications (such as CT angiography, kidney stone CT) that can tolerate higher image noise, the user can select a lower image quality requirement with AEC to achieve further dose reduction.

Despite several encouraging reports, there are several limitations to AEC techniques. Notably, selection of desired image quality for AEC must be performed carefully, as selection of higher quality can lead to higher radiation exposure. Further studies are necessary to define reference image quality requirements for different clinical applications of MDCT so that AEC techniques can then be applied in a more scientific manner.

Tube Potential (kVp)

Tube potential determines the energy of incident X-ray beams. Variation in the tube potential causes a substantial change in CT dose as well as image noise and contrast. Reduction in kVp leads to dose reduction and an increase in image noise as well as image contrast. Most MDCT examinations are performed at either 120 or 140 kVp, with little change to lower values. Some recent reports suggest substantial dose reduction with use of low kVp (80–100) for CT angiography studies in the head, chest, and abdomen [14–16]. In the abdomen, compared with 120 kVp, use of a 100-kVp protocol resulted in about a 37% dose reduction for MDCT angiography of the abdominal aorta and iliac arteries [16]. Likewise, substantial dose reduction (30–56%) has also been reported in cerebral and pulmonary MDCT angiography studies with use of lower tube potential (80 kVp). Use of lower kVp (80–100) for dose reduction has also been recommended for chest and abdominal MDCT in newborns and infants [7]. As reduction in kVp can result in substantial increase in image noise, image quality maybe impaired if the patient is too large or the tube current is not appropriately increased to compensate for the lower tube voltage. Thus, for very large patients, higher tube voltage is generally more appropriate.

Scanning Modes

Overranging of the X-ray beam with helical scanning on MDCT scanners leads to some amount of unused radiation extending beyond the beginning and ending of the region of interest. Due to this phenomenon, to achieve greater dose efficiency, efforts must be directed toward use of a single helical acquisition rather than multiple helical scans in the absence of overriding clinical considerations such as breathing movements. Use of multiple contiguous helical acquisitions should be restricted with modern high-speed MDCT scanners. However, this may be unavoidable in multiregion MDCT studies such as simultaneous neck and chest CT (position of the arm) or simultaneous chest and abdomen CT (differential delay time for contrast enhancement).

Scan Length

With rapid improvement in temporal resolution of MDCT, there is a tendency to increase the scan length (including regions beyond the actual area of interest in the neck, chest, abdomen, or pelvis). This increases the effective radiation dose to the patient [3]. Proliferation of whole-body screening CT studies must be restricted. It is also essential to draw the attention of requesting physicians to dose consequences of increasing scan length and to establish guidelines to restrict the examination to what is absolutely essential. In this regard, technologists or monitoring radiologists should restrict acquisition of any "extra images" beyond the actual area of interest [17].

Scan Collimation, Table Speed, and Pitch

These factors are interlinked to each other as well as to the detector configuration used for MDCT scanning. For helical CT scanners, pitch was defined as the ratio of table feed per gantry rotation to the nominal width of the X-ray beam. With MDCT, two terminologies were introduced for pitch: slice or volume pitch (ratio of table feed per gantry rotation to the nominal slice width) and beam pitch (ratio of table feed per gantry rotation to the beam width or effective detector thickness). The latter is preferred over the former terminology. A beam pitch of 1.0:1 implies acquisition without overlap or gap, a beam pitch of less than 1.0:1 implies an overlapping acquisition, and a beam pitch of greater than 1.0:1 facilitates an interspersed acquisition. An increase in the pitch decreases the duration of exposure received by the anatomical part being scanned. Faster table speeds for a given collimation result in higher pitch, shorter exposure time, and lower dose. A narrow collimation with slow table travel speed results in lower pitch, longer exposure time, and higher dose.

This relationship between exposure and pitch does not apply to scanners that utilize effective mAs and maintain a constant value of effective mAs irrespective of pitch value so that dose does not vary when pitch is changed. Many MDCT scanners automatically recommend or make the appropriate tube current adjustment to maintain a constant image noise when pitch is changed. Pitch has relatively lower effect on image quality of MDCT scanners than on single-slice CT scanners. A higher pitch is generally more dose efficient but tends to cause helical artifacts, degradation of section sensitivity profile (slice broadening), and decrease in spatial resolution [18]. Alterations in pitch can have varying effects on image quality in different situations. For instance, in CT colonoscopy and CT angiography studies, image quality and reconstruction artifacts are less affected by the pitch value than by beam collimation, so that a higher pitch with narrow beam collimation may be preferable to reduce radiation dose [19, 20]. However, in situations such as imaging of metastatic liver lesions or pancreatic lesions, which generally require thin collimation, an increased pitch may affect detectability, as lesions may be missed due to degradation of section sensitivity profile [21].

Generally, thicker beam collimation in MDCT results in more dose-efficient examinations, as overbeaming constitutes a smaller proportion of the detected X-ray beam. However, a wider collimation can limit the thinnest reconstructed sections. Conversely, although thin-beam collimation increases overbeaming X-rays, it allows reconstruction of thinner sections. Hence, beam collimation and pitch must be carefully selected to address specific clinical requirements. For instance, a wider collimation and pitch greater than 1:1 are usually sufficient for CT angiography studies and screening CT examinations, such as CT colonography and renal calculus.

Shielding

Shielding devices can be used to protect radiosensitive organs such as the breast, eye lenses, and gonads in pediatric patients and young adults, as these structures frequently lie in the beam pathways. With lead shields, thyroid and breast radiation doses can be reduced by an average of 45 % and 76 %, respectively, in patients undergoing routine head CT [22]. The use of a shield for radioprotection of eye lenses in paranasal sinus CT has also been found to be a suitable and effective means of reducing skin radiation by 40%. Recently, thinly layered bismuth-impregnated radioprotective latex shields have been found to reduce surface dose to breast, thyroid, and lens when they lie in the area of interest. However, use of gonadal shielding during CT examinations is controversial. A testis capsule (shield) can reduce the absorbed dose to the testes in abdominal CT whereas the lead apron is not appropriate for dose reduction to the ovaries (due to their inconstant position).

Metal Artifact Reduction (MAR) Algorithm

CT image quality can be affected by streak or starburst artifacts from metallic implants, such as joint replacement prosthesis, dental implants, or surgical clips. Often, either a second series of images are acquired (for face or neck CT in case of dental implants) to reduce loss of information from these artifacts or tube current is increased in an attempt to reduce these artifacts. Linear interpolation of reprojected metal traces and multidimensional adaptive filtering of raw data have been developed to reduce starburst artifacts from metallic implants' high attenuation objects [23, 24]. The MAR algorithms reduce starburst artifacts from metallic implants and are expected to be released for clinical applications in near future.

Noise-Reduction Filters (NRFs)

Noise-reduction filters (NRFs) have been developed to reduce noise in images obtained with reduced radiation dose or in thin images. Several approaches have been used to reduce noise in scan data sets comprising linear low-pass filter, nonlinear smoothing, and nonlinear three-dimensional filters.

NRFs are based on the principle that any image consists of a set of structural pixels representative of structures of interest and a set of nonstructural pixels representative of nonstructural regions. The NRFs perform isotropic filtering of nonstructured regions with a low-pass filter and directional filtering of the structured regions with a smoothing filter, operating parallel to the edges and with an enhancing filter operating perpendicular to the edges. Two-dimensional (2-D), nonlinear NRFs reduce noise in low-radiation-dose CT images but adversely affect the image contrast and sharpness [25–27]. A recent report documented a three-dimensional (3-D) NRF technique (3-D optimized reconstruction algorithm, or 3-D ORA, Siemens Medical Solutions) that generalizes the 2-D, nonlinear smoothing technique in all three directions (in X-, Y- and Z-axes) in order to avoid loss of image contrast and sharpness [28]. These NRFs may improve image noise without affecting contrast and lesion conspicuity in low-dose CT [28].

Conclusions

Several recent surveys have shown considerable variation in radiation dose with MDCT, which can lead to a higher radiation exposure from MDCT [29, 30]. Appropriate selection of scanning protocols and newer dose reduction techniques can help in radiation dose optimization.

References

1. McNitt-Gray MF (2002) AAPM/RSNA physics tutorial for residents: topics in CT. Radiation dose in CT. Radiographics 22:1541–1553
2. Rehani MM, Berry M (2000) Radiation doses in computed tomography. The increasing doses of radiation need to be controlled. BMJ 320:593–594
3. Kalra MK, Maher MM, Toth TL et al (2004) Strategies for CT radiation dose optimization. Radiology 230:619–628
4. Hamberg LM, Rhea JT, Hunter GJ, Thrall JH (2003) Multi-detector row CT: radiation dose characteristics. Radiology 226:762–772
5. Kalra MK, Prasad S, Saini S et al (2002) Clinical comparison of standard-dose and 50% reduced-dose abdominal CT: effect on image quality. AJR Am J Roentgenol 179:1101–1106
6. Kalra MK, Maher MM, Prasad SR et al (2003) Correlation of patient weight and cross-sectional dimensions with subjective image quality at standard dose abdominal CT. Korean J Radiol 4:234–238
7. Frush DP, Soden B, Frush KS, Lowry C (2002) Improved pediatric multidetector body CT using a size-based color-coded format. AJR Am J Roentgenol 178:721–726
8. Prasad SR, Wittram C, Shepard JA et al (2002) Standard-dose and 50%-reduced-dose chest CT: comparing the effect on image quality. AJR Am J Roentgenol 179:461–465
9. Kalra MK, Maher MM, Toth TL et al (2004) Techniques and applications of automatic tube current modulation for CT. Radiology 233:649–657
10. Kalra MK, Maher MM, D'Souza RV et al (2005) Detection of urinary tract stones at low-radiation-dose CT with Z-axis automatic tube current modulation: phantom and clinical studies. Radiology 235:523–529
11. Rizzo S, Kalra MK, Schmidt B et al (2006) Combined modulation and angular modulation techniques in CT scanning of abdomen and pelvis. AJR Am J Roentgenol (*in press*)
12. Mulkens TH, Bellinck P, Baeyaert M et al (2005) Use of an automatic exposure control mechanism for dose optimization in multi-detector row CT examinations: clinical evaluation. Radiology 237:213–223
13. Kalra MK, Maher MM, Kamath RS et al (2004) Sixteen-detector row CT of abdomen and pelvis: study for optimization of Z-axis modulation technique performed in 153 patients. Radiology 233:241–249
14. Bahner ML, Bengel A, Brix G et al (2005) Improved vascular opacification in cerebral computed tomography angiography with 80 kVp. Invest Radiol 40:229–234
15. Sigal-Cinqualbre AB, Hennequin R, Abada HT et al (2004) Low-kilovoltage multi-detector row chest CT in adults: feasibility and effect on image quality and iodine dose. Radiology 231:169–174
16. Wintersperger B, Jakobs T, Herzog P et al (2005) Aorto-iliac multidetector-row CT angiography with low kV settings: improved vessel enhancement and simultaneous reduction of radiation dose. Eur Radiol 15:334–341
17. Kalra MK, Maher MM, Toth TL et al (2004) Radiation from "extra" images acquired with abdominal and/or pelvic CT: effect of automatic tube current modulation. Radiology 232:409–414
18. Abdelmoumene A, Chevallier P, Chalaron M et al (2005) Detection of liver metastases under 2 cm: comparison of different acquisition protocols in four row multidetector-CT (MDCT). Eur Radiol 15:1881–1887
19. Power NP, Pryor MD, Martin A et al (2002) Optimization of scanning parameters for CT colonography. Br J Radiol 75:401–408
20. Laghi A, Iannaccone R, Mangiapane F et al (2003) Experimental colonic phantom for the evaluation of the optimal scanning technique for CT colonography using a multidetector spiral CT equipment. Eur Radiol 13:459–466
21. Rehani MM, Bongartz G, Kalender W et al (2000) Managing X-ray dose in computed tomography. ICRP Special Task Force Report. Annals of the ICRP 30:7–45
22. Beaconsfield T, Nicholson R, Thornton A, Al-Kutoubi A (1998) Would thyroid and breast shielding be beneficial in CT of the head? Eur Radiol 8:664–667
23. Mahnken AH, Raupach R, Wildberger JE et al (2003) A new algorithm for metal artifact reduction in computed tomography: in vitro and in vivo evaluation after total hip replacement. Invest Radiol 38:769–775
24. Watzke O, Kalender WA (2004) A pragmatic approach to metal artifact reduction in CT: merging of metal artifact reduced images. Eur Radiol 14:849–856

25. Kalra MK, Maher MM, Blake MA et al (2004) Detection and characterization of lesions on low-radiation-dose abdominal CT images postprocessed with noise reduction filters. Radiology 232:791–797

26. Kalra MK, Maher MM, Sahani DV et al (2003) Low-dose CT of the abdomen: evaluation of image improvement with use of noise reduction filters pilot study. Radiology 228:251–256

27. Kalra MK, Wittram C, Maher MM et al (2003) Can noise reduction filters improve low-radiation-dose chest CT images? Pilot study. Radiology 228:257–264

28. Rizzo SM, Kalra MK, Schmidt B (2005) CT images of abdomen and pelvis: effect of nonlinear three-dimensional optimized reconstruction algorithm on image quality and lesion characteristics. Radiology 237:309–315

29. Hollingsworth C, Frush DP, Cross M, Lucaya J (2003) Helical CT of the body: a survey of techniques used for pediatric patients. AJR Am J Roentgenol 180:401–406

30. Cohnen M, Poll LJ, Puettmann C et al (2003) Effective doses in standard protocols for multi-slice CT scanning. Eur Radiol 13:1148–1153

SECTION II

MDCT of the Abdomen

II.1

Dual-Phase Liver MDCT

Dushyant V. Sahani and Anandkumar H. Singh

Introduction

The advent of multidetector computed tomography (MDCT) scanners has provided an impetus for various changes in applications of computed tomography (CT) principles and their implementation in the design of CT protocols. The advanced MDCT scanners can produce isotropic voxel resolution, which can improve detection of subtle lesions in the organ. It thus remains the major imaging modality for detection of hepatic pathologies [1-4].

The main area of improvisation by MDCT for liver imaging appears to be in detection and characterization of small liver malignancies with better characterization of benign pathologies and vascular flow details [5]. Studies have shown that thinner images with MDCT provides some benefits, such as reduced volume-averaging artifacts, thereby improving diagnosis of focal hepatic lesions and hepatic vascular pathologies [6,7]. Also, due to shorter hepatic arterial acquisition time and thin collimation with MDCT, multiplanar imaging and CT angiography are much better [8].

Basic Concepts for Liver Imaging

The enhancement pattern of the arterial phase is dependent on the contrast medium injection rate, injection duration, and the time of the scan performed relative to the contrast bolus. The arterial opacification can primarily be controlled by the iodine administration rate, which is further dependent on the flow rate and the concentration of medium administered. It is important that the injection duration be longer than the scanning time to ensure strong vascular enhancement by the recirculation of contrast.

On the other hand, the parenchymal enhancement is independent of the injection flow rate and depends on the total volume (dose) of contrast administered. Thus, to obtain optimal liver parenchymal enhancement, a sufficient volume of contrast medium is required (approximately 120–150 cc of 370 mgI contrast agent). The iodine dose is directly proportional to the contrast volume administered and/or the iodine concentration of the contrast medium. Thus, increasing either would lead to an increase in dose. For example, for vascular mapping of the liver [computed tomographic arteriography (CTA)], arterial phase imaging is of paramount importance, and administration of a smaller volume of high-concentration contrast medium at a higher rate would suffice.

Contrast material later enters the extracellular space by diffusion, and this reduces the conspicuity of the liver lesion and its contrast with the surrounding parenchyma, later causing obscuration of the lesion. This is called the equilibrium phase, and it is important that the scan be completed well before this stage sets in.

Dual-Phase Imaging

Normally, the liver derives only 25% of its blood supply from the hepatic arterial flow and the remaining 75% from the portal venous system [9]. After the administration of iodinated contrast medium, opacification of hepatic arteries is encountered first, usually at 15–25 s (arterial phase). Liver enhancement in the portal venous system usually occurs between 45 and 55 s, followed by hepatic venous opacification at 60–70 s after contrast injection (portal venous phase). Based on the contrast circulation, the hepatic arterial phase (HAP) can be further divided into an early (true) arterial phase in which there is opacification of the hepatic arterial system without much parenchymal enhancement and a following late (dominant) arterial phase, which not only permits optimal opacification of the hepatic arteries but also higher parenchymal enhancement. This information is important in designing MDCT protocols, as hypervascular lesions are best visualized in the late arterial phase. In other words, better hepatic parenchymal contrast in the HAP is produced as a consequence of greater enhancement of hypervascular lesions and relatively less enhancement of the background liver parenchyma (Fig. 1). In the subsequent portal venous phase, these lesions are less conspicuous due to the higher enhancement of background liver parenchyma. Studies have demonstrated that HAP images reveal more numerous benign and malignant hypervascular liver lesions than portal venous phase (PVP) images [10], where most hypovascular lesions are evident (Table 1). Hence, dual-phase CT of the liver is performed in the late HAP and the PVP. Although initial reports supported the use of triple-phase scanning (early and late HAP and PVP) for evolution of hypervascular lesions, subsequent studies revealed no additional benefits of the early phase. Because of this and because of additional concerns relating to excess radiation dose, the early HAP is losing importance (Fig. 2) [11].

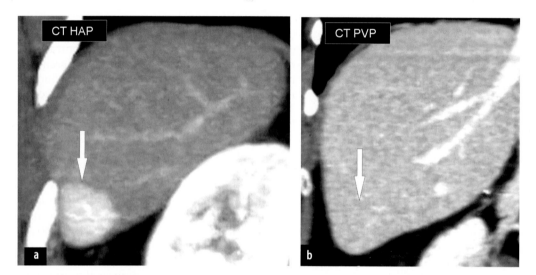

Fig. 1a, b. Hepatocellular carcinoma detection: coronal reformatted computed tomographic (CT) images of the liver in the arterial phase (**a**) showing intensely enhancing hepatocellular carcinoma (HCC) (*arrow*). Note better lesion-to-parenchymal contrast in the arterial-dominant phase in comparison with the portal venous phase image (**b**) where the lesion is not appreciated

Table 1. List of common hypervascular and hypovascular lesions encountered in the liver

Hypervascular lesions (arterial phase)	Hypovascular (PVP) lesions
Malignant	Metastases
• Primary malignancy	• Lung carcinoma
• Hepatocellular carcinoma	• Colon carcinoma
	• Breast carcinoma
Metastases	Benign
• Carcinoid	• Cysts
• Islet cell tumors	• Biliary hamartoma
• Renal cell carcinoma	
• Melanoma	
Benign	
• Hemangioma	
• Focal nodular hyperplasia	
• Hepatocellular adenoma	

PVP portal venous phase

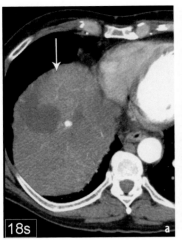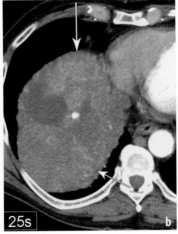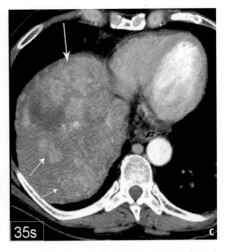

Fig. 2a-c. Improved detection of hepatocellular carcinoma (HCC) in the late arterial phase: serial images obtained at 18 s (**a**), 25 s (**b**), and 35 s (**c**) following initiation of contrast injection. Although arterially enhancing lesions are seen on images **a** and **b**, better enhancement and more lesions (*arrows*) are evident on the late arterial phase image (**c**)

Rationale for High-Concentration Contrast Medium

When a CT scan was performed with old scanners (conventional, helical, and dynamic), the liver was predominantly scanned during the preequilibrium phase due to slower scan speed and lengthened bolus time. With the evolution of MDCT, due to the reduction in scanning time, the scans can be performed during optimal phases with near perfection. One way of achieving this is by increasing the injection speed. The other way is to increase the concentration of the iodinated contrast mediun.

There should be an optimal balance between iodine concentration in the contrast and the volume of material injected for the desired hepatic parenchymal enhancement. The use of high iodine concentration contrast medium has gained importance in patients with decreased cardiac output, obesity, in conditions such as cirrhosis of the liver or portal vein thrombosis, and other conditions where there is decreased liver perfusion. It has been observed that the maximum hepatic enhancement in obese patients is significantly lower than in those who are lighter in weight. This could be attributed to the decreased level of perfusion of the liver in obese patients [12]. Also, in cases of liver cirrhosis, due to decreased portal perfusion, the peak contrast enhancement in liver is late, and usually, the plateau of contrast enhancement occurs in the late portal phase. This is again secondary to decreased portal perfusion seen in these patients [13]. The injection of contrast medium with standard iodine concentration could increase the possibility of missing hypovascular metastases during the late phase in heavy patients or in patients with cirrhosis or chronic hepatitis.

The use of high concentration contrast medium enables better visualization of the heterogeneous enhancement pattern in cirrhotic patients. The use of high concentration contrast medium for MDCT enables greater enhancement of the aorta in the early and the late arterial phases [14, 15]. It also results in higher mean attenuation of the liver in the portal phase than would be achieved by use of contrast medium of lesser iodine concentration. Therefore, the lesion-to-liver contrast can be improved when high iodine concentration contrast medium is used (Fig. 3).

Other Technical Considerations for Liver Imaging

Appropriate selection of the delay for scan initiation is essential, along with modification of the contrast administration protocol. Various technical and physiological factors affect MDCT contrast enhancement of the liver [16, 17].

Scan Delay and Contrast Delivery

With increasing detector rows in CT scanners, scan delays and contrast delivery in liver protocols need to be altered accordingly. As discussed, if the volume of contrast to be administered is kept constant and the rate is increased, the delay for peak aortic enhancement decreases [16]. Also, in patients with decreased cardiac output or more body weight, a longer time is required for the contrast to demonstrate peak aortic enhancement and thereby liver parenchymal enhancement. Thus, optimal enhancement in larger patients can be achieved by

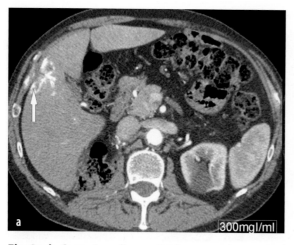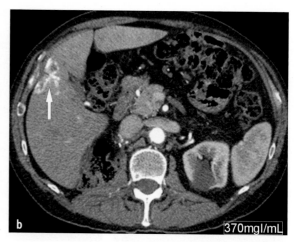

Fig. 3a, b. Comparison of low- and high-concentration contrast for characterization of a hemangioma: Arterial phase axial computed tomographic (CT) images of the liver performed with 300 mgI/ml (**a**) and 370 mgI/ml (**b**) concentration contrast media in a patient with a liver lesion. There is improved enhancement of the aorta and the liver hemangioma on the image obtained with the higher-concentration contrast medium

increasing the injection rate, and the time required for each of the phase acquisitions varies from patient to patient.

Techniques for Contrast Delivery Optimization

Timing of the hepatic arterial phase following contrast administration is of vital importance, and with the availability of computer-automated scanning technology (CAST), fixed time delays can be planned. However, fixed time delays do not take into account the patient-to-patient variability in cardiac output or the contrast circulation time.

Almost all recent scanners are now equipped with automated scanning trigger software wherein a threshold enhancement [Hounsfield units (HU)] in a vessel or an organ is preselected to initiate a scan after injection of contrast. A few initial images are obtained at a static table position, and after the contrast bolus arrives and the threshold of enhancement in the region of interest is reached, scans can be initiated either manually or automatically. Alternatively, a test bolus can be used wherein a small amount of contrast (10–15 ml at 3-4 cc/s) is injected and serial images are obtained through the upper aorta to judge its maximal opacification and determine the appropriate delay time for the patient. A test bolus is accurate but does entail additional contrast and time . With both the test bolus and automatic triggering techniques, the scan should be performed at the point of maximal opacification of the hepatic arterial system. This should enable creation of excellent images of the vascular anatomy of the liver.

However, for venous phase imaging, delays of 65–70 s, 60 s or less from the start of injection, are usually planned in 4-slice, 16-slice, and 64-slice scanners, respectively. This ensures optimal opacification of the portal vein and the hepatic veins.

Contrast Volume

Reduced volumes of contrast injection are not favored for liver imaging due to concerns about image quality. Unlike thoracic and vascular CT imaging, the authorities still recommend 120–150 ml of contrast medium of concentrations up to 300–370 mg of iodine [18]. However, in larger patients, an increased volume of up to 180 ml has been administered. In particular, patients with cirrhosis require a higher volume of contrast to achieve optimal parenchymal enhancement due to decreased liver perfusion.

Also, the volume of contrast to be injected varies depending on the iodine concentration in the contrast medium. Usually in cases of MDCT liver imaging, 120–150 cc of 300 mgI/ml of nonionic contrast is injected at a rate of 4 cc/s. On the other hand, if 370 mgI/ml is used, only 80–100 cc would be required, but this needs to be balanced with a slightly higher injection rate of 4–5 cc/s. Thus, with use of higher or lower iodine concentration contrast media, appropriate adjustments in injection rate and contrast volume are needed.

Pitch and Scan Collimation

The use of thinner collimations with increases in detector configuration of CT scanners has revolutionized the role of CT scans in imaging of liver pathologies. It has been shown that the use of 2.5 mm collimation markedly improves the detec-

Table 2. Multidetector computed tomography (MDCT) liver protocols on different computed tomography (CT) scanners

Parameters	4 channel	16 channel	64 channel
DC (mm)	4×1.25	16×0.625	64×0.6
TS (mm/s)	15	18.75	38
Pitch	1.0–2.0	0.938	0.984
Slice thickness (mm)			
Arterial phase (CTA)	1.25	1.0	1.0
Arterial phase (liver)	2.5–5.0	2.5	2.5
Venous phase (CTA)	2.5	2.0	2.0
Venous phase (liver)	5.0	5.0	5.0
Arterial Delay (s)	Bolus tracking/automated trigger Empirical delay:25–30 s		
Venous Delay (s)	65–70 s	60 s	50–60 s

DC detector collimation, *TS* table speed, *CTA* computed tomographic arteriography

tion of liver lesions compared with imaging on scanners with higher collimation such as 10 mm, 7.5 mm, and 5 mm [6]. For hepatic parenchymal imaging, 2.5 mm collimation is typically selected with a 4-row MDCT, but with increasing detector rows, such as 16- and 64-slice CT, collimations as thin as 1.25 mm and 0.625 mm can be obtained.

One of the most important factors that determines the pitch is the table speed (Table 2). New-generation MDCT scanners provide better coverage using the maximum table speed, which is due to the presence of their respective detector configurations and more data elements (Table 2). However, it is possible that this may result in unacceptable noise in the images.

Reconstruction Interval

It was shown by Kawata et al. [19] that there is no significant difference in the images obtained by using intervals of 2.5 mm, 5 mm, and 7.5 mm for detection of hypervascular hepatocellular carcinomas. It is essential that overlap of reconstructions be at least 50% to obtain optimal image quality particulary for hepatic CT angiography. Although thinner slices are desirable, reconstruction intervals of less than 2 mm can add to the noise in the image and thus affect the rate of detection of liver lesions. However, retrospective reconstruction from thinner collimated images of isotropic voxel resolution promotes reduction of partial-volume artifacts.

Role of MDCT in Imaging of Liver Tumors

The advent of MDCT scanners has ensured the availability of fast data acquisition, thinner collimations, and near-isotropic voxel resolution, but along with this has come alterations in scan delay and rate of contrast administration as well as emphasis on the importance of contrast concentration.

The two most important factors that influence the detection of lesions is lesion size and its intrinsic vascularity. Lesions as small as 1 mm have been detected by MDCT. It is generally believed that a minimum of 10 HU difference between lesion and normal liver parenchyma is required for the lesion to be detected. Different tumors may enhance at different phases of the scans depending on tumor vascularity. It must be noted that most tumors derive their blood supply from the hepatic artery and its branches. However, some may be more vascular than others and thus show increased enhancement on the hepatic arterial phase of the scan. Such tumors are classified as hypervascular tumors. Examples are hepatocellular carcinomas, metastases from melanoma, breast cancer, carcinoid, thyroid medullary carcinoma, islet cell tumors, and renal cell carcinoma.

Certain benign lesions also show increased vascularity in the hepatic arterial phase of the scan, such as focal nodular hyperplasia and hemangiomas less than 1 cm. This advantage of tiny lesion detection by MDCT scanners revealed that benign tumors in conditions such as cysts, focal nodular hyperplasia, hemangiomas, and adenomas occur in up to one third of the population without known malignancy [20]. In addition, MDCT detects tiny lesions, such as metastases in the liver, at an early stage, thereby ensuring early surgery, ablation therapy, or chemotherapy.

As we have moved to the era of 16- and 64-slice CT scanners, a study of the subtle enhancement pattern of tiny hypodense liver lesions in the hepatic arterial phase can be performed [21]. MDCT can detect the peripheral rim enhancement in hypovascular lesions and can very well depict involvement of the adjacent vasculature by the tu-

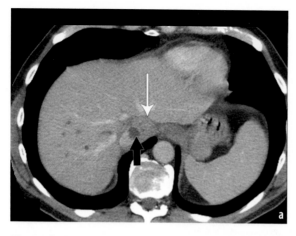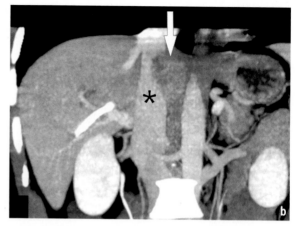

Fig. 4a, b. Preoperative planning of cholangiocarcinoma: contrast-enhanced axial image (**a**) shows an infiltrative mass in the dome of the liver with suspicion of inferior vena cava (IVC) invasion (*arrow*) seen as a filling defect. However, the corresponding coronal subvolume maximum intensity projection (MIP) image (**b**) confirmed only extrinsic compression and not invasion of the IVC (*asterisk*) by the tumor (*arrow*), and thereby surgery was feasible

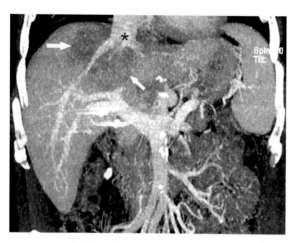

Fig. 5. Coronal reformat subvolume maximum intensity projection (MIP) image demonstrates an infiltrative cholangiocarcinoma (*arrows*) encasing the hepatic venous confluence and inferior vena cava (IVC) (*asterisk*) that makes the tumor unresectable

mor mass. It is also an important imaging modality for tumor staging (Figs. 4 and 5).

An important feature of the hepatic arterial phase for such lesions is the search for arterioportal shunting. Certain malignant lesions reveal the presence of arterioportal shunts (Fig. 6). This is due to the compression of portal or hepatic veins, which causes development of hepatic artery to portal venous collateral vessels. However, such shunts can also be visualized in the arterial phase in cases of abscess, small hemangiomas, and cirrhosis [22].

Importance of Early Tumor Detection by MDCT

Early detection of small hypervascular metastases and primary tumors by MDCT is important for

early treatment planning. Due to the inherent capability of MDCT scanners to outline smaller and more subtle lesions much earlier in the disease process, routine screening for hepatitis B patients is performed to detect early development of neoplasia in the liver. In such patients, the ability of MDCT to pick up tiny lesions in different phases of the scan proves to be a crucial imaging modality. Patients with small tumors of less than 5-cm diameter may be candidates for liver transplantation. Studies have shown the importance of late arterial phase scans for detection of tiny liver tumors [23, 24]. But due to constraints posed by inaccurate bolus tracking methods, which may read to significant hepatic venous enhancement in the late arterial phase, the use of both phases is justified [25].

Hepatic artery catheter MDCT is an invasive procedure that involves injection of lipiodol into the hepatic artery. It can detect subtle intra-arterial enhancement, which may not be revealed on intravenous contrast injection. This procedure could thus have a significant impact on tumor treatment options.

Detection of Small Benign Lesions

The differentiation between tiny benign and malignant lesions poses a challenge for MDCT. The only factor that is of vital importance to consider is the pattern of enhancement following administration of contrast. Thinner collimation with MDCT helps in accurate detection of attenuation in tiny lesions such as simple cysts. MDCT also aids in better differentiation of hemangiomas from hypervascular metastasis. Attenuation of small hemangiomas is more or less like that of the aorta in the arterial phases and similar to the hepatic veins

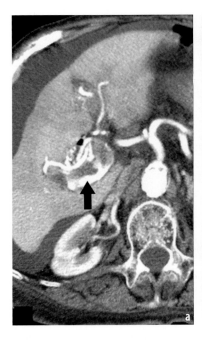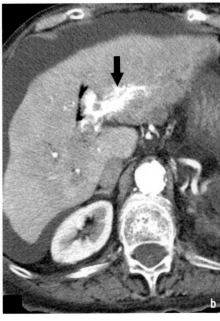

Fig. 6a, b. Tumor invasion in the portal vein from hepatocellular carcinoma (HCC). Two arterial phase axial images of the liver are shown. **a** Tumor thrombus is seen in the right portal vein (*arrow*). Also note the enhancement/contrast in the portal vein in the arterial phase. **b** Intensely enhancing arterioportal shunts from the tumor (*arrow*) around the left portal vein. Also seen is evidence of liver cirrhosis and ascites

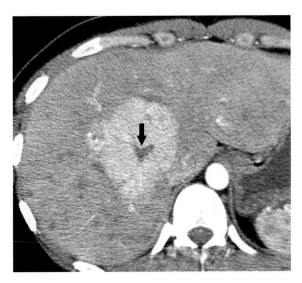

Fig. 7. Focal nodular hyperplasia: a dynamic late arterial phase axial image showing a well-defined, heterogeneously enhancing liver lesion with central scar (*arrow*), which appears as a hypoattenuating area

MDCT in Liver Cirrhosis

With the availability of smart prep technology in the recent 16- and 64-slice scanners, the arterial and venous phases can be optimally timed, which is of paramount importance in cirrhotic patients who have decreased liver perfusion. In addition, the use of high-concentration contrast medium enables better visualization of the heterogeneous enhancement pattern in cirrhotics, which is mainly due to regenerative nodules, periportal fibrosis, and microcirculatory shunts between the portal venous and hepatic venous systems. Due to the thin slice collimation and accurate definition of the arterial and venous phase with MDCT scanners, better image quality and CTA reconstructions from data sets are possible. The collateral circulation in cases of portal hypertension is also seen more clearly and with prominent paraumbilical collaterals, esophageal varices, and periportal circulation.

MDCT for Preoperative Planning

Preoperative knowledge of the variations in vascular anatomy could help avoid complications such as inadvertent ligation or injury of various hepatic arteries, hepatic ischemia, and hemorrhage and biliary leak. Variations in the celiac axis anatomy are common, and preoperative knowledge is useful for surgery, especially in obese patients who have large amounts of lymphatic and fatty tissue in the duodenal hepatic ligament and the porta hepatis [28]. CT angiography images can provide excellent outlining of the vascular struc-

in the venous phase. As MDCT can better define arterial and venous phases, detection of tiny hemangiomas is simplified to some extent.

Due to the capability of MDCT to highlight liver contrast in different phases of the scan, the detection of focal nodular hyperplasia (FNH) is also simplified. The hallmark of FNH on dual-phase MDCT is its intense enhancement pattern, with or without a low attenuation central area, on arterial phase images and rapid wash out on venous phase images, in which it becomes more or less isoattenuating with the liver [26, 27] (Fig. 7).

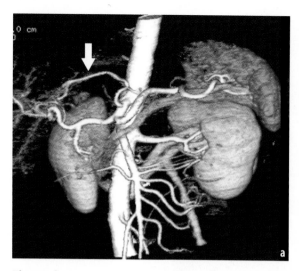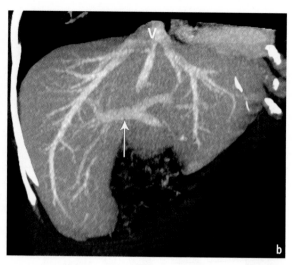

Fig. 8a, b. Preoperative planning for living-related liver transplantation: Color-coded volume-rendered computed tomographic arteriography (CTA) (**a**) demonstrates an anomalous origin of the left hepatic artery from the left gastric artery (*thick arrow*). A venous phase, subvolume maximum intensity projection (MIP) image in coronal oblique plane in venous phase (**b**) demonstrates normal portal and hepatic venous anatomy (*thin arrows*)

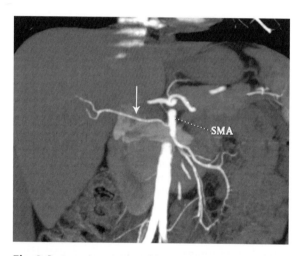

Fig. 9. Preoperative mapping of the arterial anatomy for intra-arterial chemotherapy pump placement. A coronal maximum intensity projection (MIP) computed tomographic arteriograph (CTA) displaying a replaced right hepatic artery (*arrow*) arising from the superior mesenteric artery (SMA)

have a greater longitudinal coverage with about 50 % overlap, and sufficient signal-to-noise ratio. These prerequisites are well provided by recent MDCT scanners [31].

The usual techniques for CT angiography of the liver are VR and MIP [32]. The MIP images provide no clue as to the depth of the structure but project the brightest structure, which in the hepatic arterial phase is the vascular detail (Fig. 9). Hence, optimal delay time, contrast medium concentration, and opacification are important. Due to the inherent capability of MDCT to provide desirable volumetric data and the required overlap, the reconstructed MIP images are of better quality than those obtained from older CT scanners. Some MDCT vendors allow users to save simplified scanning protocols on the user interface in the scanner so that exquisite MIP images can be obtained directly at the console.

Conclusion

MDCT offers several advantages, such as increased scanning speed and better definition of lesion conspicuity and characterization. However, to realize the maximum benefit, optimization of the acquisition parameters in different scanner types is important. Dual-phase imaging of the liver on MDCT is usually performed in the late arterial and portal venous phases, which not only enables better detection of small hypervascular lesions (in the arterial phase) at an early stage, but also plays an important role for early treatment planning. The availability of high-iodine concentration contrast medium ($\geq$370 mgI/ml) is an added benefit in

tures and demonstrate the exact extent of involvement by lesions. CTA images are especially useful for understanding vascular variations prior to hepatic resection and the extent of vascular involvement by tumors before liver surgery (Fig. 8).

The newer MDCT scanners enable routine acquisition of submillimeter sections (up to 0.5 mm) with isotropic resolution [29, 30]. The quality of the three-dimensional (3-D) images is largely dependent on the source images for reconstruction. As with other forms of visualization, such as multiplanar reformation (MPR), volume rendering (VR), and maximum intensity projections (MIP), the source images should be of thin collimation,

such settings. These contrast media not only provides better opacification of vascular structures but also add to the quality of reconstruction images, especially for preoperative planning and placement of intra-arterial pumps [33-35]. To ensure better-quality images, technical details pertaining to planning scan delays and the right time of arterial contrast delivery are important.

References

1. Tsurusaki M, Sugimoto K, Fujii M, Sugimura K (2004) Multi-detector row helical CT of the liver: quantitative assessment of iodine concentration of intravenous contrast material on multiphasic CT–A prospective randomized study. Radiat Med 22(4): 239–245

2. Kanematsu M, Oliver JH 3rd, Carr B, Baron RL (1997) Hepatocellular carcinoma: the role of helical biphasic contrast-enhanced CT versus CT during arterial portography. Radiology 205(1):75–80

3. Hollett MD, Jeffrey RB Jr, Nino-Murcia M et al (1995) Dual-phase helical CT of the liver: value of arterial phase scans in the detection of small (< or = 1.5 cm) malignant hepatic neoplasms. AJR Am J Roentgenol 164(4):879–884

4. Abdelmoumene A, Chevallier P, Chalaron M et al (2005) Detection of liver metastases under 2 cm: comparison of different acquisition protocols in four row multidetector-CT (MDCT). Eur Radiol 15(9):1881–1887

5. Fishman EK, Jeffrey RB Jr (2004) Multidetector CT: Principles, techniques and clinical applications. Lippincott Williams & Wilkins, Philadelphia, p 85

6. Weg N, Scheer MR, Gabor MP (1998) Liver lesions: improved detection with dual-detector-array CT and routine 2.5-mm thin collimation. Radiology 209(2):417–426

7. Wang G, Vannier MW (1999) The effect of pitch in multislice spiral/helical CT. Med Phys 26(12): 2648–2653

8. Spielmann AL (2003) Liver imaging with MDCT and high concentration contrast media. Eur J Radiol 45 [Suppl 1]:50–52

9. Bader TR, Prokesch RW, Grabenwoger F (2000) Timing of the hepatic arterial phase during contrast-enhanced computed tomography of the liver: assessment of normal values in 25 volunteers. Invest Radiol 35(8):486–492

10. Hollett MD, Jeffrey RB Jr, Nino-Murcia M et al (1995) Dual-phase helical CT of the liver: value of arterial phase scans in the detection of small (< or = 1.5 cm) malignant hepatic neoplasms. AJR Am J Roentgenol 164(4):879–884

11. Ichikawa T, Kitamura T, Nakajima H et al (2002) Hyper vascular hepatocellular carcinoma: can double arterial phase imaging with multidetector CT improve tumor depiction in the cirrhotic liver? AJR Am J Roentgenol 179(3):751-758

12. Furuta A, Ito K, Fujita T et al (2004) Hepatic enhancement in multiphasic contrast-enhanced MD-CT: Comparison of high- and low-iodine-concentration contrast medium in same patients with chronic liver disease. AJR Am J Roentgenol 183(1):157–162

13. Vignaux O, Legmann P, Coste J et al (1999) Cirrhotic liver enhancement on dual-phase helical CT: Comparison with non-cirrhotic livers in 146 patients. AJR Am J Roentgenol 173(5):1193–1197

14. Murakami T, Kim T, Takamura M et al (2001) Hyper vascular hepatocellular carcinoma: detection with double arterial phase multi-detector row helical CT. Radiology 218(3):763–767

15. Awai K, Takada K, Onishi H, Hori S (2002) Aortic and hepatic enhancement and tumor-to-liver contrast: Analysis of the effect of different concentrations of contrast material at multi-detector row helical CT. Radiology 224(3):757–763

16. Saini S (2004) Multi-detector row CT: principles and practice for abdominal applications. Radiology 233(2):323–327

17. Kalra MK, Maher MM, Toth TL et al (2004) Techniques and applications of automatic tube current modulation for CT. Radiology 233(3):649–657

18. Choi BI, Han JK, Cho JM et al (1995) Characterization of focal hepatic tumors. Value of two-phase scanning with spiral computed tomography. Cancer 76(12):2434–2442

19. Kawata S, Murakami T, Kim T et al (2002) Multidetector CT: diagnostic impact of slice thickness on detection of hypervascular hepatocellular carcinoma, AJR Am J Roentgenol 179(1):61–66

20. Jones EC, Chezmar JL, Nelson RC, Bernardino ME (1992) The frequency and significance of small (less than or equal to 15 mm) hepatic lesions detected by CT. AJR Am J Roentgenol 158(3):535–539

21. Schwartz LH, Gandras EJ, Colangelo SM et al (1999) Prevalence and importance of small hepatic lesions found at CT in patients with cancer. Radiology 210(1):71–74

22. Kim KW, Kim TK, Han JK et al (2001) Hepatic hemangiomas with arterioportal shunt: findings at two-phase CT. Radiology 219(3):707–711

23. Li L, Liu LZ, Xie ZM et al (2004) Multi-phasic CT arterial portography and CT hepatic arteriography improving the accuracy of liver cancer detection. World J Gastroenterol 10(21):3118–3121

24. Laghi A, Iannaccone R, Rossi P et al (2003) Hepatocellular carcinoma: detection with triple-phase multi-detector row helical CT in patients with chronic hepatitis. Radiology 226(2):543–549

25. Kim T, Murakami T, Hori M et al (2002) Small hyper vascular hepatocellular carcinoma revealed by double arterial phase CT performed with single breath-hold scanning and automatic bolus tracking. AJR Am J Roentgenol 178(4):899–904

26. Mortele KJ, Praet M, Van Vlierberghe H et al (2000) CT and MR imaging findings in focal nodular hyperplasia of the liver: Radiologic-pathologic correlation. AJR Am J Roentgenol 175(3):687–692

27. Carlson SK, Johnson CD, Bender CE, Welch TJ (200) CT of focal nodular hyperplasia of the liver. AJR Am J Roentgenol 174(3):705–712

28. Stemmler BJ, Paulson EK, Thornton FJ et al (2004) Dual-phase 3D MDCT angiography for evaluation of the liver before hepatic resection. AJR Am J Roentgenol 183(6):1551–1557

29. Hu H, He HD, Foley WD, Fox SH (2000) Four multidetector-row helical CT: image quality and volume coverage speed. Radiology 215(1):55–62

30. Flohr T, Prokop M, Becker C, Schoepf UJ et al (2002)

A retrospectively ECG-gated multislice spiral CT scan and reconstruction technique with suppression of heart pulsation artifacts for cardio-thoracic imaging with extended volume coverage. Eur Radiol 12(6):1497–1503

31. Kalender WA (1995) Thin-section three-dimensional spiral CT: is isotropic imaging possible? Radiology 197(3):578–580

32. Johnson PT, Halpern EJ, Kuszyk BS et al (1999) Renal artery stenosis: CT angiography comparison of real-time volume rendering and maximum intensity projection algorithms. Radiology 211(2):337–343

33. Takahashi S, Murakami T, Takamura M et al (2002) Multi-detector row helical CT angiography of hepatic vessels: depiction with dual-arterial phase acquisition during single breath hold. Radiology 222(1):81

34. Sahani D, Saini S, Pena C et al (2002) Using multidetector CT for preoperative vascular evaluation of liver neoplasms: Technique and results. AJR Am J Roentgenol 179(1):53–59

35. Sahani DV, Krishnamurthy SK, Kalva S et al (2004) Multidetector-row computed tomography angiography for planning intra-arterial chemotherapy pump placement in patients with colorectal metastases to the liver. J Comput Assist Tomogr 28(4):478–484

II.2

Hepatobiliary Imaging by Multidetector Computed Tomography (MDCT)

Sebastian T. Schindera and Rendon C. Nelson

Introduction

Hepatobiliary imaging by computed tomography (CT) has advanced impressively since the introduction of multidetector CT (MDCT) scanners in the late 1990s. Over the last few years, the number of detector rows has increased progressively from four, to eight, to 16, and then up to 64. Two important advantages of MDCT are the routine use of thinner, submillimeter sections, which yield higher spatial resolution, along the Z-axis and decrease in gantry rotation time, which result in a significantly reduced scan time. Sixteen-, 32- and 64-slice scanners allow the acquisition of data sets with nearly isotropic voxels for multiplanar imaging (e.g., coronal and sagittal plane), which has similar spatial resolution compared with axial planes. These off-axis reformations are particularly helpful for evaluating the hepatic vascular anatomy, the biliary system, and the segmental distribution of hepatic lesions. Since thin-section collimation also reduces partial volume averaging, sensitivity and specificity for detecting and characterizing increases, especially for small focal hepatic lesions, whether benign or malignant. Furthermore, evaluation of the biliary tract improves, not only at the level of the porta hepatis and extrahepatic bile ducts, but all the way to the hepatic periphery.

Shorter scan durations make it possible to include the entire upper abdomen during a single, comfortable breath hold. This reduces motion artefacts, especially in critically ill patients. Another advantage of reduced scan duration is more precise timing of different hepatic enhancement phases following bolus administration of iodinated contrast material, thus improving depiction and differentiation of focal hepatic lesions.

The main indication for MDCT examination of the liver is the detection and characterization of hepatic lesions. The crucial part of a diagnostic work-up of focal hepatic lesions is the differentiation between benign and malignant disease. Characterization of small incidental lesions still remains a challenging task for hepatic MDCT because of an overall lack of features. Schwartz et al. [1] has shown, however, that approximately 80% of small hepatic lesions (smaller than 1 cm) in patients with cancer diagnosed on MDCT are benign.

Urgent indications for MDCT scan of the liver include blunt and penetrating trauma, abscesses, and postoperative complications (e.g., bleeding, infection). Moreover, multiphasic MDCT plays an important role for pre- and postoperative evaluation of liver resection and transplant patients. MDCT is also highly useful for diagnosing hepatic parenchymal abnormalities (e.g., fatty infiltration, cirrhosis, iron deposition) and in some cases can provide quantitative information.

The gold standard for imaging the biliary tree is still endoscopic retrograde cholangiopancreatography (ERCP) even though this procedure is invasive, expensive, and physician intensive. In the last several years, magnetic resonance cholangiopancreatography (MRCP) has gained wide acceptance for noninvasive biliary imaging. In some practices and many academic centers, MRCP even functions as the first-choice technique for biliary tract imaging. Although spatial resolution of MDCT is superior to that of MRCP, MDCT, either with or without a cholangiographic agent, serves only as an alternative clinical tool for noninvasive evaluation of the biliary system.

In this chapter, we discuss technical principles and improvements of hepatobiliary MDCT. In addition, the principles of contrast media application and different phases of liver enhancement, including the typical enhancement pattern of various liver lesions, are reviewed.

Parameters and Technical Principles of Hepatobiliary MDCT

After introduction of the first 4-row MDCT scanner in 1998, the radiological community quickly accepted the new technology. With the development of 16-, 32-, and 64-slice scanners, data acquisition time has been further reduced. Coupling of wide collimation with large beam pitches and faster gantry rotation times has allowed for routine use of submillimeter collimation to acquire data sets with isotropic voxels. Rapid technological development, though, has increased the complexity of imaging options and scanning parameters. Radiologists using MDCT for hepatobiliary imaging should understand the imaging parameters and technical principles needed to acquire images with superior quality. The key parameters are:

- Acquisition parameters
- Reconstruction parameters
- Contrast media application
- Different phases of hepatic vascular and parenchymal enhancement.

Acquisition Parameters

As the number of detector channels increases, application of thin collimation has become a routine part of MDCT. The minimum section collimation of 16-, 32-, and 64-slice scanners is 0.625 mm (GE, Philips), 0.60 mm (Siemens), or 0.50 mm (Toshiba). This submillimeter feature allows for isotropic data acquisition. An isotropic voxel is cubic, having equal dimensions in the X-, Y- and Z-axis. Since the X- and Y-axes are determined by both field-of-view (FOV) and matrix size, isotropic voxels can be acquired only when slice thickness (Z-axis) measures 0.75 mm or less. The major advantage of these nearly isotropic data sets is the ability to reformat images in any desired plane, having similar spatial resolution to that of the axial plane. In recent studies, our group found multiplanar reformations particularly helpful for diagnosis of acute appendicitis and for evaluation of small-bowel obstruction [2, 3]. Further work is needed to evaluate the contribution of MDCT to hepatobiliary imaging.

Owing to increased spatial resolution and reduced partial volume averaging, thinner-slice collimation also results in an improved ability to detect small hepatic lesions. However, there is no consensus in the literature about the optimal collimation needed to detect small hepatic lesions [4–7]. The study performed by Haider et al. [7] using a 4-slice MDCT scanner did not find an improvement in the detection of hepatic metastases measuring 1.5 cm or smaller at collimation widths of less than 5 mm. Similar results were reported by Abdelmoumene et al. [5] when comparing four protocols with different slice collimations (5.0 and 2.5 mm) to detect small liver metastases (<2 cm). No improvement in lesion detection was found with a collimation width less than 2.5 mm. Furthermore, hepatic imaging with thinner sections caused an increase in image noise, with significantly lower performance in the detection of hepatic lesions [5]. To reduce noise associated with thinner sections, radiation dose to the patient should be increased. Typical scanning protocols for hepatobiliary imaging by MDCT are shown in Table 1. Section collimation should be tailored to the indication for hepatobiliary CT scan.

Reconstruction Parameters

With the development of 16-slice scanners, it became possible to scan the entire abdomen during a single, comfortable breath hold at a resolution of less than 1 mm in the X-, Y-, and Z-axes, resulting in a nearly isotropic data set. This three-dimen-

Table 1. Scan parameter for PVP and HAP using 4-, 16-, and 64- slice MDCT (developed for GE scanners)

	4-slice MDCT		16-sclice MDCT		64-slice MDCT	
	HAP	*PVP*	*HAP*	*PVP*	*HAP*	*PVP*
Detector configuration(mm)	4×3.75	4×2.5	16×1.25	16×0.625	64×0.625	64×σ0.625
Pitch	1.5	1.5	1.38	1.75	1.38	1.38
Table speed (mm/rotation)	22.5	15	27.5	17.5	55.0	55.0
Rotation time (s)	0.8	0.8	0.6	0.5	0.5	0.5
kV	140	140	140	140	140	140
mA	220	220	300	380	450	450
Slice thickness (mm)	5.0	5.0	5.0	5.0	5.0	5.0
Axial slice thickness for MPR and 3D-reconstruction (mm)	2.5	2.5	1.25	0.625	1.25	0.625

sional (3-D) volume can be used for further two-dimensional (2-D) and 3-D postprocessing. The most important rendering techniques for hepatobiliary MDCT are straight or curved multiplanar reformation (MPR), maximum intensity projection (MIP), minimum intensity projection (minIP), and volume rendering (VR). The type of reconstruction primarily depends on the indication for the study.

MPR, representing a 2-D reformatted plane other than the axial plane, is mainly used as a tool to visualize complex hepatic anatomic and pathological findings. Using a 4-slice CT scanner, Hong et al. [8] evaluated image quality and diagnostic value of abdominal MPRs. There was superior visualization of liver segments and lesions with MPRs compared with axial images alone; however, no significant difference in liver lesion detection between axial and MPR images could be found. The key to optimizing image quality of MPRs is to increase the reconstruction thickness to several millimeters. Recently, our group demonstrated in a qualitative analysis that 2- and 3-mm-thick coronal reformations provide the best image quality [9]; 1-mm-thick sections were too noisy whereas 4- to 5-mm slice thickness was too smooth, yielding little anatomical detail, especially for blood vessels and lymph nodes.

MIPs are routinely used to evaluate hepatic arteries and the portal veins since these projections display the greatest attenuation difference between vessels and adjacent tissue. Another indication for MIP is CT cholangiography, which is well suited to visualization of the biliary tract anatomy and the presence of congenital anomalies [10–12]. In patients with bile duct obstruction, minIPs may be helpful for demonstrating the biliary tract when MDCT is performed without a cholangiographic agent [13–15]. To improve image quality of MIPs and minIPs, partial volume averaging effects can be reduced by choosing the volume of interest as small as possible.

The VR technique allows the user to view the entire volume data set in an appropriate 3-D context, including a range of different types of abdominal tissues (Fig. 1). Various opacity values can be applied to simultaneously display both the surface and the interior of the volume. These images are well appreciated by surgeons since they offer a true 3-D view of the hepatic vascular anatomy. Other indications for VR are estimation of liver volume and virtual hepatectomy prior to living-related liver transplantation.

Contrast Media Application

Nonionic iodinated contrast agents are small molecular weight extracellular agents that are most

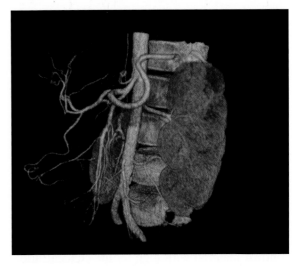

Fig. 1. Volume rendering technique of the hepatic arterial system. Note the anatomic variation of the celiac axis arising from the SMA

commonly used with hepatobiliary MDCT to delineate blood vessels and hepatic parenchyma, as well as to detect and characterize focal and diffuse hepatic abnormalities. The degree of maximum enhancement of liver parenchyma during the portal venous phase (PVP) is directly proportional to the *total amount* of iodine administered. There is no difference between contrast material injection protocols specifying 100 ml of an agent with an iodine concentration of 370 mg/ml (37 g of iodine) and 125 ml of an agent with an iodine concentration of 300 mg/ml (37.5 g of iodine). Furthermore, the introduction of faster 16- and 64-slice CT scanners did not significantly reduce the necessary volume of injected contrast media for hepatobiliary imaging since the speed of the scanner did not improve enhancement during the venous phase. For most applications, 38–44 g of iodine is recommended since 44 g has not been shown to statistically significantly improve hepatic enhancement [16]. Total iodine doses less than 30 g are also not recommended, as the duration and magnitude of hepatic enhancement will decrease, resulting in a lower detection rate of focal liver lesions.

Contrast materials with an iodine concentration up to 400 mg/ml are currently available. Most institutions administer a fixed amount of contrast agent (120–150 ml) when using iodine concentration of 300 mg/ml. However, previous studies have recommended tailoring the volume of contrast material to body weight [17–19]. Yamashita and coworkers achieved the best hepatic parenchymal enhancement with a dose of 2.0–2.5 ml/kg adjusted for body weight [18].

Opacification of the hepatic arterial system and detection of hypervascular hepatic lesions are improved primarily by the *rate* of iodine delivery and the *timing* of imaging relative to the contrast media bolus. Improved lesion-to-liver contrast can be attained either by an accelerated injection rate or by an increased iodine concentration. While the injection rate of contrast media (3–6 ml/s) may be physiologically limited, the use of contrast agents with higher iodine concentration (350–400 mgI/ml) is compelling. Regardless of iodine concentration, faster injection rates are superior in detection of hypervascular liver lesions. A recent study, Itoh et al. [20] reported improved arterial enhancement with contrast agents having high iodine concentration (350 mgI/ml) by shortening the injection duration. Awai et al. [21] found a significantly higher tumor-to-liver contrast with hepatocellular carcinoma (HCC) in the arterial phase after administration of contrast material with high iodine concentration (370 mgI/ml) compared with moderate iodine concentration (300 mgI/ml). However, there was no significant difference in hepatic enhancement during the PVP since the same iodine load was administered to both groups. There may be a potential cost saving when using a contrast material with a higher iodine concentration since the volume of contrast can be decreased to maintain the same number of grams of iodine per milliliter per second.

In the case of MDCT angiography, when only arterial enhancement is of interest, Ho et al. [19] reported a significant reduction of contrast material dose with the use of an interactive injection protocol that included an immediate interruption of the contrast injection after the aorta enhanced qualitatively. Contract media dose was reduced because of the increased speed of the MDCT scanner.

The recent development and introduction of double-syringe mechanical power injectors simplified the saline flush technique. Immediate injection of a saline bolus after contrast agent administration avoids accumulation of the contrast agent in the injection tubing and the venous system. The new injector results in superior contrast enhancement. Schoellnast et al. [22] noted a significantly higher parenchymal and vascular enhancement of the liver in a group of patients receiving a 20-ml saline flush with a double-syringe power injector compared with the same patient population using a single-syringe power injector without flush. The same contrast media protocol (100 ml of contrast agent with iodine concentration of 300 mgI/ml) was used in both groups. By using the saline flush technique, the same group showed a decrease in contrast media dose by 17% without a significant decrease in enhancement of hepatic parenchyma and vessels [23]. This injection technique may reduce total yearly amounts of contrast agent and individual patient doses, for example, for patients with renal insufficiency; however, the additional costs of a second syringe must be taken into account.

To opacify the biliary tree for diagnostic imaging with MDCT (CT cholangiography), either oral or intravenous cholangiographic contrast agents can be administered. The intravenous cholangiographic contrast agent is infused over 30 min and is followed by a CT scan within 15–30 min. Most institutions administer intravenous diphenhydramine prior to infusion of cholangiographic contrast material to diminish the incidence of allergic reactions. For CT cholangiography with oral contrast medium, the patient has to ingest 6 g of iopanoic acid after a low-fat meal the night before. Several studies have shown that intravenous MDCT cholangiography is feasible for noninvasive evaluation of the biliary anatomy [11, 12, 24]. Nonetheless, intravenous cholangiography is rarely used in the United States, not only due to the high rate of allergic reactions and of renal and hepatic toxicity, but also due to the fact that there is suboptimal visualization of the biliary tract in up to 36% of patients [12, 25].

Different Phases of Hepatic Vascular and Parenchymal Enhancement

The increasing speed of MDCT scanners has improved the ability to perform multiphasic examinations of the liver. Most of the recently introduced 64-slice MDCT scanners image the whole liver in less than 2 s. Since acquisitions are becoming closer to a snapshot, timing of contrast-material bolus is even more important. Most of the recently introduced 64-slice MDCT scanners image the whole liver in less than 2 s, which may result in superior hepatic scans during multiple phases with more optimal enhancement. Table 2 demonstrates the indication for dynamic hepatobiliary MDCT imaging.

There are selected cases in which an unenhanced CT scan of the liver is helpful and recommended. Reasonable clinical indications for a noncontrast hepatic CT include:
- Depiction of acute hemorrhage of the liver
- Delineation of siderotic nodules
- Detection and characterization of hepatic calcification (e.g., calcified metastases, epithelioid hemangioendothelioma, hydatid cysts)
- Evaluation of parenchymal liver diseases (e.g., fatty infiltration, hepatic cirrhosis, hemochromatosis)
- Follow-up CT scan after embolization of hypervascular liver lesions

Contrast-enhanced MDCT of the liver is complicated by the liver's dual blood supply (parenchyma receives 75% of its blood via the portal vein and 25% via the hepatic artery), resulting in various phases of enhancement. Figure 2 demonstrates

Table 2. Indication for dynamic hepatobiliary MDCT imaging

	Noncontrast	EAP	LAP	PVP	EQP
Hypovascular liver metastases				X	
Hypervascular liver metastases			X	X	
Hepatocellular carcinoma	X		X	X	X
Focal nodular hyperplasia			X	X	
Hepatocellular adenoma	X		X	X	
Evaluation hepatic arterial system		X			
Cholangiocarcinoma				X	X
Primary sclerosing cholangitis				X	X
Cholecystitis				X	
Gallbladder carcinoma				X	X

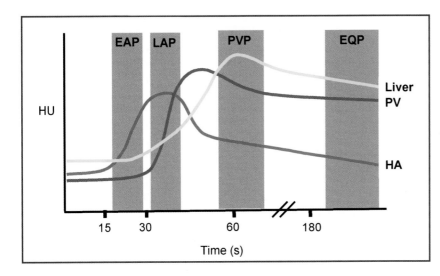

Fig. 2. Different phases of enhancement in dynamic hepatobiliary MDCT imaging (*EAP*: early arterial phase, *LAP*: late arterial phase, *PVP*: portal venous phase, *EQP*: equilibrium phase, *PV*: portal vein, *HA*: hepatic artery)

the typical enhancement curves of the hepatic artery, the portal vein, and liver parenchyma. Following an intravenous bolus of contrast material, the hepatic artery enhances first at approximately 15 s and reaches peak attenuation at approximately 30 s. After the contrast medium returns from the splanchnic system, the portal vein starts to enhance at around 30 s. Enhancement of liver parenchyma begins later, reaching a plateau at 60–70 s. The plateau may last up to 20–30 s. Finally, there is the equilibrium phase (EQP) (3 min and later), which occurs when the amount of contrast material in the intra- and extravascular extracellular space is essentially the same. Arterial hepatic enhancement is regulated mainly by cardiovascular circulation time and iodine delivery rate whereas parenchyma enhancement of the liver is related to total iodine dose administered. According to the different enhancement curves of the hepatic artery, portal vein, and hepatic parenchyma, four phases can be distinguished:

1. *Early arterial phase* (EAP) appears 20–25 s after administration of contrast material when there is conspicuous enhancement in the hepatic arteries

compared with almost no enhancement of liver parenchyma or hypervascular lesions. This phase typically provides the least information for imaging the liver, since the contrast media at that time has accumulated neither in hypervascular liver lesions nor in liver parenchyma. Nevertheless, this phase is well suited for CT angiography when used to evaluate the anatomical configuration of hepatic arteries prior to liver transplantation, hepatic tumor resection, or arterial chemoembolization.

To achieve optimum timing for EAP scanning for hepatic CT angiography, an automated triggering system may be used. This technique is superior to a fixed-delay or a test bolus. The scanner is typically set at the top of the liver with the trigger placed in the descending thoracic aorta. Following a 15-s delay after initiation of contrast material administration, a low-dose image is acquired every 3 s. When the trigger, which monitors the descending aorta, reaches a predefined attenuation (typically 90–100 HU), the scan begins for the EAP.

2. *Late arterial phase* (LAP) appears at about 30–35 s following initiation of contrast material administration. For optimum timing using the au-

tomated triggering technique, to avoid the EAP, an additional 8- to 10-s delay is required. The LAP is also referred to as the portal vein inflow phase since the portal vein is already starting to enhance during this phase. The hepatic arterial systems as well as prominent neovasculature of hypervascular hepatic neoplasms continue to enhance during the LAP while there is only minimal enhancement of hepatic parenchyma. At this point, there is a maximum attenuation difference between hypervascular liver lesions and the surrounding liver parenchyma (Fig. 3). Thus, LAP is the optimal phase for detecting hypervascular neoplasms of the liver. Foley et al. [26] was one of the first groups to propose three different hepatic circulatory phases using MDCT and showed that there was a significantly better delineation of hypervascular liver lesions during the LAP compared with the EAP. A few years later, Laghi et al. [27] investigated whether the use of the two arterial phases in combination improves the detection of hypervascular HCC with MDCT. Their data showed no significant difference between the late and the two combined arterial phases for depiction of HCC, so they concluded that acquisition of the LAP together with the PVP is considered sufficient for detection of HCC with MDCT.

3. *Portal venous phase* (*PVP*), or hepatic venous phase, appears at about 60–70 s following initiation of a contrast media bolus, when the enhancement of liver parenchyma reaches its peak and the portal vein and hepatic veins are well enhanced. For accurate timing of the PVP in a single-phase exam, we again recommend automated scanning technology instead of a fixed time delay. The trigger is placed in liver parenchyma to track the enhancement curve, and when attenuation reaches a

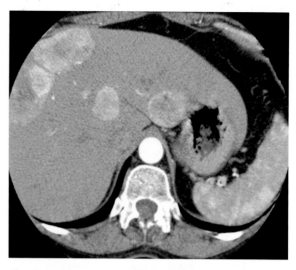

Fig. 3. Hyperenhancing or hypervascular liver metastases from a neuroendocrine tumor of pancreas during the LAP

predefined threshold (e.g., 50–70 HU), the table is moved to the top of the liver and the diagnostic scan initiated. For a dual-phase exam, there is a fixed time delay of 40 s following the end of the LAP.

Hypovascular tumors are optimally detected during the PVP when enhancement of liver parenchyma is maximal and there is the greatest liver-to-lesion attenuation difference (Fig. 4). For detection of these tumors, a single scan during the PVP is sufficient since there is no further advantage performing unenhanced or arterial-phase imaging. The PVP is also the appropriate phase for visualization and evaluation of intrahepatic bile ducts, when there is the greatest difference of attenuation between the maximally enhanced liver parenchyma and the hypoattenuating intraductal bile.

4. *Equilibrium phase* (*EQP*), or interstitial phase, appears at approximately 3 min postinjection, when there is an increased diffusion of contrast media into liver parenchyma and attenuation difference between parenchyma and vessels is minimal. Washout of the contrast material in different liver lesions may vary vastly depending on their histological nature. One clear indication for acquiring images during the EQP includes intrahepatic cholangiocarcinoma. This tumor when desmoplastic may accumulate the contrast agent and show a delayed washout compared with surrounding liver parenchyma. This delay causes hyperattenuating lesions (Fig. 5). In a study by Keogan et al. [28], 36% of proven cholangiocarcinomas on the EQP demonstrated as hyperattenuating lesions compared with the liver. By comparison, HCC may show a faster washout during the EQP relative to the surrounding liver parenchyma, representing a hypoattenuating mass (Fig. 6).

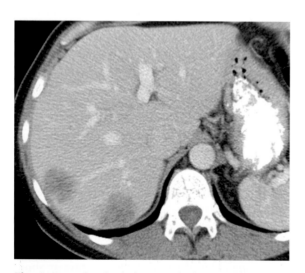

Fig. 4. Hypoenhancing or hypovascular liver metastases in the right hepatic lobe from a colon cancer detected during portal venous phase

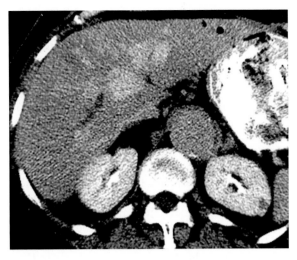

Fig. 5. Hyperattenuating lesion or delayed washout in the left hepatic lobe during the EQP in a patient with cholangiocarcinoma

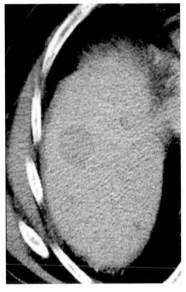

Fig. 6. Hypoattenuating mass representing faster washout of the HCC during EQP

Applications of Hepatobiliary MDCT

Liver

MDCT of the liver plays a crucial role in the detection of focal hepatic lesions as well as characterization of the mass as benign or malignant. Besides that, MDCT often functions as the technique of choice for tumor staging, monitoring response to treatment, diagnostic work-up prior to hepatic resection or liver transplantation, or guidance of percutaneous biopsy and ablation. Superior detection of liver lesions with 16-slice or 64-slice MDCT scanners is a result of their increased speed, which

allows routine use of thinner collimation to increase spatial resolution and decrease acquisition time. The diagnostic impact of the technical advances of MDCT will be discussed for different hepatic tumors.

Liver Metastases

One of the major indications for hepatic MDCT is the detection of metastatic liver disease, which is by far the most common malignant hepatic tumor in patients without cirrhosis. The CT image appearance of liver metastases may vary widely depending on the histologic nature of the lesion and its vascularity. The type of MDCT protocol for depiction of liver metastases mainly depends on the degree of primary tumor vascularization.

Hypovascular Metastases

Most hepatic metastases are hypovascular and arise from primary tumors of the gastrointestinal tract (e.g., colon, rectum, stomach), pancreas, urothelium, lung, and head and neck, as well as from gynecologic tumors. During the PVP, these lesions are typically hypoattenuating owing to superior enhancement of adjacent liver parenchyma. In the periphery of these metastases, there may be increased enhancement during either the arterial phase or the PVP, represented by a hypervascular rim or halo. Most authorities recommend a single-phase CT during the PVP for evaluation of hypovascular metastases. Several studies have shown that the additional use of unenhanced or hepatic arterial-phase images does not detect more lesions [29–31]. However, the adjunct use of arterial-phase images may be valuable in the depiction of hypovascular metastases with a hypervascular rim, for example, colon cancer. A recent study, which investigated the enhancement pattern of focal liver lesions during the arterial phase, reported a complete ring enhancement in about 85% of hypovascular metastases [32]. Although dual-phase MDCT may be beneficial for special cases, for routine imaging of hypovascular liver metastases, arterial-phase imaging is not necessary. The reported detection rate of hypovascular liver metastases for MDCT during the PVP is between 85% and 91% [29, 33]. In a study performed by Soyer et al. [29], CT depicted all hypovascular metastases with a diameter greater than 1 cm during the PVP but only two out of six metastases (33%) with a diameter smaller than 0.5 cm. None of these small metastases could be detected on the unenhanced images or during the hepatic arterial phase.

Hypervascular Metastases

Primary tumors that tend to be associated with hypervascular liver metastases include neuroendocrine tumors (e.g., islet cell carcinoma, carcinoid tumor), renal cell carcinoma, thyroid carci-

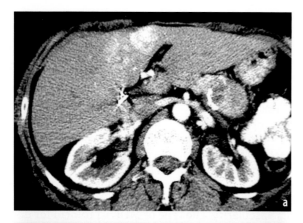

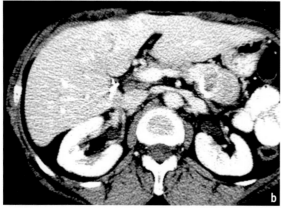

Fig. 7a, b. Hypervascular metastases from a neuroendocrine tumor of the pancreas during the LAP (**a**) and the PVP (**b**). Note that the tumors are much less apparent during the PVP

noma, melanoma, and occasionally breast cancer. The imaging protocol for hypervascular metastases is significantly different from hypovascular metastases. Hypervascular lesions are typically hyperattenuating during the late hepatic arterial phase due to an earlier and increased contrast media up-take compared with adjacent hepatic parenchyma. Blake et al. [34] investigated the sensitivity of different multiphasic contrast-enhanced CT protocols for the detection of liver metastases from melanoma. The study reported that the detection rate decreased by 14% when using only the PVP instead of obtaining an additional arterial phase. The MDCT protocol of choice for the detection of hypervascular metastases currently includes the LAP and PVP (Fig. 7a, b) [26, 27]. Other techniques that help improve the detectability of focal hypervascular liver lesions during biphasic MDCT are a contrast medium with a higher iodine concentration and a higher injection rate [20, 35]. At our institution, we evaluate hypervascular liver metastasis with a flow rate of 3.5 ml/s and contrast medium with an iodine concentration of 370 mgI/ml. The reported sensitivity of dual-phase CT for hypervascular liver metastases ranges between 78% and 96% [34, 36].

Hepatocellular Carcinoma

HCC is by far the most common primary malignant hepatic neoplasm as well as one of the most prevalent malignancies worldwide. The main predisposing factor in the Western Hemisphere is cirrhosis due to alcohol abuse whereas in Africa and Asia, the most common underlying causes are hepatitis B and C infections and exposure to aflatoxin A. While surgical resection and liver transplantation provide the best long-term outcome and are the treatments of choice for HCC, most patients are not candidates for surgical therapy [37, 38]. Before considering these treatment options, early diagnosis of HCC in a more curable stage as well as detection of the precise number of nodules must be determined.

Multiphasic MDCT plays a central role in HCC screening of high-risk cirrhotic patients. The CT appearance of HCC is extremely variable and depends on the neoplasm's growth pattern (solitary mass, multifocal masses, or diffusely infiltrating neoplasm), size, histological nature, and vascularity. Up to 36% of HCCs are associated with fatty change, which may aid detection on unenhanced images [39]. The majority of HCCs are hypoattenuating on precontrast images; however, some tend to be isoattenuating compared with adjacent liver parenchyma (Fig. 8a-d). Many HCCs are hypervascular neoplasms, which enhance significantly during the LAP because of increased blood supply from the hepatic artery (Fig. 8b). Small HCCs (<3 cm) generally demonstrate a more homogenous enhancement during the arterial phase whereas larger tumors show a heterogeneous enhancement pattern due to necrosis or hemorrhage. During the PVP, HCC usually becomes iso- to hypoattenuating to liver parenchyma depending on the extent of washout of the mass (Fig. 8c). During the EQP, the tumors themselves wash out more rapidly than hepatic parenchyma (Fig. 8d), but a tumor capsule and fibrous septation, if present, may be hyperattenuating due to delayed washout of the contrast material.

Detection of HCCs within cirrhotic liver parenchyma is challenging because of large amounts of fibrosis, distorted anatomy, and atrophy of various portions of the liver. Peterson et al. [40] investigated the sensitivity of preoperative helical CT for detecting HCC in cirrhotic patients undergoing liver transplantation [41]. In 320 patients with advanced cirrhosis, only 59% of the lesions confirmed by surgical pathology were detected on helical triphasic CT scans. In pretransplantation patients with cirrhosis, Valls et al. [41] reported a sensitivity of 94% for the detection of HCC (larger than 2 cm) with biphasic helical CT. However, the detection rate of HCC less than 2 cm was just 61%. Hence, the detection of HCCs in the setting of cirrhosis seems to depend largely on the size of the neoplasm.

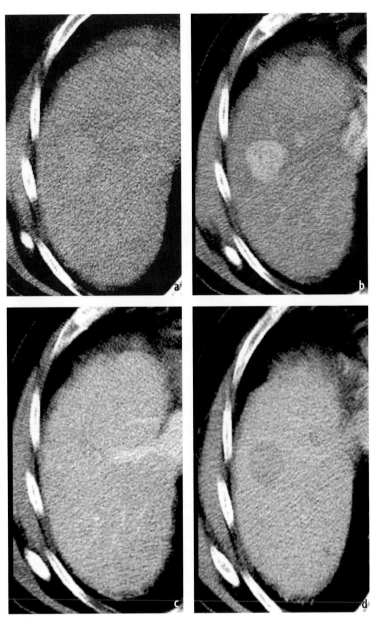

Fig. 8a-d. HCC in a cirrhotic patient during the unenhanced state (**a**), LAP (**b**), PVP (**c**) and EQP (**d**). Note that the tumor is most conspicuous during the LAP and EQP

In the last few years, several investigators have demonstrated that the use of a biphasic MDCT protocol, a LAP followed by a PVP, significantly improves the depiction of HCC [26, 27, 42]. Additional EAP images in conjunction with bi- or triplephasic MDCT protocol did not improve detection of HCC [27, 42]. Furthermore, the role of unenhanced and delayed phase images for detection of HCC with MDCT remains controversial. A recent investigation reported a significant increase in HCC detection in cirrhotic patients, with the addition of a delayed or EQP (180 s postinjection) acquisition in conjunction with a biphasic MDCT protocol [43]. Moreover, 10% of detected HCCs showed a tumor capsule, which again could only be visualized on the EQP images. Regarding the use of

unenhanced images, the study did not present any significant advantages for depiction of HCC; however, the authors believe that unenhanced images are particularly helpful in the differentiation of hyperattenuating siderotic nodules from hyperenhancing HCC nodules. At our institution, the CT protocol for detection of HCC includes all four phases: unenhanced, LAP, PVP, and EQP.

Several studies have indicated that the administration of higher-concentration contrast material (370–400 mgI/ml) significantly increases liver-to-lesion contrast during the arterial phase. This method may improve depiction of HCC [21, 44, 45]. However, it is noteworthy that a study performed by Marchiano et al. [45] did not observe a significant increase in the overall number of HCCs

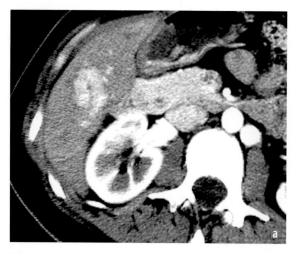 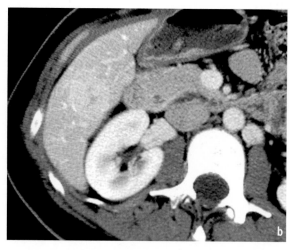

Fig. 9a, b. Focal nodular hyperplasia with a central scar during the LAP (**a**) and PVP (**b**). Note that the central scar enhances slowly

detected after the injection of a high concentration of iodinated contrast material. There is also a clear trend toward the use of faster injection rates (4–5 ml/s), which may improve conspicuity of HCCs due to superior liver-to-lesion contrast in the arterial phase [20, 46]. Oliver et al. [47] reported about a 74% detection rate for HCC with a flow rate of 4–5 ml/s during the hepatic arterial phase compared with a 58% detection rate with a flow rate of 3 ml/s. While only 19% of the detected lesions in this study showed an increase in enhancement with a flow rate of 3 ml/s, up to 83% of HCCs demonstrated as hyperattenuating on arterial-phase images using the higher flow rate.

Focal Nodular Hyperplasia
Focal nodular hyperplasia (FNH) is the second most common benign neoplasm of the liver after hemangioma. FNH arises predominately in women. The tumors are usually solitary, in a sub-capsular location and are often discovered incidentally during radiological imaging. The pathogenesis of FNH is believed to be a congenital vascular malformation having an increased arterial blood flow. A recent study by Mathieu et al. [48] suggested that FNH is not associated with the use of oral contraceptives. The neoplasm often contains a stellate central scar surrounded by small nodules of proliferating hepatocytes, bile ducts, and malformed vessels of different caliber [49, 50]. Recently, a significantly higher prevalence of hemangiomas in patients with FNH was reported by Vilgrain et al. [51], perhaps because both neoplasms are vascular malformations. The differential diagnosis of FNH includes other hypervascular liver lesions, such as hepatocellular adenoma, HCC, and hypervascular metastases. Therefore, distinction between FNH and other hypervascular

liver tumors is crucial to ensure proper therapy.

Multiphasic MDCT is an excellent imaging technique for the accurate diagnosis of FNH [50, 52]. On unenhanced CT, FNH is typically either hypoattenuating or isoattenuating to surrounding liver parenchyma. During the LAP, FNH becomes homogenously hyperattenuating with the exception of the central scar (Fig. 9a). This is felt to be the most reliable CT sign. During the portal venous and equilibrium phases, the neoplasm usually becomes isoattenuating relative to hepatic parenchyma (Fig. 9b). On EQP images, the central scar may demonstrate delayed washout. This characteristic dynamic enhancement pattern is mainly due to a prominent arterial supply of the tumor and its large draining veins. On the basis of this enhancement pattern, most authorities recommend multiphasic MDCT, including LAP and PVP images [50, 52].

Hepatocellular Adenoma
Hepatocellular adenoma is a rare benign neoplasm that is usually detected incidentally in women of childbearing age who have taken oral contraceptives for a long period. Other risk factors for hepatocellular adenoma include type 1 glycogen storage disease and, in men, the ingestion of anabolic steroids. Most hepatic adenomas are solitary; however, it is not unusual to detect two or three adenomas in one patient, particularly in patients with glycogen storage disease [53, 54]. The histological features of hepatocellular adenomas are sheets of proliferated hepatocytes surrounded by numerous dilated sinusoids with poor connective tissue support. The tumor tissue may contain a few Kupffer cells but usually lacks bile ducts. Deposition of lipid and glycogen in hepatic adenomas is not uncommon and may be valuable in diagnosing these

neoplasms. Hepatocellular adenomas have a tendency to spontaneously hemorrhage, which can be fatal. Since these lesions may also undergo malignant transformation to an HCC, they are considered surgical [53, 54].

Because of different therapeutic management, accurate differentiation of FNH and HCC is crucial. Unfortunately, the appearance on CT is variable and not specific. On unenhanced CT images, hepatocellular adenomas demonstrate either a hypoattenuating mass because of lipid and glycogen accumulation in the tumor or a hyperattenuating mass due to fresh hemorrhage (Fig. 10a). During the LAP, hepatocellular adenomas enhance rapidly and are hyperattenuating relative to the normal liver (Fig. 10b). Small lesions tend to demonstrate a more homogenous enhancement whereas larger lesions tend to enhance heterogenously [53]. During portal-venous- and equilibrium-phase imaging, most adenomas are nearly isoattenuating compared with surrounding liver parenchyma (Fig. 10c). Due to the variable CT appearances of hepatocellular adenoma, a triphasic MDCT protocol, including unenhanced, LAP and PVP images, has been recommended for detection and characterization [54, 55].

The Biliary System

Although MDCT is not generally considered to be a first-line imaging technique for patients with suspected biliary pathology, advances in MDCT scanners have resulted in an increased capability to detect and characterize various biliary diseases. The advantages of MDCT of the biliary tract are increased speed and reduction of acquisition time and respiratory motion artefacts. Furthermore, the thinner slices of MDCT result in reconstructed data sets with isotropic voxels for multiplanar reformations and 3-D displays. Straight and curved multiplanar reformations are especially valuable for visualization and evaluation of the biliary tree, which is typically oriented either perpendicular or tangential to the axial plane.

The intrahepatic bile ducts, which are linear structures accompanying the portal vein and hepatic arterial branches, can be best visualized during the PVP when there is an optimal attenuation difference between hypodense bile ducts and the adjacent enhanced vessels and parenchyma. Using thin collimation, normal intrahepatic bile ducts with a diameter of up to 2 mm can be visualized routinely, even out to the periphery of the liver. On unenhanced images, the diameter of the intrahepatic bile ducts must measure at least 2 mm to be distinguished from adjacent vascular structures and liver parenchyma. The low-attenuation extrahepatic bile ducts (common hepatic duct and com-

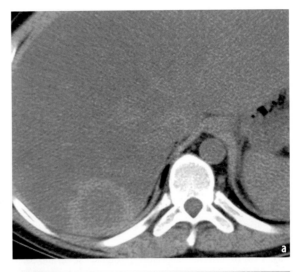

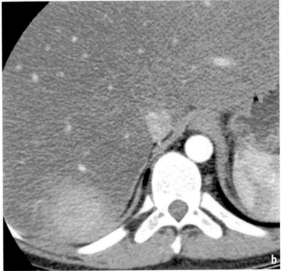

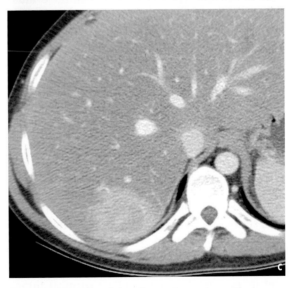

Fig. 10a-c. Hepatocellular adenoma in a patient with glycogen storage disease type 1A (von Gierke's disease) during the unenhanced state (**a**), LAP (**b**) and PVP (**c**). The liver is enlarged and there is diffuse fatty infiltration. While this particular tumor has no internal hemorrhage, there is a thin fibrous capsule

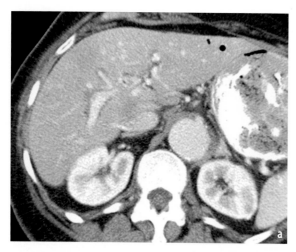 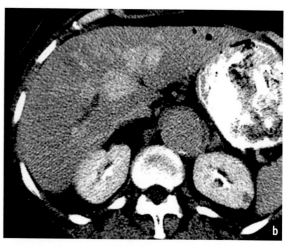

Fig. 11a, b. Hilar cholangiocarcinoma during PVP (**a**) and EQP (**b**). Delayed washout in the tumor during the EQP is apparent and indicates a high fibrous content

mon bile duct), which measure between 3 mm and 6 mm, are routinely visualized on thin-section MDCT images. Their thin walls (1 mm) usually enhance after administration of contrast media, which helps to differentiate them from the adjacent vessels. The normal gallbladder wall, which is 1- to 3-mm thick, also enhances postcontrast. The enhancement and thickness of the gallbladder wall may vary depending on luminal distension and on pathologic conditions (e.g., inflammation, tumor). There are several pathological situations in which density of bile in the gallbladder increases significantly. Examples include deposition of sludge and milk of calcium. The role of MDCT in the evaluation of different biliary pathologies and their characteristic imaging findings will be discussed below.

Cholangiocarcinoma
Cholangiocarcinoma is the most common primary malignancy of the intra- and extrahepatic biliary tract. Patients usually present with painless jaundice due to biliary obstruction. The majority of cholangiocarcinomas, adenocarcinomas, are found in the extrahepatic ducts. A tumor originating at the confluence of the left and right hepatic duct is referred to as a Klatskin tumor. Predisposing factors for cholangiocarcinoma include ulcerative colitis, sclerosing cholangitis, and congenital biliary anomalies (choledochal cyst and Caroli's disease). MDCT imaging of cholangiocarcinoma is usually employed to evaluate the extent of the neoplasm and its resectability since radical surgical tumor removal with negative histologic margins is the only curative option.

The CT appearance of cholangiocarcinoma varies depending on the site of origin – peripheral intrahepatic, hilar, and extrahepatic. Peripheral cholangiocarcinoma appears as either a well-defined or an irregular mass along the course of dilated intrahepatic ducts. On MDCT, during both the LAP and PVP, intrahepatic cholangiocarcinoma usually demonstrate as a hypoattenuating mass with incomplete peripheral enhancement (Fig. 11a) [56, 57]. The central portion of the tumor may show prolonged enhancement and be hyperattenuating on EQP images (10–15 min postinjection) due to slow washout of the contrast material by the abundant fibrous tissue in the tumor (Fig. 11b). Up to 36% of cholangiocarcinomas demonstrate hyperattenuation during the EQP [28]. A time delay of 10–20 min after contrast media administration is optimal for EQP images [28]. With infiltrating hilar cholangiocarcinoma – the most common type of hilar cholangiocarcinoma – contrast-enhanced CT images may detect focal duct wall thickening, which appears hyperattenuating relative to liver parenchyma during the PVP [58]. A supplementary CT finding of hilar cholangiocarcinomas includes lobar atrophy due to either severe, long-standing ductal obstruction or portal venous encasement and obstruction [59, 60]. Contrast-enhanced CT appearances of infiltrating extrahepatic cholangiocarcinoma are hyperenhancing thickened walls in the common bile duct or a small hyperattenuating intraluminal mass at the point of abrupt termination of bile duct dilatation. Unfortunately, all the above CT findings may also occur with benign diseases that cause bile duct strictures. The CT protocol for diagnosing suspected cholangiocarcinoma should contain at least two enhancement phases (portal venous and equilibrium phases) acquired with thin collimation to obtain multiplanar reconstructions [61].

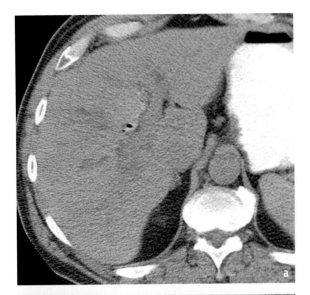

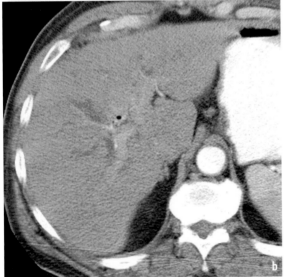

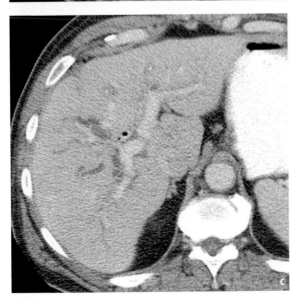

Fig. 12a-c. Early primary sclerosing cholangitis during the unenhanced state (**a**), LAP (**b**), PVP (**c**). Note the scattered intrahepatic ductal dilatation

Primary Sclerosing Cholangitis

Primary sclerosing cholangitis (PSC) is a rare chronic inflammatory condition of the intra- and extrahepatic bile ducts. It is associated with ulcerative colitis, Sjögren's syndrome, Riedel's thyroiditis, retroperitoneal fibrosis, and, occasionally, Crohn's disease. The etiology of PSC is unknown although it is probably autoimmune. PSC occurs predominantly in men during the third to fifth decade of life. The typical presentation is intermittent jaundice and recurrent episodes of cholangitis.

CT findings in PSC usually reflect pathological changes, such as ductal and periductal fibrosis, that result in segmental stricturing and dilatation of the bile ducts. In the majority of cases, both the intra- and extrahepatic bile ducts are involved. Long-standing biliary obstruction may lead to cirrhosis. Morphological changes of PSC-induced cirrhosis include fibrosis, regenerative nodules, parenchymal atrophy, and marked hypertrophy of the caudate lobe.

MDCT in patients with PSC may demonstrate closely alternating dilatation and strictures of the intrahepatic bile ducts, thereby giving them a beaded appearance (Fig. 12a-c). Other characteristic CT findings of PSC include skip dilatation, a solitary dilatation of a peripheral duct, and pruning of the bile ducts representing dilated segmental duct without any dilatation of the side branches. According to Teefey et al. [62], none of these CT findings are specific to PSC except skip dilatations.

Since ERCP and biopsy are still the gold standard for diagnosing PCS, MDCT plays a central role in the evaluation of the extent of cirrhosis, portal hypertension, and cholangiocarcinoma and their complications. In a study by MacCarty et al. [63], 13% of 104 patients with PCS developed a cholangiocarcinoma, proven either by biopsy or autopsy. In a more recent investigation, Campbell et al. [64] demonstrated that CT provides higher sensitivity than cholangiography in detecting cholangiocarcinoma complicated by PCS.

Acute and Chronic Cholecystitis

Acute cholecystitis is mainly caused by an impacted stone in the cystic duct, resulting in bile stasis and gallbladder distension. Ultrasound is the diagnostic method of choice for the initial work-up of suspected gallbladder pathologies. Since the clinical symptoms of acute cholecystitis are usually nonspecific, MDCT often serves as the initial imaging modality for evaluation of the acute abdomen. MDCT is also the preferred technique for diagnosing acute cholecystitis complications. The most common features on CT in acute cholecystitis include gallstones, thickening of the gallbladder wall (>3 mm), gallbladder distension or hy-

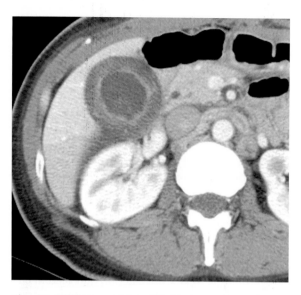

Fig. 13. MDCT image of the gallbladder in a patient with acute cholecystitis. Note the hyperenhancement of adjacent liver parenchyma

drops (>5 cm), hyperattenuating bile, and pericholecystic fluid and stranding (Fig. 13) [65]. Furthermore, contrast-enhanced MDCT may reveal increased enhancement of the gallbladder wall, though this is a nonspecific finding. Yamashita et al. reported hyperenhancement in liver parenchyma adjacent to the gallbladder, likely due to hyperemia and to early venous drainage (Fig. 13) [66]. Common complications of acute cholecystitis include emphysematous cholecystitis, gangrene, and perforation of the gallbladder. In emphysematous cholecystitis, which occurs more commonly in elderly and diabetic patients, intramural gas secondary to gas-producing bacteria such as *Clostridium perfringens* can be detected on CT. No intravenous contrast material is required for a CT scan, which is the most accurate imaging technique to depict gas within the gallbladder wall [67].

Chronic cholecystitis may demonstrate many of the same findings on CT as acute cholecystitis. However, patients with chronic cholecystitis do not tend to have significant pericholecystic inflammation or fluid. The most common findings include calculi and mild to moderate thickening of the gallbladder wall. Since gallbladder carcinoma may show radiological features similar to chronic cholecystitis, to ensure adequate therapeutic management, it is important to differentiate between neoplasia and a chronic inflammatory process. Yun et al. [68] evaluated enhancement of the gallbladder wall during arterial and PVP CT images in patients with chronic cholecystitis and gallbladder carcinoma. With inflammation, the inner layer of the gallbladder wall was isoattenuating during the arterial phase and PVP. With neoplasia, the inner layer of the gallbladder wall was hyperattenuating

during both phases. Furthermore, the gallbladder wall tends to be thicker and more irregular in patients with carcinoma.

Gallbladder Carcinoma
Gallbladder carcinoma is the most common biliary tract neoplasm, being the fifth most common malignancy of the GI tract, and it occurs predominantly in elderly women. Adenocarcinoma is the main histological type, accounting for up to 90% of cases. Predisposing factors for gallbladder carcinoma include chronic cholecystitis, inflammatory bowel disease, familial adenomatous polyposis, and porcelain gallbladder. The reported incidence of gallbladder carcinoma found in patients with calcified or porcelain gallbladders ranges from 12% to 61% [69]. However, a more recent study demonstrated a lower incidence of 5%, and another group found no association between gallbladder carcinoma and porcelain gallbladder [69, 70]. Both clinical symptoms and CT appearances of gallbladder carcinoma are nonspecific, and as a result, most tumors are detected at an unresectable stage.

There are three different morphological types of gallbladder carcinoma: (1) a mass replacing the gallbladder, (2) an intraluminal mass, and (3) thickening of the gallbladder wall [71]. The mass in the gallbladder bed, the most common type, appears on unenhanced scans as a nodular hypoattenuating mass, which often infiltrates adjacent liver parenchyma (Fig. 14a). After administration of intravenous contrast material, the tumor demonstrates variable but heterogeneous enhancement (Figs. 14b, c). The soft tissue mass may also show enclosed gallstones and central necrosis. The intraluminal mass type, which is less invasive, usually presents as a polypoid mass, which must be differentiated from a benign polyp. Polyp size is an indicator of malignancy since benign lesions are usually smaller than 1 cm [72]. CT diagnosis of the least common type of gallbladder carcinoma, thickening of the gallbladder wall, is challenging due to this carcinoma's similar CT appearance to cholecystitis [73]. Additional CT findings of gallbladder carcinoma include biliary obstruction, direct invasion into adjacent liver parenchyma, liver metastases, lymphadenopathy, and peritoneal carcinomatosis.

Several investigators have recently demonstrated that CT is a very useful tool in preoperative evaluation of the resectability of gallbladder carcinoma [74, 75]. The accuracy for staging ranges from 83% to 93%. Detection of gallbladder carcinoma in the early stage, however, remains a challenge [74, 75].

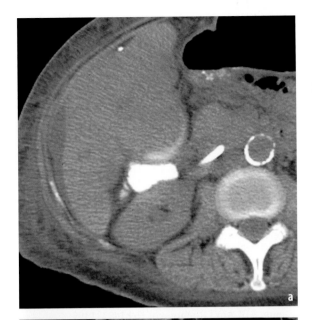

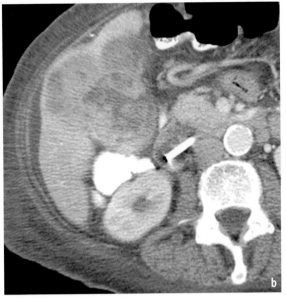

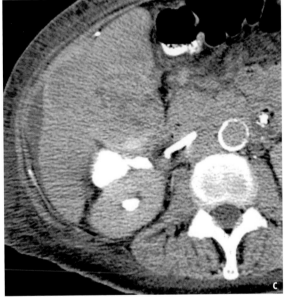

Fig. 14a-c. Gallbladder carcinoma during unenhanced state (**a**), PVP (**b**) and EQP (**c**). Note that the tumor has invaded adjacent liver parenchyma, seen best during the PVP

References

1. Schwartz LH, Gandras EJ, Colangelo SM et al (1999) Prevalence and importance of small hepatic lesions found at CT in patients with cancer. Radiology 210:71–74
2. Paulson EK, Harris JP, Jaffe TA et al (2005) Acute appendicitis: added diagnostic value of coronal reformations from isotropic voxels at multi-detector row CT. Radiology 235:879–885
3. Caoili EM, Paulson EK (2000) CT of small-bowel obstruction: another perspective using multiplanar reformations. AJR Am J Roentgenol 174:993–998
4. Kawata S, Murakami T, Kim T et al (2002) Multidetector CT: diagnostic impact of slice thickness on detection of hypervascular hepatocellular carcinoma. AJR Am J Roentgenol 179:61–66
5. Abdelmoumene A, Chevallier P, Chalaron M et al (2005) Detection of liver metastases under 2 cm: comparison of different acquisition protocols in four row multidetector-CT (MDCT). Eur Radiol 15:1881–1887
6. Weg N, Scheer MR, Gabor MP (1998) Liver lesions: improved detection with dual-detector-array CT and routine 2.5-mm thin collimation. Radiology 209:417–426
7. Haider MA, Amitai MM, Rappaport DC et al (2002) Multi-detector row helical CT in preoperative assessment of small (< or = 1.5 cm) liver metastases: is thinner collimation better? Radiology 225:137–142
8. Hong C, Bruening R, Schoepf UJ et al (2003) Multiplanar reformat display technique in abdominal multidetector row CT imaging. Clin Imaging 27:119–123
9. Jaffe TA, Nelson RC, Johnson GA et al (2006) Optimization of multiplanar reformations from isotrop-

ic datasets acquired on a 16-element multidetector helical CT scanner. Radiology (*in press*)

10. Stabile Ianora AA, Memeo M, Scardapane A et al (2003) Oral contrast-enhanced three-dimensional helical-CT cholangiography: clinical applications. Eur Radiol 13:867–873

11. Wang ZJ, Yeh BM, Roberts JP et al (2005) Living donor candidates for right hepatic lobe transplantation: evaluation at CT cholangiography – initial experience. Radiology 235:899–904

12. Caoili EM, Paulson EK, Heyneman LE et al (2000) Helical CT cholangiography with three-dimensional volume rendering using an oral biliary contrast agent: feasibility of a novel technique. AJR Am J Roentgenol 174:487–492

13. Zandrino F, Benzi L, Ferretti ML et al (2002) Multislice CT cholangiography without biliary contrast agent: technique and initial clinical results in the assessment of patients with biliary obstruction. Eur Radiol 12:1155–1161

14. Kim HC, Park SJ, Park SI et al (2005) Multislice CT cholangiography using thin-slab minimum intensity projection and multiplanar reformation in the evaluation of patients with suspected biliary obstruction: preliminary experience. Clin Imaging 29:46–54

15. Rao ND, Gulati MS, Paul SB et al (2005) Three-dimensional helical computed tomography cholangiography with minimum intensity projection in gallbladder carcinoma patients with obstructive jaundice: comparison with magnetic resonance cholangiography and percutaneous transhepatic cholangiography. J Gastroenterol Hepatol 20:304–308

16. Brink JA, Heiken JP, Forman HP et al (1995) Hepatic spiral CT: reduction of dose of intravenous contrast material. Radiology 197:83–88

17. Heiken JP, Brink JA, McClennan BL et al (1995) Dynamic incremental CT: effect of volume and concentration of contrast material and patient weight on hepatic enhancement. Radiology 195:353–357

18. Yamashita Y, Komohara Y, Takahashi M et al (2000) Abdominal helical CT: evaluation of optimal doses of intravenous contrast material – a prospective randomized study. Radiology 216:718–723

19. Ho LM, Nelson RC, Thomas J et al (2004) Abdominal aortic aneurysms at multi-detector row helical CT: optimization with interactive determination of scanning delay and contrast medium dose. Radiology 232:854–859

20. Itoh S, Ikeda M, Achiwa M et al (2005) Multiphase contrast-enhanced CT of the liver with a multislice CT scanner: effects of iodine concentration and delivery rate. Radiat Med 23:61–69

21. Awai K, Takada K, Onishi H, Hori S (2002) Aortic and hepatic enhancement and tumor-to-liver contrast: analysis of the effect of different concentrations of contrast material at multi-detector row helical CT. Radiology 224:757–763

22. Schoellnast H, Tillich M, Deutschmann HA et al (2004) Improvement of parenchymal and vascular enhancement using saline flush and power injection for multiple-detector-row abdominal CT. Eur Radiol 14:659–664

23. Schoellnast H, Tillich M, Deutschmann HA et al (2003) Abdominal multidetector row computed tomography: reduction of cost and contrast material dose using saline flush. J Comput Assist Tomogr 27:847–853

24. Chopra S, Chintapalli KN, Ramakrishna K et al (2000) Helical CT cholangiography with oral cholecystographic contrast material. Radiology 214:596–601

25. Ott DJ, Gelfand DW (1981) Complications of gastrointestinal radiologic procedures: II. Complications related to biliary tract studies. Gastrointest Radiol 6:47–56

26. Foley WD, Mallisee TA, Hohenwalter MD et al (2000) Multiphase hepatic CT with a multirow detector CT scanner. AJR Am J Roentgenol 175:679–685

27. Laghi A, Iannaccone R, Rossi P et al (2003) Hepatocellular carcinoma: detection with triple-phase multi-detector row helical CT in patients with chronic hepatitis. Radiology 226:543–549

28. Keogan MT, Seabourn JT, Paulson EK et al (1997) Contrast-enhanced CT of intrahepatic and hilar cholangiocarcinoma: delay time for optimal imaging. AJR Am J Roentgenol 169:1493–1499

29. Soyer P, Poccard M, Boudiaf M et al (2004) Detection of hypovascular hepatic metastases at triple-phase helical CT: sensitivity of phases and comparison with surgical and histopathologic findings. Radiology 231:413–420

30. Miller FH, Butler RS, Hoff FL et al (1998) Using triphasic helical CT to detect focal hepatic lesions in patients with neoplasms. AJR Am J Roentgenol 171:643–649

31. Ch'en IY, Katz DS, Jeffrey RB Jr et al (1997) Do arterial phase helical CT images improve detection or characterization of colorectal liver metastases? J Comput Assist Tomogr 21:391–397

32. Nino-Murcia M, Olcott EW, Jeffrey RB Jr et al (2000) Focal liver lesions: pattern-based classification scheme for enhancement at arterial phase CT. Radiology 215:746–751

33. Valls C, Andia E, Sanchez A et al (2001) Hepatic metastases from colorectal cancer: preoperative detection and assessment of resectability with helical CT. Radiology 218:55–60

34. Blake SP, Weisinger K, Atkins MB, Raptopoulos V (1999) Liver metastases from melanoma: detection with multiphasic contrast-enhanced CT. Radiology 213:92–96

35. Furuta A, Ito K, Fujita T et al (2004) Hepatic enhancement in multiphasic contrast-enhanced MD-CT: comparison of high- and low-iodine-concentration contrast medium in same patients with chronic liver disease. AJR Am J Roentgenol 183:157–162

36. Oliver JH 3rd, Baron RL, Federle MP et al (1997) Hypervascular liver metastases: do unenhanced and hepatic arterial phase CT images affect tumor detection? Radiology 205:709–715

37. Figueras J, Jaurrieta E, Valls C et al (2000) Resection or transplantation for hepatocellular carcinoma in cirrhotic patients: outcomes based on indicated treatment strategy. J Am Coll Surg 190:580–587

38. Island ER, Pomposelli J, Pomfret EA (2005) Twenty-year experience with liver transplantation for hepatocellular carcinoma. Arch Surg 140:353–358

39. Kutami R, Nakashima Y, Nakashima O (2000) Pathomorphologic study on the mechanism of fatty

change in small hepatocellular carcinoma of humans. J Hepatol 33:282–289

40. Peterson MS, Baron RL, Marsh JW Jr (2000) Pretransplantation surveillance for possible hepatocellular carcinoma in patients with cirrhosis: epidemiology and CT-based tumor detection rate in 430 cases with surgical pathologic correlation. Radiology 217:743–749

41. Valls C, Cos M, Figueras J et al (2004) Pretransplantation diagnosis and staging of hepatocellular carcinoma in patients with cirrhosis: value of dual-phase helical CT. AJR Am J Roentgenol 182:1011–1017

42. Kim SK, Lim JH, Lee WJ et al (2002) Detection of hepatocellular carcinoma: comparison of dynamic three-phase computed tomography images and four-phase computed tomography images using multidetector row helical computed tomography. J Comput Assist Tomogr 26:691–698

43. Iannaccone R, Laghi A, Catalano C et al (2005) Hepatocellular carcinoma: role of unenhanced and delayed phase multi-detector row helical CT in patients with cirrhosis. Radiology 234:460–467

44. Sultana S, Morishita S, Awai K et al (2003) Evaluation of hypervascular hepatocellular carcinoma in cirrhotic liver by means of helical CT: comparison of different contrast medium concentrations within the same patient. Radiat Med 21:239–245

45. Marchiano A, Spreafico C, Lanocita R et al (2005) Does iodine concentration affect the diagnostic efficacy of biphasic spiral CT in patients with hepatocellular carcinoma? Abdom Imaging 30:274–280

46. Kim T, Murakami T, Takahashi S et al (1998) Effects of injection rates of contrast material on arterial phase hepatic CT. AJR Am J Roentgenol 171:429–432

47. Oliver JH, Baron RL (1999) High flow injection rates versus low flow injection rates: does increasing the injection rate result in greater detection of enhancement of hepatocellular carcinoma during hepatic arterial phase CT? 213:92–96

48. Mathieu D, Kobeiter H, Maison P et al (2000) Oral contraceptive use and focal nodular hyperplasia of the liver. Gastroenterology 118:560–564

49. Hussain SM, Terkivatan T, Zondervan PE et al (2004) Focal nodular hyperplasia: findings at state-of-the-art MR imaging, US, CT, and pathologic analysis. Radiographics 24:3–19

50. Brancatelli G, Federle MP, Grazioli L (2001) Focal nodular hyperplasia: CT findings with emphasis on multiphasic helical CT in 78 patients. Radiology 219:61–68

51. Vilgrain V, Uzan F, Brancatelli G (2003) Prevalence of hepatic hemangioma in patients with focal nodular hyperplasia: MR imaging analysis. Radiology 229:75–79

52. Carlson SK, Johnson CD, Bender CE, Welch TJ (2000) CT of focal nodular hyperplasia of the liver. AJR Am J Roentgenol 174:705–712

53. Grazioli L, Federle MP, Brancatelli G et al (2001) Hepatic adenomas: imaging and pathologic findings. Radiographics 21:877–892

54. Ichikawa T, Federle MP, Grazioli L, Nalesnik M (2000) Hepatocellular adenoma: multiphasic CT and histopathologic findings in 25 patients. Radiology 214:861–868

55. Ruppert-Kohlmayr AJ, Uggowitzer MM, Kugler C et

al (2001) Focal nodular hyperplasia and hepatocellular adenoma of the liver: differentiation with multiphasic helical CT. AJR Am J Roentgenol 176:1493–1498

56. Kim TK, Choi BI, Han JK et al (1997) Peripheral cholangiocarcinoma of the liver: two-phase spiral CT findings. Radiology 204:539–543

57. Valls C, Guma A, Puig I et al (2000) Intrahepatic peripheral cholangiocarcinoma: CT evaluation. Abdom Imaging 25:490–496

58. Han JK, Choi BI, Kim AY et al (2002) Cholangiocarcinoma: pictorial essay of CT and cholangiographic findings. Radiographics 22:173–187

59. Vazquez JL, Thorsen MK, Dodds WJ et al (1985) Atrophy of the left hepatic lobe caused by a cholangiocarcinoma. AJR Am J Roentgenol 144:547–548

60. Jarnagin WR, Fong Y, DeMatteo RP et al (2001) Staging, resectability, and outcome in 225 patients with hilar cholangiocarcinoma. Ann Surg 234:507–517

61. Zech CJ, Schoenberg SO, Reiser M, Helmberger T (2004) Cross-sectional imaging of biliary tumors: current clinical status and future developments. Eur Radiol 14:1174–1187

62. Teefey SA, Baron RL, Schulte SJ et al (1992) Patterns of intrahepatic bile duct dilatation at CT: correlation with obstructive disease processes. Radiology 182:139–142

63. MacCarty RL, LaRusso NF, May GR et al (1985) Cholangiocarcinoma complicating primary sclerosing cholangitis: cholangiographic appearances. Radiology 156:43–46

64. Campbell WL, Peterson MS, Federle MP et al (2001) Using CT and cholangiography to diagnose biliary tract carcinoma complicating primary sclerosing cholangitis. AJR Am J Roentgenol 177:1095–1100

65. Grand D, Horton KM, Fishman EK (2004) CT of the gallbladder: spectrum of disease. AJR Am J Roentgenol 183:163–170

66. Yamashita K, Jin MJ, Hirose Y et al (1995) CT finding of transient focal increased attenuation of the liver adjacent to the gallbladder in acute cholecystitis. AJR Am J Roentgenol 164:343–346

67. Grayson DE, Abbott RM, Levy AD, Sherman PM (2002) Emphysematous infections of the abdomen and pelvis: a pictorial review. Radiographics 22:543–561

68. Yun EJ, Cho SG, Park S et al (2004) Gallbladder carcinoma and chronic cholecystitis: differentiation with two-phase spiral CT. Abdom Imaging 29:102–108

69. Stephen AE, Berger DL (2001) Carcinoma in the porcelain gallbladder: a relationship revisited. Surgery 129:699–703

70. Towfigh S, McFadden DW, Cortina GR et al (2001) Porcelain gallbladder is not associated with gallbladder carcinoma. Am Surg 67:7–10

71. Itai Y, Araki T, Yoshikawa K et al (1980) Computed tomography of gallbladder carcinoma. Radiology 137:713–718

72. Koga A, Watanabe K, Fukuyama T et al (1988) Diagnosis and operative indications for polypoid lesions of the gallbladder. Arch Surg 123:26–29

73. Kim BS, Ha HK, Lee IJ et al (2002) Accuracy of CT in local staging of gallbladder carcinoma. Acta Radiol 43:71–76

74. Kumaran V, Gulati S, Paul B et al (2002) The role of dual-phase helical CT in assessing resectability of carcinoma of the gallbladder. Eur Radiol 12: 1993–1999

75. Yoshimitsu K, Honda H, Shinozaki K et al (2002) Helical CT of the local spread of carcinoma of the gallbladder: evaluation according to the TNM system in patients who underwent surgical resection. AJR Am J Roentgenol 179:423–428

II.3

Soft Organ MDCT Imaging: Pancreas and Spleen

Dushyant V. Sahani and Zarine K. Shah

Introduction

Imaging is now integral for diagnosing pancreatic disease and neoplasms. The use of multidetector computed tomography (MDCT) scanners has dramatically reduced scan acquisition time, with resultant improvement in patient compliance and image quality. Fast scanning time enables the acquisition of multiple phases of enhancement, which is of paramount importance in imaging the pancreas. The improved Z-axis resolution permits excellent image reconstructions, which play a critical role in diagnosis and staging of pancreatic neoplasms due to the anatomic layout of the pancreas and its vasculature. The cross-sectional imaging of splenic pathology has also improved due to the improvement in MDCT technology. MDCT can rapidly image the spleen and is valuable in the diagnosis of a variety of congenital, neoplastic, inflammatory, and traumatic lesions of the spleen.

Concepts in Pancreatic Imaging

Detection of lesions within the pancreas on CT depends largely on the enhancement pattern of the lesion and the alteration in contour of the normal pancreas. Before initiation of contrast-enhanced MDCT of the pancreas, administration of negative oral contrast medium is performed to distend the stomach and duodenum, which facilitates detection of abnormalities in the pancreatic bed. The use of negative oral contrast medium has an added advantage in that it does not mask radiopaque stones in the common bile duct, and it may aid in the evaluation of gastric and duodenal wall lesions [1].
Enhancement of the pancreatic parenchyma and lesions is influenced by volume, iodine concentration, and injection rate of the contrast medium. Contrast-enhanced imaging of the pancreas can

be performed in three distinct phases [2]. The early arterial phase, which is seen at approximately 20 s after contrast administration, demonstrates contrast uptake preferentially within the arterial tree with almost no enhancement of the pancreatic parenchyma. The next phase is the delayed arterial phase or the pancreatic phase, which is acquired at about 35–40 s following contrast administration. In this phase, there is optimal enhancement of the pancreatic parenchyma and excellent delineation of the arterial vascular system [2]. The third phase is the portal venous phase, which is usually acquired at 65–70 s after contrast administration. This phase offers the highest contrast uptake by the portal venous vessels, with good enhancement of the liver parenchyma. The exact timing of scan delay is variable based on the individual patient and can be optimized using bolus tracking techniques, where the initiation of the scan is based on the time when arterial enhancement peaks to a predetermined Hounsfield unit (HU) value. The Smart Prep technique used at our institute involves placing the region of interest (ROI) in the aorta just above the level of the pancreas and setting an HU value between 120 and 130 as the trigger. Scanning for the pancreatic phase starts 15 s after this threshold is reached.

Rationale for High-Concentration Contrast Media

An important determinant of image quality is contrast medium dynamics. The use of intravenous iodinated contrast media is routine with MDCT, and the dose and rate of contrast injection must be adapted to the higher scanning speeds of multidetector systems. The recommended maximum amount of iodine is 35–45 g, which should not change based on the concentration of the contrast medium used [3].

Higher concentrations of contrast in the ROI can be achieved by either an increase in injection rate or increase in the iodine concentration of the contrast medium. Since the contrast injection rate is limited by IV access and vessel diameter, the concentration of iodine (total iodine dose being kept constant) becomes an important factor. For a description of contrast enhancement of organs, a computer-generated, two-compartment model was used [4]. According to this model, organ enhancement is a result of enhancement of intravascular and extracellular–extravascular spaces. Contrast enhancement of the extracellular–extravascular space depends on the concentration gradient between intravascular and extracellular–extravascular spaces, the volume of the extracellular–extravascular space, the permeability of organ microvasculature and cellular interfaces, and surface area and time. A high concentration gradient between intravascular and extracellular–extravascular spaces allows a high influx of contrast material into the extracellular–extravascular space and contributes to high organ enhancement.

In a study by Fenchel et al. [5], the use of 400 mgI/ml of contrast medium concentration (Iomeprol 400) led to a significantly higher arterial and portal venous phase enhancement as compared with 300 mgI/ml concentration, the rate of contrast injection and the total dose of iodine being kept constant. It is likely that the use of high concentrations of contrast medium would improve conspicuity of hypovascular and hypervascular lesions in the pancreas.

Scanning Technique

A noncontrast CT of the upper abdomen is performed using 10-mm slice collimation to cover the pancreas. Depending on the scanner type, a pancreatic phase is performed using 1- to 2-mm slice collimation. Acquisition of the pancreatic phase is usually at a delay of 35–40 s following a bolus of 125–150 cc of iodinated contrast medium injected at a rate of 4–5ml/s. The scanned area extends from the diaphragm to below the transverse duodenum in a single breath hold [6]. A weight-based approach to IV contrast medium administration is now considered more appropriate in order to optimize the iodine dose for a study. An iodine dose of 550 mg/kg body weight can be used for both pancreatic and vascular enhancement that translates into 1.8–2.0 cc/kg body weight.

For the next phase, the patient is instructed to breathe deeply following the pancreatic phase acquisition, and a second spiral acquisition is performed at a 70–80 s scan delay. This is the portal venous phase, which covers the entire upper abdomen using 2.5- to 5-mm slice collimation, depending on the patient's body habitus (Table 1). This phase is critical for the detection of small hypodense liver metastases and in the diagnosis of venous encasement by a tumor. Early arterial phase scans can be performed if a CT angiogram is desired.

Dual-Phase Imaging for the Pancreas

Dual-phase MDCT of the pancreas is typically undertaken in the late arterial (pancreatic) phase and the portal venous phase and is considered optimal for assessment of pancreatic adenocarcinoma [2]. The gland enhances avidly during the pancreatic phase, thus, most pancreatic adenocarcinomas appear as low-density lesions compared with the normal enhancing pancreatic parenchyma, making tumor conspicuity maximal during this phase [7, 8] (Figs. 1a, b and 2a, b) The pancreatic phase also facilitates visualization of major arterial structures and permits staging the tumor and determining resectability based on vascular involvement (Fig. 3a, b). The criteria of unresectability of

Table 1. Multidetector computed tomography (MDCT) parameters for the pancreas: Protocols for GE Scanners at our institute

Parameters	4 channel	16 channel	64 channel
DC (mm)	1.25	0.625	0.6
TS (mm/s)	15	18.75	38
	Beam Pitch 1.0–2.0		
Slice thickness (mm)			
Arterial (CTA)	1.25	1.0	1.0
Arterial (liver)	2.5–5.0	2.5	2.5
Venous (CTA)	2.5	2.0	2.0
Venous (liver)	5.0	5.0	5.0
	Delay arterial bolus tracking empirical delay 25–30 s		
Venous Delay (s)	65–70	65–70	65–70

DC detector collimation, TS table speed, CTA computed tomographic arteriography

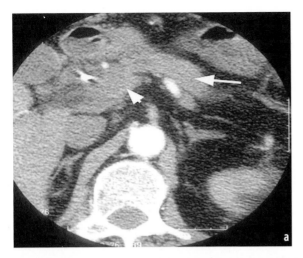

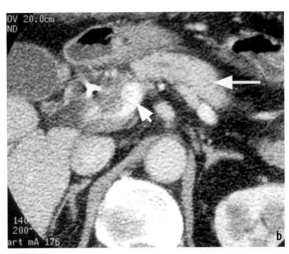

Fig. 1a, b. Importance of optimal phase imaging: **a** Early arterial phase axial multidetector computed tomography (MDCT) image in a patient with adenocarcinoma of the pancreatic head. Suboptimal enhancement of the normal pancreas (*long white arrow*) and portal vein (*short white arrow*). **b** Pancreatic phase helical computed tomography (CT) in the same patient, demonstrating optimized parenchymal (*long white arrow*) and vascular enhancement. Furthermore, the tumor is clearly identified and encases the portal vein (*short white arrow*)

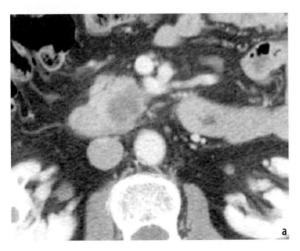

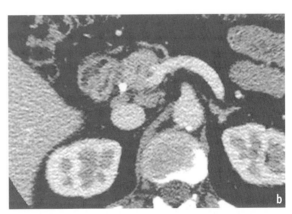

Fig. 2a, b. Importance of optimal "pancreatic phase" imaging: **a** Image acquired in the pancreatic phase clearly reveals the relatively hypodense mass in the pancreatic head. **b** Axial multidetector computed tomography (MDCT) image in a different patient taken later than the pancreatic phase shows a soft tissue invading into the superior mesenteric vein (SMV); however, the mass is not conspicuous on this phase due to equal enhancement of the mass and the normal pancreatic parenchyma

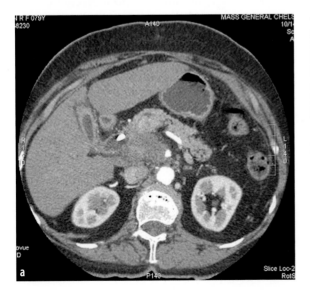

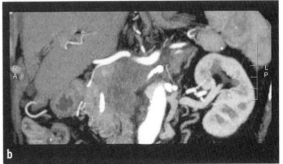

Fig. 3a, b. Axial contrast-enhanced 16-channel multidetector computed tomography (MDCT) image in a 79-year-old woman demonstrates an infiltrating mass involving the head and uncinate process of the pancreas, which encases the origin of the celiac axis, superior mesenteric vein (SMA), and invades into the inferior vena cava (IVC). (a) Coronal reformatted image in the same patient gives a better idea of the true extent of the tumor in the vertical dimension (b)

Table 2. Comparative results for detection and respectability of pancreatic adenocarcinoma

Image mode	Sensitivity	Specificity	Accuracy
Single-slice CT	81–89%	81–89%	69–87%
	Nishiharu T et al [11]	Nishiharu T et al [11]	Trede M et al [12]
MDCT	96%	77%	85–90%
	Ellsmere J [13]	Grenacher L [14]	Kulig J et al [15]
EUS	89–100%	100%	69–87%
	DeWitt J et al [16]	Wiersema MJ [17]	Trede M et al [12]

CT computed tomography, *MDCT* multidetector computed tomography, *EUS* endovascular ultrasound

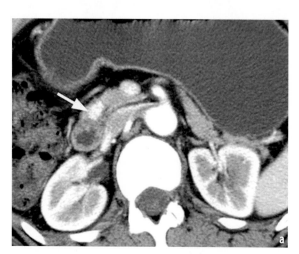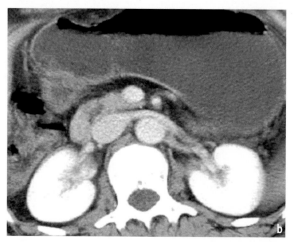

Fig. 4a, b. Pancreatic arterial phase helical computed tomography (CT) demonstrating a hypervascular tumor (*white arrow*) in the head of the pancreas. (**a**) Portal venous phase image reveals a hypodensity in the region of the tumor. It is imperative to perform an arterial phase CT in a patient with suspected endocrine tumor to allow adequate characterization of the mass, which is well demonstrated in this case (**b**)

pancreatic adenocarcinoma now includes extra-pancreatic invasion of major vessels (defined as tumor-to-vessel contiguity >50%) such as celiac artery, hepatic artery, portal vein, superior mesenteric artery or superior mesenteric vein, or massive venous invasion with thrombosis (Fig. 3a, b). Likewise, the presence of distant metastasis to the liver, regional lymph nodes, or omentum is a contraindication for surgical resection. However, partial venous invasion (tumor-to-vessel contiguity <50%) without thrombosis or obliteration of the venous lumen can still be classified as resectable adenocarcinoma [9, 10]. (Table 2).

Functioning or hormone-producing neuroendocrine tumors are typically hypervascular, and they enhance in the early arterial phase (20–25 s). Therefore, the scanning protocol for these tumors should be optimized to include arterial phase imaging. Neuroendocrine tumors are often seen as homogenously enhancing discrete lesions in the arterial phase [18] (Fig. 4a, b). Gouya et al., in their study comparing endovascular ultrasound (EUS) and CT, observed that MDCT alone has 94.4% di-

agnostic sensitivity for detecting insulinomas using the multiphasic protocol. EUS had a sensitivity of 93.8% and a combination of MDCT and EUS a sensitivity of 100% [19]. Although other modalities such as gadolinium-enhanced magnetic resonance imaging (MRI), somatostatin-receptor imaging, and EUS have emerged as possible diagnostic modalities for pancreatic endocrine neoplasm, multiphasic MDCT is far superior in both detection and staging of pancreatic islet-cell tumors [20]. The presence of hypervascular metastatic deposits to the pancreas can be detected in the arterial phase (Fig. 5). Arterial-enhancing liver metastasis from neuroendocrine tumors is also well seen during this phase.

Cystic Lesion Detection and Characterization

Cystic lesions in the pancreas are now frequently diagnosed due to the increased utilization of CT. These lesions encompass true neoplasms as well as

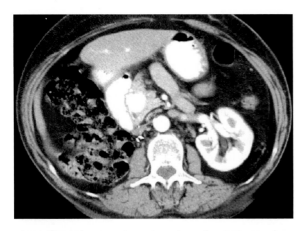

Fig. 5. Axial contrast-enhanced 16-channel multidetector computed tomography (MDCT) image reveals a hypervascular lesion in the head of pancreas. This patient is status postright nephrectomy for a renal call carcinoma. The lesion in the pancreas is an enhancing metastatic deposit from the renal cell carcinoma

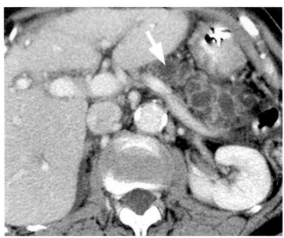

Fig. 6. Portal venous phase helical computed tomography (CT) in a 77-year-old man with chronic abdominal pain, demonstrating diffuse dilatation of the pancreatic duct (*white arrow*) with numerous side-branch cysts, consistent with a diagnosis of combined main duct and side branch intrapancreatic mucinous neoplasm (IPMN)

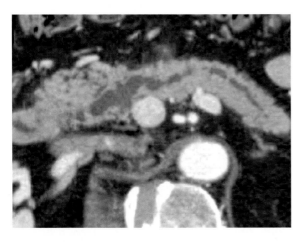

Fig. 7. Curved reformatted image in a middle-aged woman reveals segmental dilatation of the pancreatic duct without transition. These findings are consistent with main duct intrapancreatic mucinous neoplasm (IPMN)

pancreatic mucinous neoplasms (IPMN) arise from the epithelium of the main pancreatic duct and its side branch and may be benign or malignant. Demonstration of communication between the ductal system and the cystic neoplasm is diagnostic of IPMNs [25] (Fig. 6). MDCT with postprocessing is now considered excellent for the comprehensive evaluation of cystic lesions. Pancreatic ductal anatomy and pathology, including cyst communications, can be reliably detected with CT (Fig. 7).

Inflammatory Pathologies of the Pancreas

Although inflammatory pathologies in the pancreas are primarily diagnosed from clinical and laboratory findings, such as serum amylase, lipase, etc., CT is often used to confirm the diagnosis, determine the severity, and evaluate for any associated complication. There have been some minor changes in the protocol for imaging patients suspected of having pancreatitis with the use of MDCT. The use of positive oral contrast is no longer required to distinguish collections from hollow viscus since the high resolution of the MDCT scanners and the availability of reformatted images allow easy differentiation of the two. Intravenous contrast-enhanced multiphasic MDCT can detect all but the mildest forms of pancreatitis. The subtle findings of relatively poor enhancement of the pancreatic parenchyma, either diffusely or focally, and the loss of normal parenchymal lobulations can be a clue to the diagnosis of this condition

inflammatory lesions. The accurate characterization of a cystic lesion is critical to triage a treatment decision in these patients. Serous cystadenoma is seen as a solid lesion, with a "honeycomb" appearance due to presence of microcysts [21]. The previously described appearance of a large mass with a central scar and "sunburst" calcification is uncommonly seen, as these lesions are being detected at early stages. Central scar when present is considered characteristic for serous cystadenoma. Mucinous neoplasms, on the other hand, are macrocystic, with few discrete compartments [22]. The classical septal or peripheral eggshell calcification, which is diagnostic of mucinous cysts, is an uncommon feature [23, 24]. Intra-

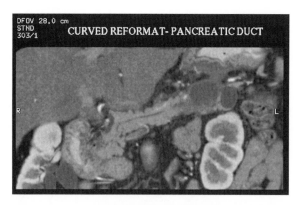

Fig. 8. Curved reformatted image along the pancreatic duct in a patient who presented with abdominal pain reveals an area of poor enhancement of the pancreatic parenchyma at the body due to parenchymal edema and presence of two pseudocysts in the tail of the pancreas. These features are typical of pancreatitis. The excellent resolution of 16-channel multidetector computed tomography (MDCT) permits accurate diagnosis of even subtle pancreatic inflammatory processes

(Fig. 8). Dual phase imaging for pancreatitis can be beneficial if a vascular complication, such as a pseudoaneurysm, is suspected clinically.

Autoimmune pancreatitis is a rare form of diffuse or focal enlargement of the pancreas. Diffuse "sausage-shaped" enlargement of the pancreas with a rim or "halo" around it is considered a characteristic finding for this entity. Also, lack of vascular encasement may aid in distinguishing the focal form of autoimmune pancreatitis or focal chronic pancreatitis from adenocarcinoma of the pancreas [26].

Chronic pancreatitis, on the other hand, occurs due to repeated episodes of inflammation, which can lead to glandular atrophy and subsequent glandular scarring and fibrosis. The presence of calcifications within part or whole of the gland or intraductal calculi may be associated with these features. These findings may occur alone or with pancreatic ductal dilatation.

Image Processing and Display

Various types of image postprocessing can be used for the evaluation of tumor resectability. The advantage of MDCT is the ability to obtain a volumetric data set with near-isotropic voxels. This improves the quality of two-dimensional (2-D) and three-dimensional (3-D) reformations. The evaluation of peripancreatic vasculature is of paramount importance in the diagnosis of locally advanced pancreatic adenocarcinoma. The addition of 2-D and 3-D reformatted images provides information regarding tumor extent, which may be difficult to evaluate on axial images alone. The pres-

ence of reconstructed images allows rapid identification of salient features by surgeons and gastroenterologists [27].

It is important to perform overlapping reconstructions at one half the slice thickness of the scan acquisition so as to ensure optimal spatial resolution [6]. A variety of image processing options are available, such as curved reformatted images, minimum-intensity projections, volume-rendered images, standard coronal and sagittal plane reformations, and coronal oblique reformations. Curved reformations are easily understood by surgeons and gastroenterologists. These are routinely obtained in two orthogonal planes. Curved-transverse and curved-coronal reformations are both useful. Since soft tissues are displayed with the ductal and vascular structures, curved reformations are important in determining vascular involvement and ductal abnormalities [28].

Minimum-intensity projections are used to visualize low-attenuation structures, such as pancreatic and common bile ducts [29]. Maximum-intensity projections evaluate high attenuation structures, such as peripancreatic vasculature. Volume-rendered images aid in peripancreatic vessel and tumor encasement.

MDCT Imaging of the Spleen

Evaluation of the spleen is most often done in conjunction with the liver and pancreas. Focal lesions in the spleen are encountered in patients with or without a risk of malignancy. There exists a significant overlap in the imaging features of these lesions, and thus accurate characterization of a lesion into benign or malignant histopathologic subtypes is often difficult.

When MDCT is performed specifically for imaging the spleen, images are obtained at 50–70 s after contrast injection, which is the phase of homogenous parenchymal enhancement of the spleen. When the splenic parenchyma is imaged in the arterial phase, a typical inhomogeneous "tigroid" enhancement pattern is noted due to differential enhancement of the white and red pulp [3] (Fig. 9a, b). At least 50% of normal spleens demonstrate heterogenous enhancement on dynamic CT, which is more pronounced on MDCT due to high levels of bolus contrast opacification [30]. Ideally, thin-detector collimation (2.5 mm) is preferred for evaluation. Image reconstructions are performed at 1–2 mm, which improves the quality of the 3-D images. Three-dimensional and multiplanar reconstructions are very helpful in detecting splenic and perisplenic processes.

Splenomegaly can be due to a variety of conditions. MDCT can determine whether the spleen is

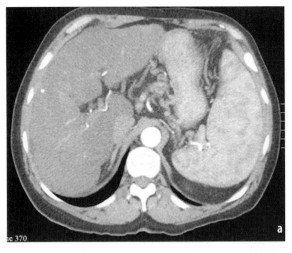
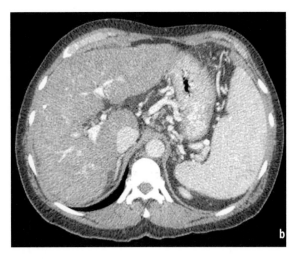

Fig. 9a, b. Arterial phase multidetector computed tomography (MDCT) of the abdomen shows the typical heterogenous enhancement pattern of the spleen sometimes called "tigroid" enhancement. (**a**) Equilibrium (venous) phase confirms the absence of pathology in the splenic parenchyma with homogenous enhancement of the spleen (**b**)

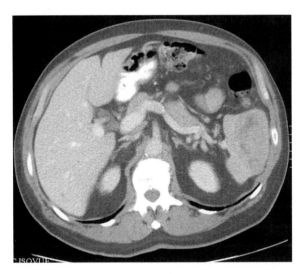

Fig. 10a, b. Axial multidetector computed tomography (MDCT) image of the abdomen demonstrates an exophytic heterogeneously enhancing mass within the spleen. (**a**) Abnormal periportal and portocaval lymphadenopathy is also visualized. These findings were suspicious of lymphoma on MDCT scan. Pathology examination proved this to be a non-Hodgkin's lymphoma (**b**)

enlarged and the degree of enlargement. Infiltrating conditions, such as malignancy, lymphoma (Fig. 10), and leukemia; and infectious processes, such as infective endocarditis and mononucleosis, can result in splenomegaly. Systemic processes, such as Gaucher's disease and sarcoidosis, can present with splenomegaly with or without focal masses. Angiosarcoma is the most common malignant primary nonlymphoid tumor of the spleen [31]. It has an aggressive growth pattern on CT, with cystic and necrotic areas seen within the tumor.

Splenic cysts may be congenital-epithelial true cysts, acquired posttraumatic pseudocysts, or parasitic cysts (echinococcal cysts). True epithelial-lined cysts are relatively uncommon (20%) [32]. Congenital cysts are well-defined, low-density lesions with sharply defined borders and no enhancement following contrast administration.

Splenic hemangiomas are often cavernous lesions, which may be from a few millimeters to several centimeters in size. Central punctate calcifications in the solid component and curvilinear peripheral calcifications may be seen. MDCT can identify these lesions as low density with enhancing periphery due to the vascular nature of the pathology. Lymphangiomas may be single or multiple and filled with proteinaceous material. Cystic variants may contain thin-walled, septated cysts, which do not enhance on contrast administration.

Splenic metastases on MDCT are usually low attenuation single or multiple foci. Distinction of cystic splenic metastasis from benign cysts is often difficult. MDCT may detect an enhancing component within the lesion, which favors malignancy (Fig. 11a, b). Splenic abscesses are typically focal and hypodense with a thick enhancing capsule. Presence of gas is a critical feature in making the diagnosis, and MDCT with multiplanar reconstruction is useful in detection of gas when present [33]. Splenic infarcts occur due to embolic occlusion of the splenic artery. A focal wedge-shaped area of decreased attenuation is the typical CT finding of splenic infarct (Fig. 12). Traumatic involvement of the spleen results in lacerations, subcapsular hematomas, or frank splenic rupture. These conditions can be diagnosed using MDCT.

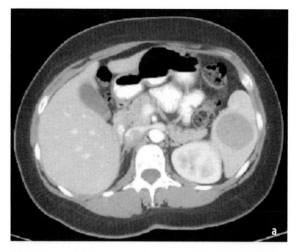
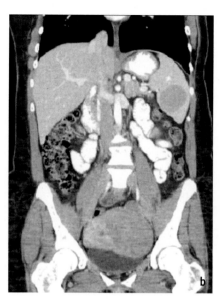

Fig. 11a, b. Axial contrast-enhanced 16-channel multidetector computed tomography (MDCT) in a 39-year-old woman with breast carcinoma reveals a predominantly hypodense mass lesion within the spleen, which has increased in size since the previous study. The presence of some enhancement within the lesion points toward a metastatic pathology as the likely cause. (**a**) Coronal reformatted image of the same patient shows the entire extent of the lesion (**b**)

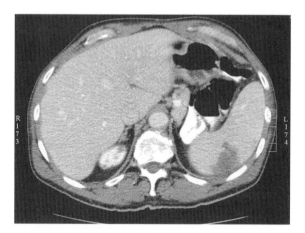

Fig. 12. Axial contrast-enhanced multidetector computed tomography (MDCT) image of the abdomen in the portal venous phase shows a wedge-shaped hypodensity in the spleen typical for a splenic infract

Conclusion

The availability of MDCT scanners has added new dimensions to spatial and temporal resolutions in CT imaging. The use of appropriately designed scanning protocols is the key issue for obtaining optimal quality studies. Availability of thinner-slice collimations leads to almost isotropic voxels and permits high-quality 2-D and 3-D reconstructions. Multiphasic imaging is especially important in the pancreas, where conspicuity of a tumor may change dramatically in the optimal phase. For pancreatic cancer detection, a pancreatic phase is considered optimal whereas for hypervascular lesion detection, early arterial phase scanning is required. Three-dimensional imaging with MDCT is now an integral part of preoperative staging and surgical planning. The use of high-concentration contrast media may further improve contrast enhancement in the tissue and vasculature.

MDCT has improved the diagnostic confidence for splenic lesions as well. Since there is considerable overlap between benign and malignant pathologies affecting the spleen, it is often difficult to accurately classify a lesion into a histopathological subtype. However, the use of multiphasic imaging and postprocessing techniques has considerably improved the scope for diagnosis of splenic pathology.

References

1. Tunaci M (2004) Multidetector row CT of the pancreas. Eur J Radiol 52:18–30
2. McNulty NJ, Francis IR, Platt JF et al (2001) Multidetector row helical CT of the pancreas: effect of contrast enhanced multiphasic imaging on enhancement of the pancreas, peripancreatic vasculature, and pancreatic adenocarcinoma. Radiol 220:97–102
3. Fenchel S, Boll DT, Fleiter TR (2003) Multislice helical CT of the pancreas and spleen. Eur J Radiol 45:S59–S72
4. Bae KT, Heiken JP, Brink JA (1998) Aortic and hepatic contrast medium enhancement at CT. Part I. Prediction with a computer model. Radiology 207:647–655

5. Fenchel S, Fleiter TR, Aschoff AJ et al (2004) Effect of iodine concentration of contrast media on contrast enhancement in multislice CT of the pancreas. Br J Radiol 77:821–830

6. Elliot K Fishman, Jeffrey RB Jr (2004) Multidetector CT: Principles, techniques and clinical applications. Lippincott Williams & Wilkins, Philadelphia, pp 85

7. Boland GW, O'Malley ME, Saez M et al (1999) Pancreatic-phase versus portal vein-phase helical CT of the pancreas: optimal temporal window for evaluation of pancreatic adenocarcinoma. AJR Am J Roentgenol 172:605–608

8. Lu DSK, Vedantham S, Krasny RM et al (1996) Two-phase helical CT for pancreatic tumors: pancreatic versus hepatic phase enhancement of tumor, pancreas and vascular structures. Radiology 199: 697–701

9. Warshaw AL, Fernandez-del-Castillo C (1992) Pancreatic carcinoma. N Engl J Med 326:455–465

10. LU DS, Reber HA, Krasny RM et al (1997) Local Staging of pancreatic cancer: criteria for unrectability of major vessels as revealed by pancreatic phase, thin-section helical CT. AJR Am J Roentgenol 168:1439–1443

11. Nishiharu T, Yamashita Y, Abe Y et al (1999) Local extension of pancreatic carcinoma: assessment with thin-section helical CT versus with breath-hold fast MR imaging – ROC analysis. Radiology 212:445–452

12. Trede M, Rumstadt B, Wendl K et al (1997) Ultrafast magnetic resonance imaging improves the staging of pancreatic tumors. Ann Surg 226:393–405

13. Ellsmere J, Mortele K, Sahani D et al (2005) Does multidetector-row CT eliminate the role of diagnostic laparoscopy in assessing the resectability of pancreatic head adenocarcinoma? Surg Endosc 19:369–373

14. Grenacher L, Klaus M, Dukic L et al (2004) Diagnosis and staging of pancreatic carcinoma: MRI versus multislice CT – a prospective study. Rofo 176: 1624–1633

15. Kulig J, Popiela T, Zajac A et al (2005) The value of imaging techniques in the staging of pancreatic cancer. Surg Endosc 19:361–365

16. DeWitt J, Devereaux B, Chriswell M et al (2004) Comparison of endoscopic ultrasonography and multidetector computed tomography for detecting and staging pancreatic cancer. Ann Int Med 141(10):753–763

17. Wiersema MJ (2001) Accuracy of endoscopic ultrasound in diagnosing and staging pancreatic carcinoma. Pancreatology 1:625–632

18. Sheth S, Hruban R, Fishman E (2002) Helical CT of islet cell tumors of the pancreas: typical and atypical manifestations. AJR Am J Roentgenol 179:725–730

19. Gouya H, Vignaux O, Augui J et al (2003) CT, endoscopic sonography, and a combined protocol for preoperative evaluation of pancreatic insulinomas. AJR Am J Roentgenol 181:987–992

20. Ichikawa T, Peterson M, Federle M et al (2000) Islet cell tumor of pancreas: Biphasic CT versus MR imaging in tumor detection. Radiology 216:163–171

21. Procacci C, Graziani R, Bicego E et al (1997) Serous cystadenoma of the pancreas: report of 30 cases with emphasis on the imaging findings. J Comput Assist Tomogr 21:373–382

22. Grogan JR, Saeian K, Taylor AJ et al (2001) Making sense of mucin-producing pancreatic tumors. AJM Am J Roentgenol 176:921–929

23. Curry C, John Eng, Karen M et al (2000) CT of primary cystic pancreatic neoplasms: Can CT be used for patient triage and treatment? AJM Am J Roentgenol 175:99–103

24. Wilentz RE, Albores-Saavendra J, Zahurak M et al (1999) Pathologic examination accurately predicts prognosis in mucinous cystic neoplasms of the pancreas. Am J Surg Pathol 23:132–137

25. Sugiyama M, Atomi Y (1998) Intraductal papillary mucinous tumors of the pancreas: imaging studies and treatment strategies. Ann Surg 228:685–691

26. Sahani D, Kalva SP, Farrell J et al (2004) Autoimmune Pancreatitis: Imaging Features. Radiology 233:345–352

27. Rubin GD (2000) Data explosion: the challenge of multidetector row CT. Eur J Radiol 36:74–80

28. Nono-Murcia M, Jeffrey RB Jr, Beaulieu CF et al (2001) Multidetecotr CT of the pancreas and bile duct system: value of curved planar reformations. AJR Am J Roentgenol 176:689–693

29. Raptopoulos V, Prassopoulos P, Chuttani R et al (1998) Multiplanar CT pancreatography and distal cholangiography with minimum intensity projections. Radiology 207:317–324

30. Donnelly LF, Foss JN, Frush DP et al (1999) Heterogenous splenic enhancements patterns on spiral CT images in children: minimizing misinterpretation. Radiology 210:493–497

31. Smith VC, Eisenberg Bl, McDonald EC (1985) Primary splenic angiosarcoma. Case report and literature review. Cancer 55:1625–1627

32. Warshauer DM, Koehler RE (1998) Spleen. In: Lee JKT, Sagel SS, Stanley Rj, Heiken JP (eds) Computed body tomography with MRI correlation, 3rd ed. Lippincott-Raven,1New York, pp 845–872

33. Urrutia M, Mergo PJ, Ros LH et al (1996) Cystic masses of the spleen: radiologic-pathologic correlation. Radiographics 16:107–129

II.4

Mesenteric and Renal CT Angiography

Lisa L. Wang, Christine O. Menias and Kyongtae T. Bae

Introduction

Multidetector-row computed tomography (MDCT) is changing the spectrum of vascular imaging as a result of its fast image acquisition speed and spatial resolution. When coupled with high-quality three-dimensional (3-D) image representations, MDCT angiography effectively permits the evaluation of the abdominal visceral vasculature and is preferred to conventional angiography because of its noninvasiveness.

Abdominal, applications of CT angiography (CTA) are growing. This chapter focuses on CTA evaluation of the mesenteric and renal vessels. Common indications include staging and surgical planning of tumors, evaluation for renal donor transplantation, workup of renovascular hypertension, and assessment of mesenteric ischemia and inflammatory bowel disease.

General Contrast Medium Principles

For CTA, contrast administration technique should be optimized to best delineate the vascular structure. Positive oral contrast is not administered because the anatomical separation of the intravenously enhanced vascular structures from the opacified gastrointestinal (GI) tract is difficult and can be problematic when displaying vasculature in 3-D. Prior to imaging, patients can drink approximately 1 l of water to distend the proximal GI tract. Optimal CTA contrast enhancement requires accurate timing of data acquisition with rapid and precise intravenous delivery of contrast medium. The amount of contrast medium required to achieve a desirable enhancement in CTA may be reduced because of a faster acquisition time with MDCT. An increased injection rate and high contrast medium concentration can compensate for the somewhat decreased magnitude of aortic enhancement achieved with the smaller contrast medium volume [1–3]. Contrast medium volumes ranging from 90 to 120 ml with 350–400 mgI/ml concentration are injected intravenously at rates of 4–5 ml/s. Given high injection rates, an intravenous access of at least 20 gauge or larger in the antecubital fossa should be used. In order to maintain an equivalent degree of contrast enhancement, larger patients require a larger iodine dose while smaller patients require smaller iodine dose. A saline flush improves the efficiency of contrast medium use and reduces artifact [4] and is particularly beneficial when a small total amount of contrast medium is used.

Precise arterial timing is critical to the CTA technique. Either a test bolus or bolus-tracking technique is used to determine the contrast bolus arrival time (*Tarr*). The *Tarr* is derived by placing the region of interest within the reference vessel of interest. To ensure adequate vascular opacification, the scan delay is determined with an additional delay of 5–15 s plus the *Tarr*, as described in Section I.2 [4, 5].

3-D CTA Postprocessing

CTA protocols generate a large amount of data. Interactive 3-D workstations are becoming more efficient in both managing the large data set and generating 3-D angiographic presentations [6]. Initially, reviewing axial images can be performed expeditiously by scrolling. Multiple planes can be selected on the interactive dedicated 3-D workstation to evaluate the vessel of interest. Volumetric data, reconstructed at 0.7–1.0 mm, can be reviewed using several available 3-D display techniques: maximum intensity projection (MIP), multiplanar reformatting (MPR), curve planar reformatting (CP), and volume rendering (VR).

The MIP technique displays only the maximum intensity voxel values along a viewer projection in a given volume of 3-D data. Thus, additional image processing steps are often required to remove bones and other hyperdense structures that are of high CT attenuation values and superimpose over and obscure the vascular structure of interest. MPR illustrates all structures within a particular plane. Thus, to circumvent this restriction in evaluating a vessel, curved planar reformatting, which can be also time consuming, is utilized. VR is an easily adaptable technique, as it requires minimal data editing by the operator and can dexterously display complex anatomy [7–11]. As VR preserves spatial depth and relationships, it has been proven to be better than MIP in evaluating the peripancreatic and renal vessels [9, 12, 13]. Nonetheless, MIP images readily simulate conventional angiographic images and are effective in evaluating atherosclerotic burden in the vessels. The workstation should be user friendly and flexible for radiologists to switch rapidly from one display mode to another to depict anatomy and pathology in the most informative manner.

Mesenteric Vascular Imaging

CTA of the mesenteric vasculature includes the superior mesenteric artery (SMA) (Fig. 1), the inferior mesenteric artery (IMA) (Fig. 1), the superior mesenteric vein (SMV), and the inferior mesenteric vein (IMV) (Fig. 2). MDCT can be used to delineate involvement of the mesenteric vessel from disease processes such as neoplasm, mesenteric ischemia, and inflammatory bowel disease [12].

Imaging Techniques

For any type of CTA, attention to patient preparation, intravenous contrast medium administration, scanner features, data quality, and postprocessing techniques is crucial. The mesenteric CTA protocol depends on the scanner type available. These protocols are summarized in Tables 1–3. Negative oral contrast such as water allows simultaneous detailed characterization of bowel-wall

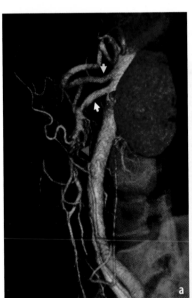
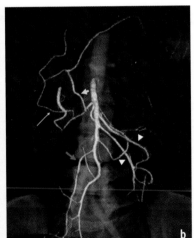
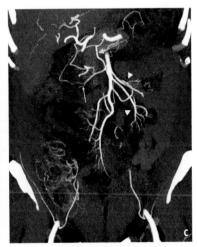
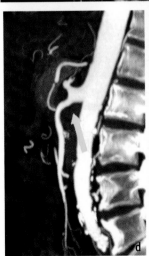
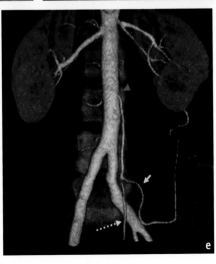

Fig. 1a-e. Normal superior and inferior mesenteric arteries. **a** Sagittal three-dimensional (3-D) volume rendering (VR) demonstrates the normal anatomy of the superior mesenteric artery (SMA) (*white arrow*) arising from near the L2 body approximately 1 cm caudal to the celiac axis (*yellow arrow*). Inferior mesenteric artery (IMA) (*red arrowhead*) arises approximately 7 cm caudal to the SMA. **b** Coronal VR and **c** coronal maximum intensity projection (MIP) demonstrating SMA branches: intestinal branches (*white arrowheads*), ileocolic artery (*red arrow*), middle colic artery (*short thick yellow arrow*), and right colic artery (*long thin yellow arrow*). **d** Uncommon variant of celiacomesenteric trunk (1%) (*yellow arrow*), which gives rise to the celiac axis and SMA in a different patient. **e** Coronal three-dimensional (3-D) VR of IMA (*red arrowhead*) with left colic artery (*short yellow arrow*) and superior rectal artery (*dashed yellow arrow*) [33]

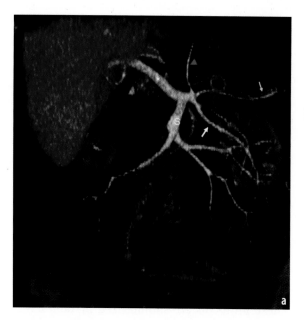 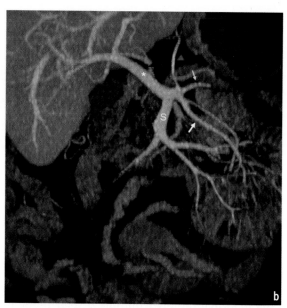

Fig. 2a, b. Normal portal venous system. Coronal volume rendering (VR) showing main portal vein (*), splenic vein (*yellow arrow*), and superior mesenteric vein (SMV) (*S*) joining at the portal confluence. The inferior mesenteric vein (IMV) (*white arrow*) and the gastroepiploic vein (*red arrowhead*) can drain into the splenic vein

Table 1. Mesenteric computed tomography angiography (CTA) parameters for 64-slice multidetector-row computed tomography (MDCT)[a]

Phase	Noncontrast	Arterial	Portal venous
kVp/effective mAs / rotation time (s)	120/240/0.5	120/240/0.5	120/240/0.5
Detector collimation (mm)	0.6	0.6	0.6
Slice thickness (mm)	5	1	2
Beam Pitch	1:1	1:1	1:1
Recon increment (mm)	5	0.7	2
Scan delay		Bolus tracking	60 s

[a] Scan parameters from Siemens Sensation 64

Table 2. Mesenteric computed tomography angiography (CTA) parameters for 16-slice multidetector-row computed tomography (MDCT)[a]

Phase	Noncontrast	Arterial	Portal venous
kVp/effective mAs/rotation time (s)	120/160/0.5	120/180/0.5	120/180/0.5
Detector collimation (mm)	1.5	0.75	1.5
Slice thickness (mm)	5	1	2
Feed/rotation (mm)	24	12	24
Recon increments (mm)	5	0.8	2
Scan delay		Bolus tracking	60 s

[a] Scan parameters from Siemens Sensation 16

Table 3. Mesenteric computed tomography angiography (CTA) parameters for 4-slice multidetector-row computed tomography (MDCT)[a]

Phase	Noncontrast	Arterial	Portal venous
kVp/effective mAs/rotation time (s)	120/180/0.5	120/180/0.5	120/180/0.5
Detector collimation (mm)	2.5	1.25	2.5
Slice thickness (mm)	5	1.25	3
Feed/rotation (mm)	10	4	10
Recon increment (mm)	5	1	2
Scan delay		Bolus tracking	60 s

[a] Scan parameters from Siemens VolumeZoom

enhancement and 3-D vascular reconstruction without interference from bowel content [14]. The noncontrast phase is used to delineate bowel hemorrhage and vascular calcifications, the arterial phase is used for arterial vascular mapping and treatment planning, and the portal venous phase is used for portal-venous vascular mapping and visceral evaluation [15].

Applications

Neoplasms

Among numerous neoplastic processes, pancreatic cancer most commonly involves the mesenteric vessels. SMA invasion (Fig. 3) precludes surgery for pancreatic cancer [16, 17]. Limited involvement of the portal vein or confluence may not be an ab-

solute contraindication for surgical resection. When a vessel is either narrowed or occluded by an adjacent soft tissue mass, vascular involvement is suspected (Fig. 4). Also, collateral vessels can be an ancillary sign of vascular involvement [12].

Other conditions such as carcinoid tumor, lymphoma (Fig. 5), or sclerosing mesenteritis (Fig. 6), can present as masses that infiltrate and encase the mesenteric vessels. The masses enveloping the mesenteric vessels are readily delineated on CTA but not on conventional digital subtraction angiography (DSA). For this reason, 3-D CTA is highly beneficial for planning surgery or biopsy.

Mesenteric Ischemia

Compromise (occlusion, thrombosis, or poor perfusion) of the major mesenteric vessels (SMV or

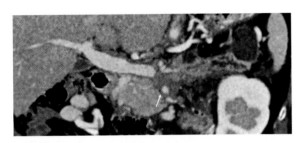

Fig. 3. Curved planar multiplanar reformat (MPR) reveals that the pancreatic adenocarcinoma (*) has totally encased the superior mesenteric artery (SMA) (*white arrow*). This finding is a contraindication for surgical treatment. Note the atrophy of the pancreatic body and tail to the *left* of the mass

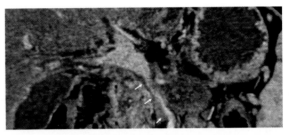

Fig. 4. Curved planar multiplanar reformat (MPR) demonstrating the pancreatic adenocarcinoma (*) severely narrowing the portal venous system at the portal confluence (*white arrows*)

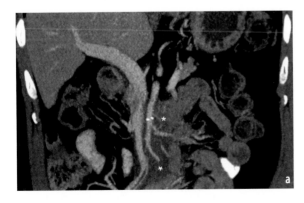

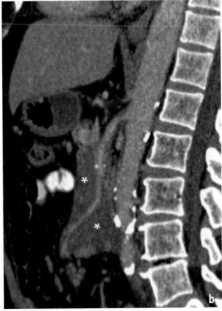

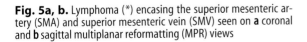

Fig. 5a, b. Lymphoma (*) encasing the superior mesenteric artery (SMA) and superior mesenteric vein (SMV) seen on **a** coronal and **b** sagittal multiplanar reformatting (MPR) views

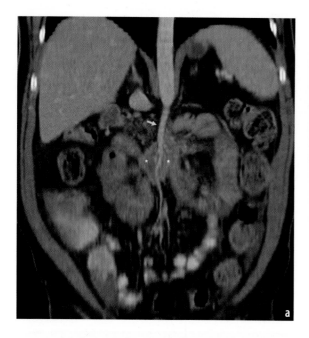

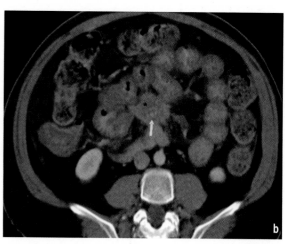

Fig. 6a, b. a Thick-section coronal and **b** axial multiplanar reformat (MPR) images demonstrate a soft tissue mass (*) encasing the superior mesenteric artery (SMA) (*yellow arrow*) with mesenteric tethering. Open surgical biopsy revealed the mass to be sclerosing mesenteritis

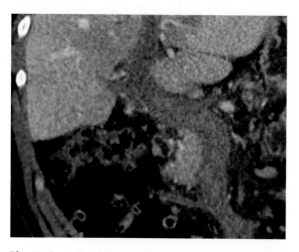

Fig. 7. Coronal multiplanar reformat (MPR) revealing acutely thrombosed portal venous system (*red arrows*). This patient, who had distal pancreatectomy and splenectomy for intraductal papillary mucinous neoplasm and subsequently developed acute pancreatitis of the remaining pancreas, now presents with thrombosed portal venous system

SMA) (Figs. 7 and 8) can lead to bowel ischemia or infarction. Thrombosis of the main mesenteric vessels can be seen on the axial images (Fig. 8c, d), and, if chronic, occlusions can present with collaterals (Figs. 9 and 10). Narrowing or occlusion of the origins of the major mesenteric vessels from atherosclerotic disease may be best seen on 3-D CTA (Figs. 9 and 10). Evaluation of the distal branches may also be improved with 3-D reformatted images.

Acute mesenteric ischemia can present with a variety of appearances. Manifestations can include thickened bowel loops with either intramural low attenuation suggesting edema or high attenuation representing submucosal/intramural hemorrhage (Fig. 8g). Bowel caliber can increase, bowel-wall enhancement can be decreased due to compromised blood supply or be increased due to hyperemia. Pneumatosis suggests irreversible infarction, but this is not specific, as it can be seen in mucosal ischemia (Fig. 8h) [14, 18–20].

Inflammatory Disease

Three-dimensional MDCTA may be helpful in assessing changes of active inflammation in patients with inflammatory bowel disease or vasculitis such as systemic lupus erythematosus (Fig. 11) and cystic medial necrosis (Fig. 12). Enlargement of the mesenteric vessels feeding the affected intestine may indicate hyperemia [12, 21].

Gastrointestinal Bleed

Oftentimes, when a patient presents with GI bleed, the source of the bleed is very difficult to find. CTA may be helpful in depicting the region or source and planning treatment of the patient's underlying disease condition (Fig. 13). Mesenteric vessel aneurysms or pseudoaneurysms (PSA) are accurately depicted with CTA (Fig. 14). CTA is particularly efficient in acquiring diagnostic information quickly for a patient in a trauma in order for surgeons and interventional radiologists to plan and expedite an appropriate treatment (Fig. 15).

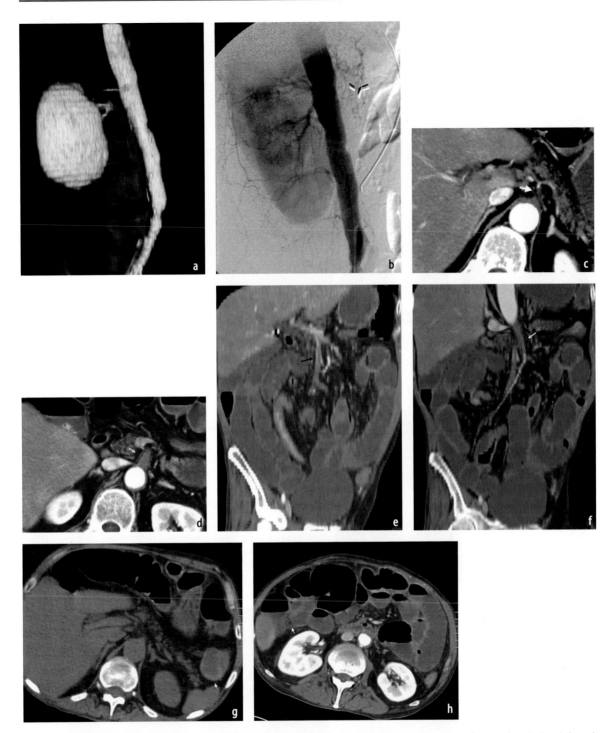

Fig. 8a-h. With history of worsening chronic abdominal pain and weight loss, this 59-year-old man was found to have ischemic bowel. All his major mesenteric vessels were occluded, as shown on **a** three-dimensional (3-D) volume rendered (VR) computed tomography angiography (CTA) and **b** conventional angiography, which demonstrate no major mesenteric vessel opacification. **c** Thrombosis of the celiac axis and **d** superior mesenteric artery (SMA) can be seen on axial plane. **e** Thick-section curved planar image demonstrates thrombus in the SMV. **f** Curve planar reformat reveals the SMA thrombosis. **g** Noncontrast axial image revealing submucosal hemorrhage (*arrow*). **h** Pneumatosis (*arrow*) in this case represents necrotic bowel

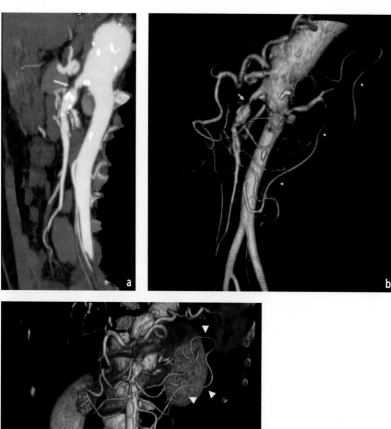

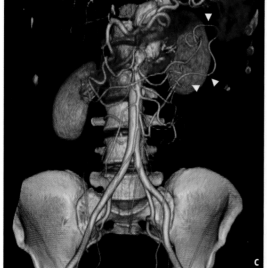

Fig. 9a-c. A 43-year-old man with thoracic and suprarenal abdominal aneurysm with an atherosclerotic superior mesenteric artery (SMA) stenosis just distal to its origin. **a** Thick-section multiplanar reformatting (MPR) and **b** and **c** three-dimensional (3-D) volume rendering (VR) reveal atherosclerotic plaque narrowing the SMA (*arrow*) with post-stenotic aneurysmal dilatation. Collaterals between the inferior mesenteric artery (IMA) and the SMA (*white arrowhead*) are formed via the arc of Riolan [33]

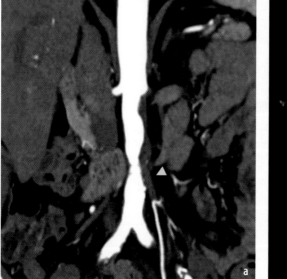

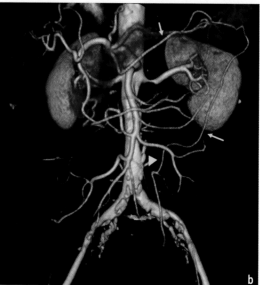

Fig. 10a, b. a Coronal multiplanar reformat (MPR) demonstrating the occluded proximal inferior mesenteric artery (IMA) (*arrowhead*) from atherosclerotic mural thrombus in a 69-year-old man with peripheral vascular disease. **b** Volume rendered (VR) image demonstrates the arc of Riolan (*yellow arrow*) that provides collateral to the IMA distal to the site of occlusion [33]

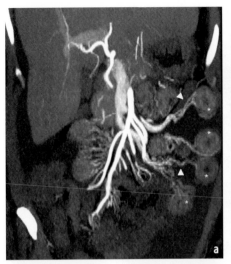
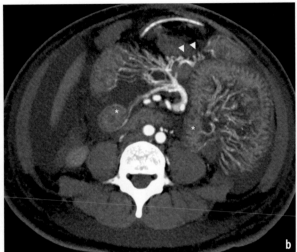

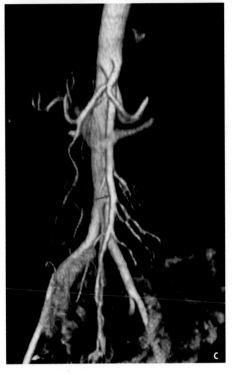

Fig. 11a-c. Thick-section multiplanar reformat (MPR) images demonstrating diffuse wall thickening (*) of the small bowel and small vessel collateralizations (corkscrew collaterals) of the jejunal branches of the superior mesenteric arteries (SMA) (*white arrowhead*) (**a, b**). Volume rendering (VR) image demonstrating the SMA (*red arrow*) (**c**) and its collateral vessels affected with vasculitis resulting in ischemia [34]. This patient is a 37-year-old woman with history of systemic lupus erythematosus who presented post-partum with several days of bloody stool. Similar arteriographic findings of corkscrew collaterals can be seen in patients with scleroderma, CREST syndrome, Buerger's disease, rheumatoid vasculitis, mixed connective-tissue disease, antiphospholipid-antibody syndrome, diabetes mellitus [35]

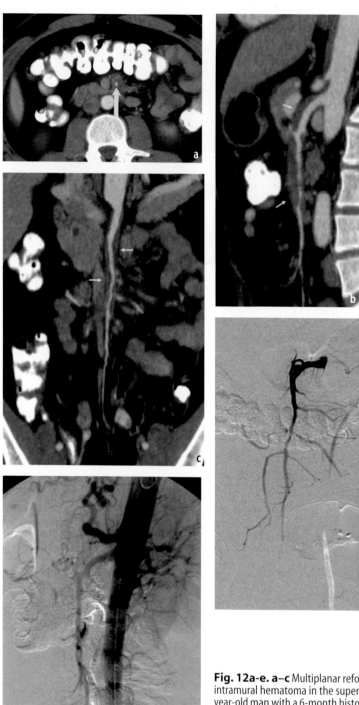

Fig. 12a-e. a–c Multiplanar reformat (MPR) images demonstrating a dissection with intramural hematoma in the superior mesenteric artery (SMA) (*yellow arrows*) in a 40-year-old man with a 6-month history of abdominal pain and a recent onset of diarrhea. **d, e** This abnormality of the SMA is not appreciated with the conventional angiogram because only opacified lumen is visualized. Surgical pathology demonstrates cystic medial necrosis as the etiology. Isolated SMA dissection is uncommon, and when it is seen, the reported causes include trauma, cystic medial necrosis, fibromuscular dysplasia, and hypertension [36]

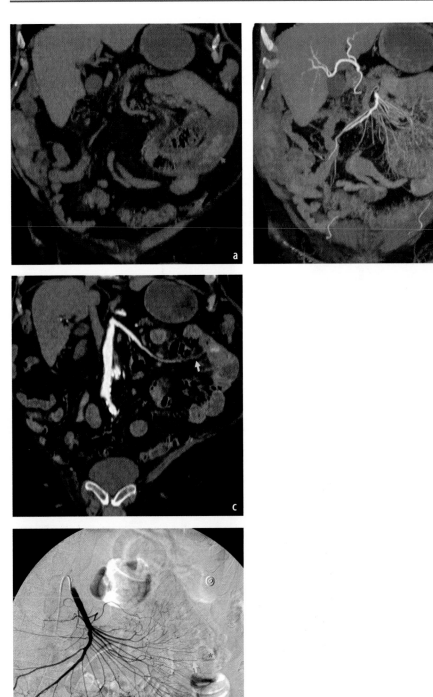

Fig. 13a-d. a Coronal thick-section multiplanar reformat (MPR) images demonstrating jejunal intraluminal hematoma (*red arrow*) on the unenhanced exam. **b, c** Active intravenous contrast extravasation (*) in a jejunal arterial branch (*yellow arrow*) on the enhanced images in a 76-year-old man with gastrointestinal (GI) bleed. **d** The leak is not as well seen on the conventional angiography

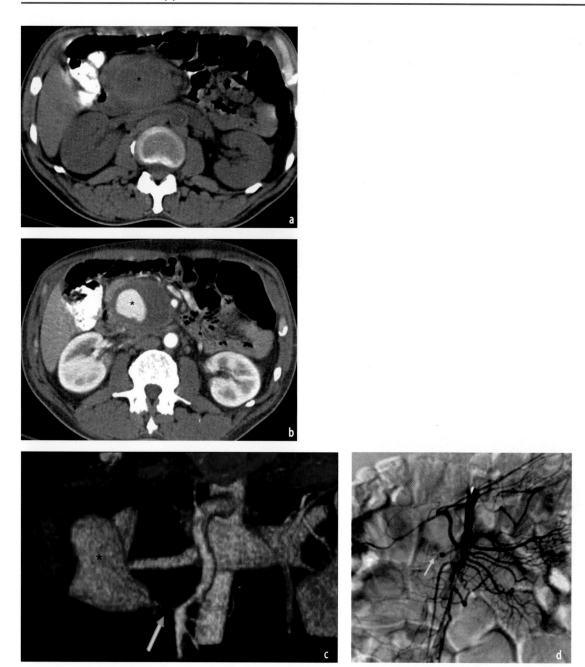

Fig. 14a-d. a A reported pancreatic "mass" (*) seen on unenhanced computed tomography (CT); **b** corresponds to a gastroduodenal artery pseudoaneurysm (*) apparent on the enhanced CT. This is a 53-year-old man with a history of alcohol-induced pancreatitis who presented with a diagnosis of a pancreatic mass. **c** Feeding vessel (*arrow*) from the superior mesenteric artery (SMA) was identified on the volume rendering (VR) image, **d** subsequently confirmed on the conventional preembolization angiogram

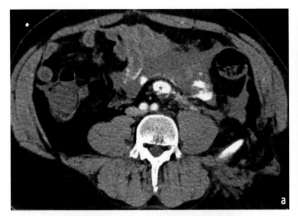

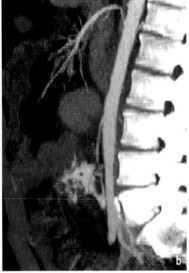

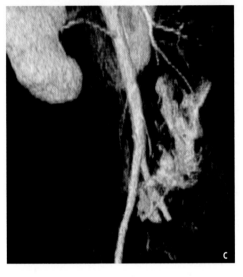

Fig. 15a-c. Active extravasation (*) from the inferior mesenteric artery (IMA) (*arrow*) depicted on the **a** axial computed tomography (CT), **b** sagittal maximum intensity projection (MIP), **c** and volume rendering (VR) images from a 44-year-old man who became hypotensive and unresponsive after suffering a motor vehicle collision

Renal Vascular Imaging

CTA is replacing conventional angiography in evaluation of renal vascular anatomy and pathology. Indications for renal CTA include renal donor transplant evaluation, renovascular hypertension workup and posttreatment assessment, oncologic perioperative staging, planning, and surveillance, and renal anomaly/variant workup. Advancement in technology, optimization of CTA protocols, and improvement of contrast application have allowed reliable and accurate depiction of renal vascular pathology [7–11, 22–24].

Imaging Techniques

After drinking approximately 1 liter of water for enteric contrast, patient should have an intravenous line at least 20 gauge or larger placed in the antecubital fossa. The patient lies supine, head first, on the CT table. Scanning is performed with the patient holding his or her breath at end inspiration. For concomitant assessment of the kidneys, including calcification and hemorrhage, unen-

hanced CT images are obtained. For assessment of renal artery anatomy for surgical planning and renovascular disease, MDCT with 16 detector rows or more should be used to acquire thin-section (<1-mm) arterial images. Nephrographic-phase renal imaging is critical for evaluation of the renal parenchyma and mass. Scanning protocols for 16- and 64-slice MDCT are shown in Table 4 and 5.

Applications

Living Renal Donor Evaluation and Renal Mass Surgical Planning

Renal CTA is extremely accurate in delineating the renal artery and vein anatomy [25] (Fig. 16). As laparoscopic surgery for renal harvesting is common, to prevent undesirable or possible life-threatening outcome, accurate preoperative knowledge of the presence of renal arterial and venous location and variant is essential for planning [26]. Almost 30% of patients may have variant renal vascular anatomy [7] (Fig. 17). Renal MDCTA has a mean accuracy of 94% in detecting accessory arteries, 95% in depicting early branching (Fig. 17c), and 98% in demonstrating renal-vein anomalies [27, 28]. Atypical location and diameter of adjacent vessels, such as lumbar, adrenal, and gonadal veins, must be identified to prevent or minimize complications during surgery [27]. Imaging is also crucial to define vascular anatomy in patients with renal anomalies for treatment planning (Fig. 18).

Renal Artery Pathology

Renovascular Hypertension (RVH) Assessment

Given its low prevalence of approximately 1%, RVH is usually screened with a minimally invasive or noninvasive imaging technique for high-risk patients [29]. Renovascular hypertension results from decrease renal perfusion secondary to a severe renal arterial lesion; the most common cause is atherosclerotic renal artery stenosis (RAS) near the origin (Fig. 19). Fibromuscular dysplasia (FMD) (Fig. 20) is the second most common cause, with the most prevalent type being medial fibroplasia, which presents with the "string-of-beads" appearance [11]. CTA is highly sensitive in the diagnosis of FMD [30]. As RVH is potentially treatable, its diagnosis is important. Because the renal arteries have a circuitous path, evaluation of these vessels is challenging and necessitates the use of a 3-D image display workstation. The caliber of the renal artery is evaluated more accurately with MPR than MIP reconstruction [31]. VR technique is reported to have a higher specificity (99%) than MIP (87%) for demonstrating RAS [9]. Indirect

Table 4. Renal computed tomography angiography (CTA) parameters for 64-slice multidetector-row computed tomography (MDCT)[a]

Phase	Noncontrast	Arterial/corticomedullary	Nephrographic
kVp/effective mAs/rotation time (s)	120/240/0.5	120/240/0.5	120/240/0.5
Detector collimation (mm)	0.6	0.6	0.6
Slice thickness (mm)	3	1	2
Beam Pitch	1	1	1
Recon increment (mm)	3	0.7	1
Scan delay		Bolus tracking	90 s

[a] Scan parameters from Siemens Sensation 64

Table 5. Renal computed tomography angiography (CTA) parameters for 16-slice multidetector-row computed tomography (MDCT)[a]

Phase	Noncontrast	Arterial/corticomedullary	Nephrographic
kVp/effective mAs/rotation time (s)	120/240/0.5	120/240/0.5	120/240/0.5
Detector collimation (mm)	1.5	0.75	1.5
Slice thickness (mm)	3	1	2
Feed/rotation (mm)	24	10	24
Recon increment (mm)	3	0.7	1
Scan delay		Bolus tracking	90 s

[a] Scan parameters from Siemens Sensation 16

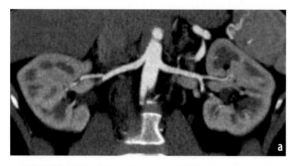
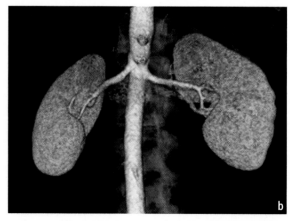

Fig. 16a, b. Single bilateral normal renal arteries seen on the **a** multiplanar reformatting (MPR) and **b** volume rendering (VR) image in a 32-year-old woman being evaluated for a potential renal donor

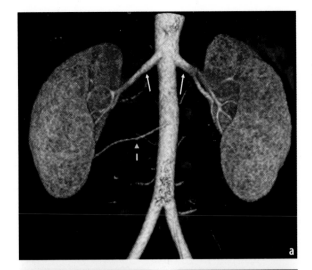

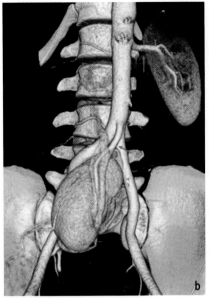

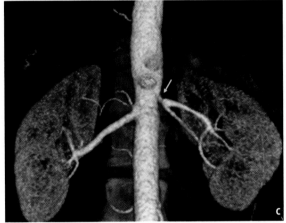

Fig. 17a, b. Volume rendering (VR) images of the renal arteries from three different patients being evaluated for potential renal donors. **a** Right-sided accessory renal artery (*dashed yellow arrow*), **b** right-sided pelvic kidney (*red arrow*), and **c** left-sided early bifurcating renal artery with incidentally discovered renal artery stenosis (*yellow arrow*) at the origin

findings of RAS include a smooth but atrophic kidney, poststenotic dilatation, delayed and prolonged nephrogram, and thinned renal cortex [7] (Fig. 21). After revascularization of RAS, CTA can be used to evaluate renal stent patency [32].

Renal Artery Aneurysms

Renal artery aneurysms (RAA) can be readily depicted with MIP and VR images. RAA is mainly due to atherosclerosis but can be seen with pregnancy, FMD, and neurofibromatosis. Pseudoaneurysms may be seen secondary to trauma, inflammation, and surgical complications (Fig. 22) [7].

Renal Venous Disorder

Renal vein thrombosis can be readily assessed with MDCTA. The etiology of renal vein thrombosis includes renal or adrenal malignancies, glomerulonephritis, collagen vascular disease, sepsis, diabetes, and severe dehydration. The renal venous enhancement typically peaks during the corticomedullary phase [7], unless the scan delay used for the corticomedullary phase is too early to allow a complete drain of the renal vein.

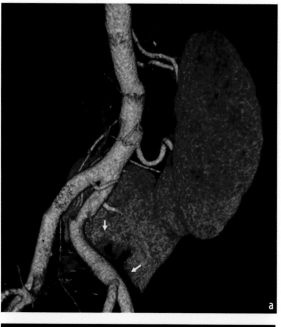

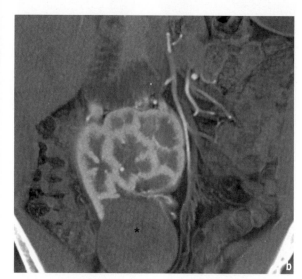

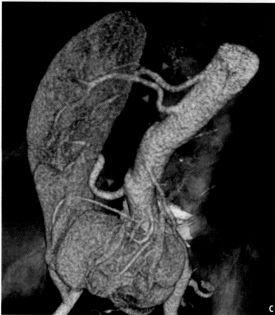

Fig. 18a-c. A 35-year-old man with crossed fused renal ectopia who was diagnosed with a renal mass suspected to be renal cell carcinoma underwent renal computed tomography angiography (CTA) to delineate the vascular anatomy for surgical planning. **a** Volume rendering (VR) in the prone projection reveals a mass (*arrows*) in the inferior aspect of the anomalous kidney. **b** On the coronal multiplanar reformatting (MPR) image, the hypovascular mass (*) is depicted. **c** Five renal arteries (*red arrows*) are identified on the oblique VR projection

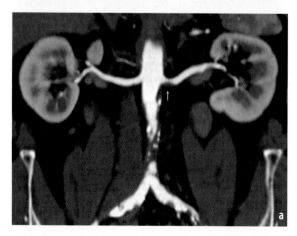

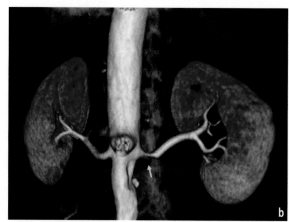

Fig. 19a, b. A significant left-sided renal artery stenosis (*arrow*) near the ostium from atherosclerotic mural plaque is seen on the **a** curved planar reformatting (CP) and **b** volume rendering (VR) images in a 68-year-old man with hypertension and peripheral vascular disease

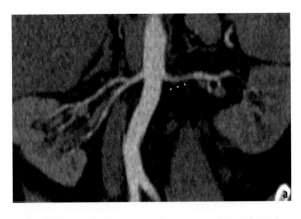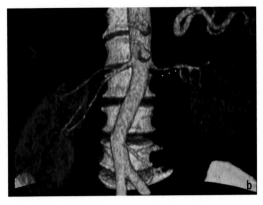

Fig. 20a,b. Irregularly beaded left renal artery (*arrows*) consistent with fibromuscular dysplasia seen on the **a** coronal curved planar re-formatting (CP) and **b** volume rendering (VR) images in a 40-year-old man with refractory hypertension

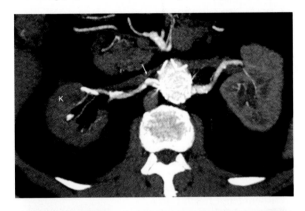

Fig. 21. Right renal artery stenosis from calcified atherosclerotic plaques (*arrow*) near the ostium as shown on this axial thick-section maximum intensity projection (MIP) with right renal atrophy and delayed perfusion

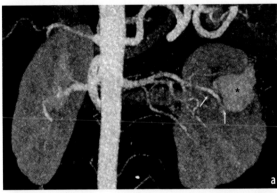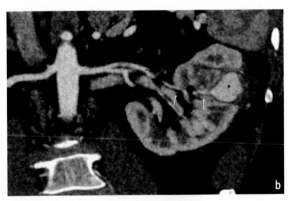

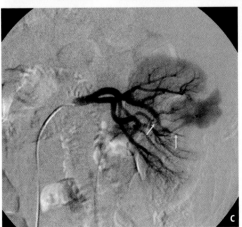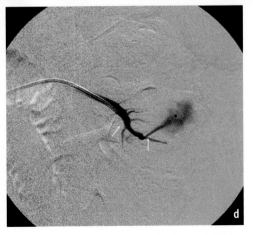

Fig. 22a-d. Pseudoaneurysm (*) with a feeding renal artery (*arrows*) in the left kidney near the postsurgical bed seen on **a** maximum intensity projection (MIP) and **b** curved planar reformatting (CP) images. This is a 47-year-old man status post a partial nephrectomy of the left kidney for renal cell carcinoma. **c, d** Computed tomography angiography (CTA) findings are confirmed on the conventional renal angiogram

Conclusion

Because of its minimal invasiveness and depiction of 3-D cross-sectional anatomy, CTA is supplanting conventional angiography for many diagnostic applications. The use of CTA to delineate the anatomy and to detect pathology of the mesenteric and renal vessels is growing. CT scanning and contrast administration protocols are rapidly evolving, as with the advance of MDCT technology. CT radiation dosage to the patient should be minimized and limited by diligently customizing the scanning protocols to adapt to each patient's clinical question. Magnetic resonance angiography can be used when radiation exposure is a concern or when iodinated contrast medium is contraindicated. The storing of immense image data sets can be a challenge. Advancing technology has kept abreast of this issue. The evaluation of 3-D vascular anatomy often involves a review of numerous images and detail anatomy and thus may take longer than the evaluation with conventional angiography. Furthermore, one must also pay attention to the extravascular findings, as alternative or additional pathology may be detected from the CT images.

References

1. Bae KT, Heiken JP, Brink JA (1998) Aortic and hepatic contrast medium at CT part I. Prediction with a computer model. Radiology 207:647–655
2. Bae KT, Heiken JP, Brink JA (1998) Aortic and hepatic contrast medium at CT part II. Effect of reduced cardiac output in a porcine model. Radiology 207:657–662
3. Fleischmann D (2002) Present and future trends in multiple detector-row CT applications: CT angiography. Eur Radiol 12[Suppl 2]:S11–S16
4. Haage P, Schmitz-Rode T, Hubner D et al (2000) Reduction of contrast material dose and artifacts by a saline flush using a double power injector in helical CT of the thorax. AJR Am J Roentgenol 174: 1049–1053
5. Van Hoe L, Marchal G, Baert AL et al (1995) Determination of scan delay-time in spiral CT-angiography: Utility of a test bolus injection. J Comput Assist Tomogr 19:216–220
6. Rubin GD (2003) 3-D imaging with multidetector CT. Eur J Radiol 45[Suppl 1]:S37–S41
7. Sheth S, Fishman E (2004) Multi-detector row CT of the kidneys and urinary tract: Techniques and applications in the diagnosis of benign disease. Radiographics 24:e20 http://radiographics.rsnajnls.org/cgi/content/full/e20v1. Cited 30 Jan 2006
8. Kuszyk BS, Heath DG, Ney DR et al (1995) CT angiography with volume rendering: imaging findings. AJR Am J Roentgenol 165:445–448
9. Johnson PT, Halpern EJ, Kuszyk BS et al (1999) Renal artery stenosis: CT angiography – comparison of real-time volume rendering and maximum intensity projection algorithms. Radiology 211:337–343
10. Kattee R, Beek F, de Lange E et al (1997) Renal artery stenosis: detection and quantification with spiral CT angiography and optimized digital subtraction angiography. Radiology 205:121–127
11. Urban BA, Ratner LE, Fishman EK (2001) Three-dimensional volume rendered CT angiography of the renal arteries and veins: Normal anatomy, variants, and clinical applications. Radiographics 21:373–386
12. Horton KM, Fishman EK (2002) Volume-rendered 3D CT of the mesenteric vasculature: normal anatomy, anatomic variants, and pathologic conditions. Radiographics 22:161–172
13. Hong KC, Freeny PC (1999) Pancreaticoduodenal arcades and dorsal pancreatic artery: comparison of CT angiography with three dimensional volume rendering, maximum intensity projection, and shaded-surface display. AJR Am J Roentgenol 172:925–931
14. Horton KM and Fishman EK (2001) Multi-detector row CT of the mesenteric ischemia: Can it be done? Radiographics 21:1463–1473
15. Foley WD (2002) Multidetector CT: abdominal visceral imaging. Radiographics 22:701–719
16. Lu DS, Reber HA, Krasny RM et al (1997) Local staging of pancreatic cancer: criteria for unresectability of major vessels as revealed by pancreatic phase, thin section helical CT. AJR Am J Roentgenol 168:1439–1443
17. Raptopoulos V, Steer ML, Sheiman RG et al (1997) The use of helical CT and CT angiography to predict vascular involvement from pancreatic cancer: correlation with findings at surgery. AJR Am J Roentgenol 168:971–977
18. Taourel PG, Deneuville M, Pradel JA et al (1996) Acute mesenteric ischemia: diagnosis with contrast enhanced CT. Radiology 199:632–636
19. James S, Balfe DM, Lee JKT et al (1987) Small bowel disease, categorization by CT examination. AJR Am J Roentgenol 148:863–868
20. Bartnicke BJ, Balfe DM (1994) CT appearance of intestinal ischemia and intramural hemorrhage. Radiol Clin North Am 32:845–860
21. Fishman EK (2001) CT Angiography: Clinical applications in the abdomen. Radiographics 21:S3–S16
22. Platt JF, Ellis JH, Korobkin M, Reige K (1997) Helical CT evaluation of potential kidney donors: findings in 154 subjects. AJR Am J Roentgenol 169: 1325–1330
23. Smith PA, Ratner LE, Lynch FC et al (1998) Role of CT angiography in the preoperative evaluation for laparoscopic nephrectomy. Radiographics 18: 589–601
24. Rubin GD, Alfrey EJ, Dake MD et al (1995) Assessment of living renal donors with spiral CT. Radiology 195:457–462
25. Rankin SC, Jan W, Koffman CG (2001) Noninvasive imaging of living related kidney donors: evaluation with CT angiography and gadolinium enhanced MR angiography. AJR AM J Roentgenol 177:349–355
26. Rydberg J, Kopecky KK, Tann M et al (2001) Evaluation of prospective living renal donors for laparoscopic nephrectomy with multisection CT: the marriage of minimally invasive imaging with minimally invasive surgery. Radiographics 21:S223–S236
27. Kawamoto S, Montgomery RA, Lawler LP et al (2003) Multidetector CT angiography for preopera-

tive evaluation of living laparoscopic kidney donors. AJR Am J Roentgenol 180:1633–1638

28. Sahani DV, Rastogi N, Greenfield AC et al (2005) Multi-detector row CT in evaluation of 94 living renal donors by readers with varied experience. Radiology 235:905–910

29. Grenier N, Trillaud H (2000) Comparison of imaging methods for renal artery stenosis. BJU International 86[Suppl 1]: 84–94

30. Beregi JP, Louvegny S, Gautier C et al (1999) Fibromuscular dysplasia of the renal arteries: comparison of helical CT angiography and arteriography. AJR Am J Roentgenol 172:27–34

31. Galanski M, Prokop M, Chavam A et al (1993) Renal artery stenoses: spiral CT angiography. Radiology 189:185–192

32. Behar JV, Nelson RC, Zidar JP et al (2002) Thin-section multidetector CT angiography of renal artery stents. AJR Am J Roentgenol 178:1155–1159

33. Lin PH, Chaikof EL (2000) Embryology, anatomy, and surgical exposure of the great abdominal vessels. Surg Clin North Am 80(1):417–433

34. Lalani TA, Kanne JP, Hatfield GA et al (2004) Imaging findings in systemic lupus erythematosus. Radiographics 24: 1069–1086

35. Olin JW (2000) Thromboangiitis obliterans (Buerger's disease). NEJM 343:864–869

36. Nakamura K, Nozue M, Sakakibara Y et al (1997) Natural history of a spontaneous dissecting aneurysm of the proximal superior mesenteric artery: Report of a case. Surg Today 27:272–274

SECTION III

MDCT of the Cardiovascular System

III.1

Imaging Protocols for Cardiac CT

Frank J. Rybicki and Tarang Sheth

The incorporation of multiple detectors into spiral computed tomography (CT) scanners has expanded the clinical role of CT in cardiac imaging, including coronary CT angiography (CTA). Advances in both the speed at which the X-ray source rotates and the number of detectors have improved the ability of CT to resolve smaller anatomic detail and have enabled imaging of the native coronary arterial tree. At present, and for at least the near future, CT is the most robust modality to noninvasively image the coronary arteries. CTA contributes largely to cardiovascular diagnoses, but one of the most important and one of the most promising contributions is its high negative predictive value for coronary artery disease (CAD). That is, using the protocol detailed in this chapter, CAD can be reliably excluded in minutes without arterial catheterization. Moreover, in a single CT acquisition, native coronary imaging can be extended to include the beating myocardium, valve motion, ventricular outflow tracks, and coronary bypass grafts. In this chapter, in addition to detailing a basic cardiac imaging protocol, examples of examinations are illustrated.

Introduction

Protocols for electrocardiogram (ECG)-gated cardiac CT have evolved with rapid improvement in technology. The technique has progressed from early cardiac CT [4-slice multidetector CT (MDCT) with 1-s gantry rotation] to current standards (ECG-gated 64-slice MDCT with gantry rotation times as low as 330 ms). Technology has developed at a rapid rate, fueled primarily by the promise of a robust, noninvasive method of performing diagnostic coronary angiography (Fig. 1). Additional MDCT imaging includes coronary bypass grafts and evaluation of cardiac valves. This chapter fo-

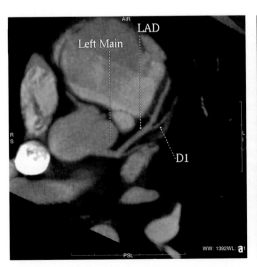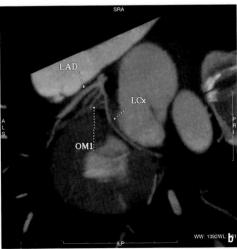

Fig. 1a, b. Multiplanar reformatted CTA images demonstrate the major branches of the left coronary arterial system. This patient presented with atypical chest pain, and coronary artery disease was excluded noninvasively

cuses on the coronary CTA protocol and also described how the basic protocol can be modified or extended for problem solving.

Temporal Resolution

Successful cardiac imaging by any modality relies on the ability of the technology to produce motion free images or to scan faster than the heart beats. Thus, cardiac CT is founded on (1) imaging faster than the heart beats, or (2) slowing cardiac motion. *Temporal resolution* is the metric that measures imaging speed. For a CT scanner with a single photon source, the temporal resolution is one half of the CT gantry rotation time. This is because image reconstruction requires CT data acquired from one half (180°) of a complete gantry rotation. At the time of publication, all manufacturers have gantry rotation times less than 500 ms, with a minimum of 330 ms. With a 330-ms gantry rotation, an ECG-gated cardiac image can be reconstructed (using single-segment reconstruction described below) with CT data acquired over 165 ms of the cardiac cycle. Thus, the reconstructed images display the average of the cardiac motion over the 165 ms during which the data was acquired. This is how ECG gating enables coronary CTA. Without gating, cardiac images are nondiagnostic because the reconstruction "averages" the motion over the entire RR interval – 1,000 ms for a patient with a heart rate of 60 beats per minute.

Temporal resolution can be improved in single-source scanners by adopting a so-called "multisegment" image reconstruction. The principle underlying multisegment reconstruction is that the acquisition over several heart beats is summed to obtain the one half gantry (i.e., 180°) CT data. For example, in a two-segment reconstruction, two heart beats are used to generate a single axial slice, and thus the temporal resolution is halved. Similarly, if four heat beats are used (four segment reconstruction), only 45° of data are used from each heart beat. This would yield a four-fold reduction in the temporal resolution. Since multiple heart beats are used to fill the 180° of gantry rotation necessary for the reconstruction, stable periodicity of the heart is essential. Moreover, multisegment reconstruction requires a lower CT pitch, resulting in greater data oversampling and a higher radiation dose. Radiation considerations and a simple formula to estimate effective patient dose are given in an upcoming section.

A recent approach to improving temporal resolution involves the use of two independent sources and two independent (64-slice) detector systems (Siemens Definition; Siemens Medical Solutions, Erlangen, Germany). The second X-ray source is positioned 90° from the first X-ray source, and the second detection system is positioned 90° from the first detection system. With respect to temporal resolution, the practical consequence of this CT configuration is that 180° of gantry rotation can be achieved in half the time (e.g., 82.5 ms as opposed to 165 ms). This improvement in the temporal resolution is expected to eliminate the need for multisegment reconstruction. In fact, in patients with a higher heart rate or a heart rate that is difficult to control with beta blockade (described below), the CT pitch can be increased without compromising image quality.

Beta Blockade for Heart-Rate Control

As suggested from the discussion on temporal resolution, beta blockade is an important component of most cardiac CT examinations. A useful rule of thumb for the target heart rate is "the first number is a 5" – i.e., an ideal heart rate between 50 and 59 beats per minute. While this goal is not achieved in every patient, it provides a useful reference frame. IV metoprolol is routinely administered at our institution; with cardiac monitoring, 5-mg increments are given every 5 min up to a total dose of 25 mg. Doses greater than 15 mg are rarely needed. Beta blockade can be safely performed by a radiologist or a cardiologist. An alternative approach involves the use of oral beta blockade. Although this approach has the disadvantage of a longer serum half life, most patients arrive for the study with a heart rate already in the target range. This can simplify patient preparation on site and has the potential to increase patient throughput. The tradeoff is the extra step of premedicating the patient and issues surrounding patient compliance.

In theory, using the multisegment reconstruction approach described above, beta blockade can often be avoided because using multiple heart beats in the reconstruction enables the scanner to have an effective temporal resolution in the range of 40–50 ms. However, when multisegment reconstruction is used, image quality becomes highly dependent on cardiac beat-to-beat variability. In our experience, multisegment reconstruction works well in patients with high heart rates who are being studied for clinical indications where the highest image quality may not be required, for example, coronary bypass graft location and patency. For coronary CT angiography, beta blockade is still recommended.

ECG Gating

ECG gating refers to the simultaneous acquisition of both the patient's electrocardiogram (ECG)

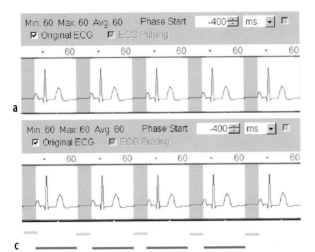
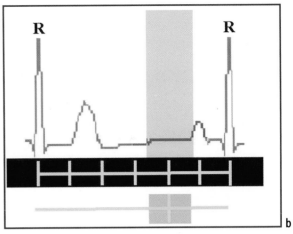

Fig. 2a-c. a Electrocardiogram (ECG) gating as demonstrated on a Somatom Sensation 64 cardiac computed tomography (CT) scanner (Siemens Medical Solutions, Erlangen, Germany). Continuous ECG tracing is displayed on the console. In this case, minimum, maximum, and average heart rate is 60 beats per minute (*top left*). Thus, the width of the RR interval is 1,000 ms. The *gray vertical bars* indicate that portion of the cardiac cycle used in the reconstruction. As discussed in the text, the width of the gray bar is the temporal resolution of the scan. For this single-segment reconstruction, the width is half the gantry rotation time, or 165 ms. The term "–400 ms" refers to the fact that the center of the gray bars is located 400 ms before the second of the two R waves in the RR interval. **b** Enlarged view of a single RR interval. To provide a simple demonstration of how the RR interval is divided, six segments are illustrated. In clinical imaging, CT scanners divide the RR interval into a number of segments between 10 and 20. The gray block at the very bottom emphasizes that each reconstructed image uses only a small portion of the cardiac cycle. The gray block is positioned in diastole; its center is approximately 65% between the R waves, i.e., 650 ms elapse between the first R wave and the center of the block. This reconstruction is the most commonly used to visualize the left coronary arterial system. If this reconstruction does not provide the most optimal images, additional reconstructions, either earlier or later phases, are performed. Since the right and left coronary arterial system are asynchronous, it is sometimes the case that evaluation of the right system is best performed using images closer to systole. **c** Electrocardiogram (ECG)-based tube current modulation or ECG pulsing. The ECG tracing is identical to the one illustrated in **a**. *Yellow bars* under the tracing correspond to the gray bars and correlate where, with current modulation, the optimal tube current (e.g., effective mAs = 650) will be used. *Red lines* show times that correspond to portions of the cardiac cycle where the X-ray CT tube current is minimized. ECG pulsing can reduced patient effective radiation dose by 30–50%

tracing and CT data (Fig. 2a, b). By acquiring both pieces of information, CT images can be reconstructed using only a short temporal segment periodically located in the same location of the RR interval over multiple cardiac cycles. The duration of the temporal segment is equal to the temporal resolution of the scanner. Each temporal segment of the RR interval is named by its "phase" in the cardiac cycle; the most commonly used nomenclature is to name the percentage of a specific phase with respect to its position in the RR interval. For example, if a manufacturer enables reconstruction of 20 (equally spaced) phases, they would typically be named 0%, 5%, 10% ... 95%, beginning with one R wave and ending with the following R wave. The period in which the heart has the least motion is usually (but not always) in mid diastole, near a phase between 55% and 75%. Thus, under the assumption that the position of the heart remains consistent over the RR intervals during which CT data is acquired, cardiac motion is minimized by producing images from the same phase over multiple cardiac cycles. This explains why ECG gating typically fails to freeze cardiac motion in patients with an irregular rhythm, such as atrial fibrillation. Consequently, atrial fibrillation patients rarely have diagnostic cardiac CT examinations,

and it is our policy to not perform coronary CTA in this population.

If only static (as opposed to cine) images are desired, image reconstruction can usually be performed over a small number of phases for which motion is minimized. (This is in contrast to cine imaging where images are reconstructed in all parts of the cardiac cycle and then played, in cine mode, to demonstrate cardiac motion.) The image reconstruction phases used for interpretation must account for differences in movement of the left and right coronary arterial systems. Because coronary arterial motion is not synchronous, the phase of the cardiac cycle that proves best for diagnosis of the left main and left anterior descending artery is often different than the phase that proves most diagnostic for the right coronary artery. Moreover, it is often necessary to view more than one phase to best assess the full extent of an individual artery and its branches (e.g., the left anterior descending and the diagonal branches).

The most complete cardiac CT examinations include cine imaging. In cine cardiac CT, images are reconstructed in periodic phases throughout the cardiac cycle to yield information regarding a moving structure. For example, cardiac CT offers an outstanding assessment of the aortic valve and

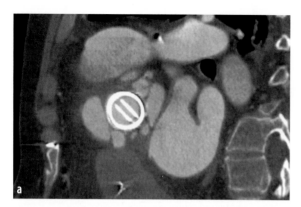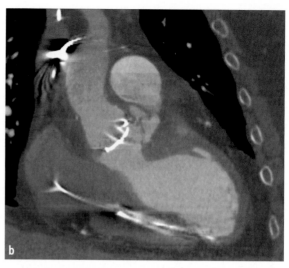

Fig. 3a, b. Reformatted ECG-gated cardiac CT images in a patient status post aortic valve replacement. Note that the patient has a pacemaker (noted by the right heart wires in 3b), and thus magnetic resonance imaging (MRI) was contraindicated. **a** Image through the mechanical valve while it is open demonstrates multiple surrounding collections of contrast, characteristic of pseudoaneurysm. **b** orthogonal view again demonstrates abnormal contrast to the right of the valve. This patient required emergent surgery with successful placement of a new valve. Images courtesy of Scott Koss, MD

aortic root (Fig. 3). In addition to the fact that cine imaging can be used to assess valve motion, CT is by far the best imaging modality to identify and quantify calcification, and thus both structure and function can be well characterized in a single breath-hold CT acquisition. Cine CT can also be used to assess ventricular-wall motion. In comparison with cardiac magnetic resonance (MR), the gold standard for global and regional-wall motion abnormalities, CT has less contrast to noise, and images typically have greater artifact owing to poorer temporal resolution. However, it is important to emphasize that cine CT is not a separate image acquisition. The entire CT data set (coronary, valve, myocardium, pericardium) is acquired in a single breath hold; cine CT is simply part of the image postprocessing. It is also important to note that the most common contraindications for cardiac CT (e.g., impaired renal function as measured by glomerular filtration rate or alternatively by serum creatinine) differ from those for MR (pacemaker), and thus CT can often be used for patients who cannot have MR.

Finally, it is important to note that future CT equipment with up to 256 slices is expected to perform whole-heart coverage with a single half-gantry (180°) rotation. This approach holds the promise of a subsecond cardiac scan. In addition to the fact that patient radiation would be decreased, this would provide the ability to perform multiple scans over the same injection of iodinated contrast material and thus create the opportunity for a host of additional studies (e.g., myocardial perfusion) that are, at present, largely in the domain of cardiac MR and nuclear cardiology.

Patient Irradiation

In some cardiac CT applications, for example, the location and patency of bypass grafts (Figs. 4 and 5), all diagnostic information can typically be obtained from reconstruction of only a single phase of the cardiac cycle in mid diastole. However, as emphasized above, in cardiac CT, image data is acquired throughout the cardiac cycle. Thus, for studies such as bypass graft analyses, the CT data (and the radiation used to acquire that data) in the remaining "unused" phases is wasted.

Because cardiac CT requires ECG gating with a CT pitch less than 1, the patient radiation in cardiac CT is higher than that for CT of any other body part. While dose should be a consideration for all patients undergoing CT, it is essential that discussions regarding CT dose are based on sound principles. The risk most commonly cited as a cause for concern is the development of a fatal radiation-induced neoplasm. While sparse, all human data and antidotal reports to date support a latency period of no less than 20 years for a radia-

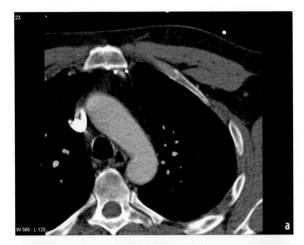

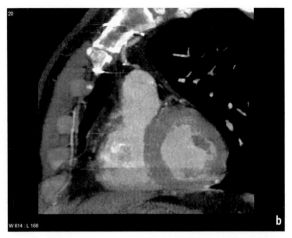

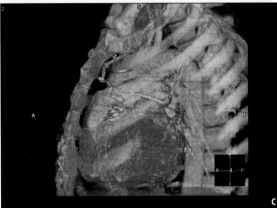

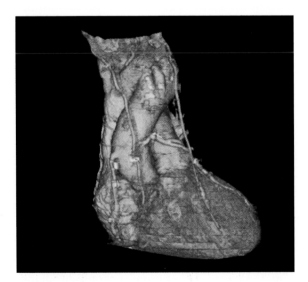

Fig. 4a-c. ECG-gated CT images from a patient status post left internal mammary artery to left anterior descending artery coronary bypass grafting. This patient was scheduled for a repeat bypass graft. CTA with reformatting is now performed routinely to detect cases such as this one where the graft becomes adherent to the posterior table of the sternum. **a** Axial image demonstrates proximity of the internal mammary to the sternum. **b** Sagittal and obliquely reformatted images are essential in the evaluation of these patients. In this case, the graft is demonstrated to be patent and too close to the sternum for a repeat thoracotomy through the sternal incision; an alternate surgical approach was required for this patient. **c** Selected image from a three-dimensional (3-D) volume rendering again demonstrates the course of the graft. Volume rendering is often more appealing to our referring clinicians and can help in the communication of important findings

Fig. 5. 3-D volume-rendered image from a patient with normal internal mammary arteries who had undergone saphenous vein coronary bypass grafting. Note that the left-sided vein graft is bifurcated. The vein graft to the right coronary territory is single. In a patient with only saphenous vein grafts, it is essential to image the entire course of the internal mammary arteries since, when normal, they will be used for redo coronary artery bypass

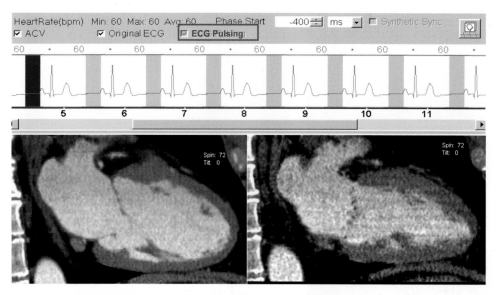

Fig. 6. ECG-based tube current modulation, or ECG pulsing. The *top* demonstrates how the operator selects current modulation from the console of the Somatom Sensation 64 cardiac computed tomography (CT) scanner (Siemens Medical Solutions, Erlangen, Germany). The image on the *left* is a two-chamber view (note the normal mitral valve that is well demonstrated with ECG gating) that is reconstructed at 65% of the RR interval. The *right-hand*, two-chamber view was reconstructed from 10% of the RR interval, where the X-ray CT tube current was dramatically reduced. Subsequently, this image suffers from high noise, the consequence of fewer photons received at the detector

tion-induced neoplasm. For this reason, for the purpose of radiation dose, it is important to separate patients into two groups: those with a life expectancy of roughly 20 years or less, and those with a longer life expectancy. In the former group, the only dose consideration of any consequence is the radiation that could cause a skin burn (the only short-term complication of any consequence). X-ray skin burns are extremely uncommon, particularly in CT (even for ECG-gated studies), and would be the consequence of multiple exams repeated at short-term intervals. Thus, for this subset of patients, radiation dose should be a lesser consideration in determining a modality for coronary imaging.

For patients with a life expectancy much greater than 20 years, ECG-based tube current modulation (also called ECG pulsing) represents one strategy to lower overall patient radiation by modulating the tube current over the course of the cardiac cycle (Fig. 2c) so that the desired diagnostic tube current is delivered in diastole while the current is reduced for the remainder of the cardiac cycle.

Current modulation is featured on newer CT scanners and is important in many cases (e.g., pediatric patients). However, the decision to incorporate current modulation should be made carefully since the potential drawbacks are significant. First, once current modulation is used, images subsequently reconstructed during phases with low tube current will be noisy (Fig. 6). That is, reducing the tube current results in the production of fewer X-rays, and subsequently fewer X-rays pass though the patient and reach the detection system. Second, current modulation eliminates the potential to reconstruct high-quality cine imaging since every phase of the cardiac cycle will not have the "full" tube current. Thus, if cine imaging is desired, current modulation cannot be utilized. Another potential drawback concerns the identification of incidental findings (e.g., bicuspid aortic valve) on static imaging acquired with current modulation. In these cases, it is impossible to perform postprocessing of a high-signal cine loop for a more complete evaluation.

While cine cardiac CT can provide a useful adjunct to high spatial resolution anatomic data, CT has poor temporal resolution and ventricular image contrast when compared with steady-state free precession (SSFP) cardiac MR (CMR). For this reason, SSFP cine CMR remains the gold standard to assess cardiac function and to evaluate cardiac masses. However, CT is far more accessible, it is easier to perform, and a cardiac pacemaker is not a contraindication. Moreover, there are many cardiac masses that can be well or better seen on CT (Fig. 7). Hence, CT has become not only an adjunct to cardiac MR but in some cases the diagnostic test of choice (Fig. 8).

Since patient dose in CT is so frequently discussed and has great potential to be misquoted, the

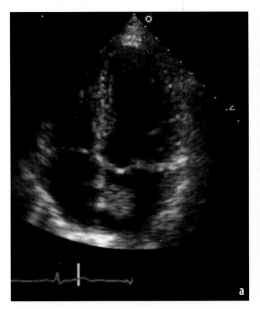
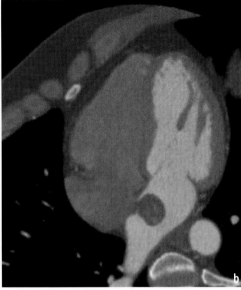

Fig. 7a, b. Left atrial myxoma. **a** Four-chamber echocardiogram demonstrates the round lesion adjacent to the intra-atrial septum. **b** ECG-gated CT shows the mass with higher spatial resolution, well depicting the attachment point of the mass with the intra-atrial septum. Note that the left heart is well opacified with contrast material and the right heart is filled with saline. This is the goal in the timing of the dual injection protocol (contrast followed by saline)

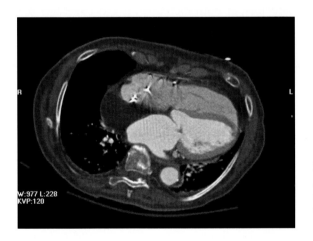

Fig. 8. Axial ECG-gated four-chamber image in a patient with a pacemaker. The patient has a history of renal cell carcinoma, and echocardiography demonstrated an ill-defined echogenic mass. This image from the single 12-s CT acquisition excludes a metastatic deposit as the source of the finding on ultrasound. Fat splays the left and right atria, diagnostic of lipomatous hypertrophy of the intra-atrial septum. CT is the most rapid and accurate imaging modality to demonstrate both fat and calcium

fundamentals of CT dose, including the dose from cardiac CT, are described here. There are three different parameters used to describe, quantify, and calculate the dose:

1. CT dose index (CTDIvol) [1]. CTDIvol units are milligray (mGy) [3].
2. Dose-length product (DLP) [2]. Units of DLP are mGy × centimeters.
3. Effective dose [3]. Units of effective dose are milliSievert (mSv).

The numerical value for CTDI is determined by measuring dose in a cylindrical phantom. Although the phantom should somehow reflect the attenuation of a human body, the CTDI is not used to make a statement regarding an individual patient's dose. Rather, it is used to compare different scan protocols, optimize scan protocols, and com-

pare protocols used on different CT scanners. In contrast to parameters such as tube current, CTDI values reflect delivered dose since parameters, such as scanner geometry and filtration, are considered.

CTDIvol describes dose for a single rotation. DLP characterizes CT exposure over a complete field of view (FOV); DLP is defined as the product of the CTDIvol and the craniocaudal extent (Z-axis length) of the scan. Even though DLP reflects most closely radiation dose for a specific CT examination, it is important to keep in mind that DLP is a function of patient size (i.e., how much Z-axis coverage is required to complete the CT scan). Therefore, CTDIvol should be used to optimize exam protocols.

While CTDIvol and DLP enable evaluation of

CT scanners and comparison of protocols across manufacturers, these values only characterize the scanner. It is the effective dose, a weighted sum over the organ doses [4], that quantifies patient dose. Since the dose to an individual organ cannot be measured directly, it is difficult to determine the effective dose of a CT scan. However, methods have been described to estimate effective dose from measurable values [5–8]. A simple estimation is that the effective dose is the product of DLP and a conversion factor, E_{DLP} that is specific to a body region. For example, for the chest, the $E_{DLP} = 0.017 \ mSv{\times}mGy^{-1}{\times}cm^{-1}$ [2].

As an example of a how this is used in clinical practice, consider the following hypothetical coronary CTA. The user console will give the CTDIvol. A typical value for a high-dose scan without current modulation would be on the order of 60 mGy. Assume that the craniocaudal extent of the scan is 15 cm, a typical value for a normal-sized heart. For this study, the DLP = 60 mGy×15 cm = 900 mGy×cm. Given that the heart is in the chest, the appropriate conversion factor is $E_{DLP} = 0.017 \ mSv{\times}mGy^{-1}{\times}cm^{-1}$, and the effective dose for this patient is 60 mGy×15 cm x 0.017 $mSv{\times}mGy^{-1}{\times}cm^{-1}$ ~ 15 mSv. Note that, as discussed above, dose values in gated exams can be reduced with "ECG pulsing". The degree of reduction is a function of the patient's heart rate but is typically 30–50%.

Image Acquisition Time

Improved temporal resolution decreases the time of the CT examination. This is important not only for decreasing the effect of cardiac motion but also for completing the examination in a breath hold. Scan time becomes a factor for cardiac and ascending aorta imaging because of the required ECG gating. The image data must be "oversampled" since, for the reconstruction of each interval, only a small portion of the cardiac cycle is used. Data oversampling for cardiovascular applications differentiates it from all other MDCT scans that can capitalize on undersampling and interpolation in image reconstruction to dramatically decrease scan time.

CT pitch (a unitless parameter) is most accurately characterized as the distance the patient moves through the scanner in a single gantry rotation divided by the width of the X-ray beam used. Because such a small part of the RR interval is used to reconstruct an entire image, significant overlap along the craniocaudal extent of the patient is required, translating into a pitch between 0.2 and 0.35, or an oversampling rate between 5:1 and roughly 3:1. In addition to cardiac imaging, ECG gating is routinely required for CTA of the ascending aorta to eliminate artifacts from aortic motion that can be confused with pathology.

The practical consequence of oversampling is that scan time (craniocaudal imaging over approximately 15 cm) is far greater than nongated scanning of the same Z-axis region of any other body part. This is one great benefit of scanners equipped with a larger number of detectors, which allow coverage of a larger craniocaudal territory per rotation. In the extreme case, craniocaudal coverage can be large enough that the entire heart is covered in a single rotation. The number of detectors and focal spots determines the number of slices obtained per gantry rotation. That is, 64-slice coronary CTA (Figs. 9 and 10) can be achieved with 32 detectors and a dual focal spot or 64 detectors and a single focal spot. The important factors are temporal resolution (determined by gantry rotation time), slice thickness, and quality of the X-ray CT tube.

Increasing either number of slices, thickness of detectors, or both increases "Z-axis coverage" per rotation and thus decreases scan time. For example, for coverage of the heart, a 4-slice scanner may require a 35-s breath hold while a 64-slice acquisition (performed with the same gantry rotation time and detector width) on the same patient may require only 15 s.

While thicker detectors decrease scan time by providing more Z-axis coverage per rotation, increasing detector width for cardiac applications is undesirable since it degrades the *spatial resolution* of the examination. In general, spatial resolution refers to the ability to differentiate two structures. In practical terms, spatial resolution refers to the thinnest axial slices that can be reconstructed from configuration of the detectors. The CT industry, driven by the promise (and the competition) of selling scanners to noninvasively image coronary arteries, has dramatically improved spatial resolution by producing detection systems that can reconstruct submillimeter images. Thinner slices (higher spatial resolution) correspond to longer scan times; however, all imaging applications do not require the highest spatial resolution. For example, myocardial and ascending aortic imaging rarely requires submillimeter slices. In particular, when a patient is expected to have difficulty with breath holding, imaging should be performed with thicker slices to maximize the diagnostic information available.

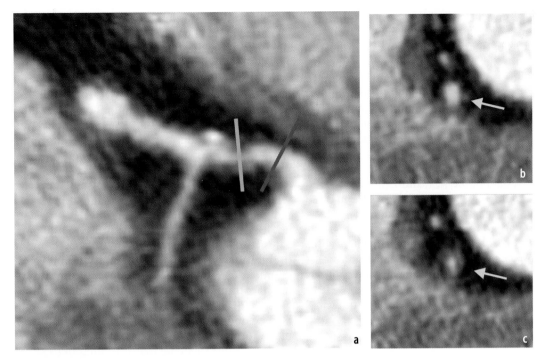

Fig. 9a-c. Diagnostic quality coronary computed tomography angiography. **a** Oblique multiplanar reformatted image of the proximal right coronary artery. One of the major advantages of coronary CTA in comparison with digital subtraction angiography is the ability to obtain an orthogonal view through any lesion. This is the most important step in image interpretation. **b** The *upper right-hand image* framed in *red* corresponds to the more proximal right coronary artery. There is no coronary artery disease at this level. **c** The *lower right-hand image* framed in *yellow* corresponds to the more distal right coronary artery lesion. This orthogonal view is obtained at the center of the noncalcified (soft) plaque and demonstrates a greater than 70% stenosis

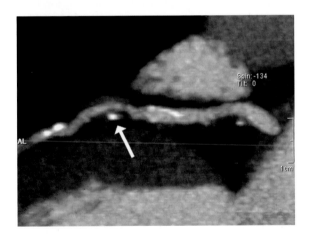

Fig. 10. Curved multiplanar reformatted image of the right coronary artery. Curved multiplanar images track (either automated, semiautomated, or manually) the center of the coronary artery though a long segment of its course and then display this long segment on a single image. While curved multiplanar reformatted images have no added information with respect to multiple short-segment standard reformatted images, they have the advantage that a large amount of data is displayed on a single image. However, it is essential to note that curved multiplanar reformatted images rely heavily on a precise placement of the center line. In our experience, interpretation of curved multiplanar reformatted images created from an imprecise center line is the most common source of error in image interpretation. This image demonstrates a complex (combination of calcified and noncalcified) plaque in the right coronary artery. At the calcified central component (*white arrow*), the stenosis was 50%

Scanning Parameters

As with ECG gating, image data oversampling, and spatial resolution, modern cardiac CT pushes the limits of technology with respect to the X-ray source. The two main scanning parameters that determine the number of photons used are the effective milliampere second (mAs) and kilovolts (kV). Effective mAs is defined as mAs divided by CT pitch and is proportional to X-ray CT tube current and scan time. Effective mAs and kV are set by the operator at the time of image acquisition. Typical values of effective mAs and kV are 550–700 and 120, respectively. However, in order to avoid reconstruction of images with significant noise, larger patients require more photons and thus higher settings. The most common way to maintain diagnostic images is to increase the effective mAs. Cardiac imaging of very obese patients is often limited. All X-ray CT tubes have a "limit" to the number of photons that can be produced, and for a particular application, all methods to decrease image noise (using the tube limit, increasing image thickness, scanning a smaller region) should be considered.

As described above, Z-axis spatial resolution is

determined by image slice thickness. For all modern scanners, the resolution is submillimeter. Although details of image interpretation are beyond the scope of this article, it is important to point out one major advantage of CT in comparison with other imaging modalities, such as catheter angiography, is the ability to perform multiplanar reconstructed images. Quality of reconstructed images is inversely related to image slice thickness, and it is beneficial to reconstruct images on so-called "isotropic data"; that is, CT data sets where spatial resolution is equal in the X, Y, and Z-directions. As an example of the impact of spatial resolution, consider native coronary CTA acquired with perfect ECG gating and no respiratory motion. In this setting, a 3-mm coronary artery reconstructed with 0.4 mm isotropic voxels spans seven or eight high-quality pixels (3 mm/0.4 mm) in any direction. This explains why properly performed CTA can differentiate between <50% and >50% stenosis but cannot grade a stenosis more precisely.

Scan Range and Image Field of View

Scan range in the Z-axis should include the anatomy of interest and allow for variations induced by both breath holding and the possibility that pathology can extend in both the cranial and caudal directions. In coronary imaging, occasionally, the left main and proximal left anterior descending arteries course superiorly over 1–2 cm, after which these vessels follow their usual path. Even in these situations, when imaging the native coronaries, the superior border of the scan should be set at the top of the carina, and the inferior border should scan through the entire inferior wall of the heart. Ideally, the planned field of view (FOV) should include several slices of the liver to account for cardiac displacement during breath holding. Since CT data is acquired in the craniocaudal direction, obtaining a small amount of CT data inferior to the heart does not affect image quality. Extended craniocaudal coverage is required for specific applications (Fig. 11). The most common applications are evaluation of coronary bypass grafts and of chest pain. For bypass grafts, imaging extends cranially to include the origins of the internal mammary arteries from the subclavian arteries. It is important to image the full extent of both sides, as course, caliber, and patency is important in the assessment of patients who have an internal mammary graft as well as those in whom the internal mammary artery is being considered for bypass.

The operator also specifies the FOV in the XY plane for coronary CT reconstruction. Choosing an FOV in the XY plane that is smaller than 24 cm is not recommended, as these images can be noisy. Typical values range between 24 cm and 30 cm, and it is almost always the case that coronary artery reconstruction will include the most important anatomy in the mediastinum.

In every case, complete CT reconstruction with a full FOV should be performed, followed by "skin-to-skin" interpretation in lung, mediastinum, and bone windows. Patients have significant "incidental" findings, including cases of acute pulmonary embolism and lung masses invading the chest wall, that can be the source of chest pain.

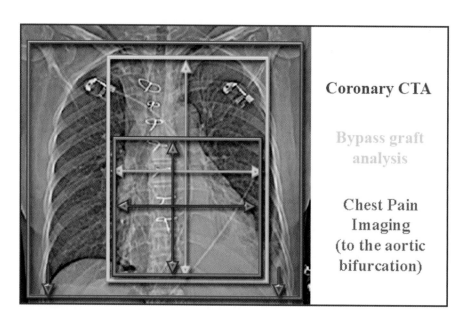

Coronary CTA

Bypass graft analysis

Chest Pain Imaging (to the aortic bifurcation)

Fig. 11. Topogram of a cardiovascular patient. For imaging of the native coronary arteries (*blue range*), imaging should extend from the top of the carina though the inferior of the heart. Ideally, imaging should include a few slices of the liver to ensure that the inferior of the heart is covered. For bypass graft imaging (*yellow range*), the superior aspect of the range is extended to include both subclavian arteries and the origin of the internal mammary arteries. In chest-pain imaging, the entire chest, as well as the full extent of the aorta, is imaged

Contrast Material

While intravenous contrast can be administered with either a single or a dual injection system, dual injection (iodinated contrast followed by saline) is recommended for coronary CTA. Saline is used to avoid dense opacification of the right heart and potential artifacts that can limit interpretation of the right coronary artery. In addition, the injection of saline after iodinated contrast pushes the iodinated contrast to its anatomic destination and helps to minimize dilution of the contrast as it passes through the central veins.

It is now standard to inject contrast material at rates of at least 5 cc/s, and most centers have an injection rate between 6 cc and 7.5 cc/s. This rate of delivery requires that the IV be placed in the antecubital vein and be at least 20 gauge (usually 18 guage is required). A right-arm injection is preferred since contrast material injected into the left arm often fills the left brachiocephalic vein at the time of image acquisition, and dense opacification of the brachiocephalic vein can be the source of artifact in the anterior mediastinum. Contrast material volume is determined by contrast injection rate and scan time required to cover the craniocaudal extent of the heart. As an example, consider an 18-s scan of the native coronaries plus bypass grafts. With an injection rate of 5 cc/s, an adequate volume of contrast media would be 90 cc (18 s × 5 cc/s). Since the administration of contrast material after completion of image acquisition is of no benefit, it is important to perform this calculation so that excessive contrast does not fill the right heart and subsequently induce image artifact.

With respect to timing the contrast injection, there are two general methods that can be used: bolus tracking and a test bolus. Both are illustrated in the setting of imaging the native coronary arteries. As previously mentioned, the superior border

of the region to be imaged is set at the top of the carina. The axial slice at this position is usually 2–4 cm above the origin of the left main coronary artery. In patients with normal cardiac output, no venous obstruction, and whose arms are positioned over the head and above the right heart, the typical transit time from the right antecubital vein to the ascending aorta at the level of the carina is between 17 s and 23 s. In bolus tracking, the contrast injection begins with the scanner prepared to repetitively image a region of interest (ROI) in the ascending aorta at the axial slice defined by the position of the carina. Roughly 10 s after the contrast injection begins, images of the same slice are acquired while enhancement of the ascending aorta is monitored; that is, the bolus is "tracked" in the ascending aorta just above the coronary ostia. Once enhancement reaches a preset threshold (typically 200 HU above baseline attenuation in the ascending aorta), craniocaudal diagnostic images are acquired, beginning at the axial location where bolus tracking was performed.

A test bolus uses a separate injection to time the diagnostic injection. For an injection rate of 6 cc/ s, a typical test bolus would be 12 cc of contrast followed by 30 cc of saline. As with bolus tracking, the ROI is chosen in the ascending aorta at the level of the carina. However, 10 s after the beginning of the test injection, scans separated by 1 s are used to plot enhancement versus time to include the time of peak enhancement (Fig. 12). Once the optimum delay is determined from the plot, the diagnostic images are obtained with a second contrast injection. When using a test bolus, it is important that the test injection mirrors the diagnostic injection. In particular, injection rates should be the same. Also, most centers routinely give nitroglycerin (0.4 mg sublingually) for coronary vasodilatation to all patients undergoing native coronary CTA. While the effect of nitroglyc-

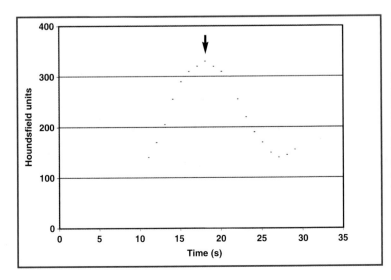

Fig. 12. Typical appearance of timing bolus plot for coronary CTA. The region of interest is approximately 3 cm above the origin of the left main coronary artery. Contrast (12 cc) followed by saline (30 cc) is administered at a rate of 6 cc/s, and images are acquired every second. There are no data points for the first 10 s of the timing bolus since imaging is not performed while the contrast passes from the venous system to the pulmonary arterial system. In this example, the contrast in the ascending aorta peaks at 18 s (*arrow*). The subsequent coronary CTA will use a 21-s delay. The rationale is that the additional 3 s will ensure that the coronary arteries have time to fill with contrast before the CT data is collected

erin on cardiac output (and thus iodinated contrast transit time) is typically negligible, the nitroglycerin should be administered before the test injection.

While using a test bolus has the disadvantage that a separate injection is required, there are distinct advantages in coronary imaging. First, unlike bolus tracking, when a test bolus is used, actual time to peak enhancement can be obtained. This will better ensure that when the diagnostic contrast injection is performed, peak enhancement will be achieved. Second, the test injection tests the quality of the intravenous access. Finally, since the test bolus can be performed with the breathing instructions that will be used in the diagnostic injection, it allows the patient to "practice" the exam, and it enables the operator to visualize variation in heart rate during a breath-hold IV contrast injection.

Image Reconstruction

Single-segment (one heartbeat) or multisegment (greater than one heartbeat) retrospective image reconstruction can be performed, the later strategy yielding an improvement in temporal resolution at the expense of greater data oversampling and more patient irradiation. In addition to choosing a single- versus multisegment algorithm, the operator can choose a reconstruction kernel for a particular application. Reconstruction with additional kernels is most often done in the evaluation of patients with one or more coronary stents

(Fig. 13). At present, stenosis within a stent cannot be quantified reliably. However, sharper imaging kernels (i.e., closer to a bone algorithm than a soft tissue algorithm) can be used to "sharpen" edges and determine that a coronary stent is not occluded. This can provide useful information in patients who present with chest pain post-stent placement.

Another technique that can be used to improve image quality is ECG editing. This refers to the ability to manually modify and/or eliminate a reconstruction phase in one or in a few RR intervals (Fig. 14). ECG editing is most commonly used when a patient has a premature ventricular contraction (PVC) during image acquisition. Since the reconstructed phase of the cardiac cycle is triggered from the high amplitude of the R wave, reconstruction software can mistake a PVC for an R wave. Reconstructed slices that correspond to RR intervals with this error will suffer from severe motion artifact since these slices will be reconstructed over a different part of the cardiac cycle than the remainder of the scan. Since coronary CTA data is oversampled (CT pitch <1), reconstruction can be performed after removal of a PVC, often yielding a dramatic improvement in image quality. This can be a critical step for patients who have a PVC, particularly for those who do not have CAD. Since the high negative predictive value of coronary CTA depends on acquiring diagnostic images through the full extent of the major coronary arteries, elimination of a short segment of severe motion artifact can enable the interpreting physician to determine that a study is normal.

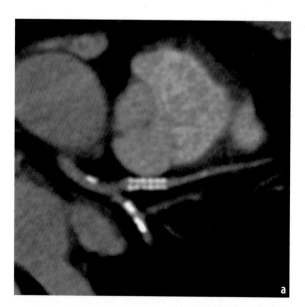
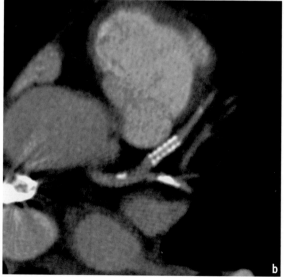

Fig. 13. For patients with coronary artery stents, both image artifacts and the spatial resolution of coronary CTA limit the interpretation. **a** Curved multiplanar reformatted image in a patient with a stent in the proximal left anterior descending artery. This image is reconstructed with a standard coronary imaging kernel. **b** Image reconstructed with a kernel closer to a bone algorithm shows sharper edges and less artifact from the high attenuation stent. The in-stent lumen is better visualized

Before ECG Editing

After ECG Editing

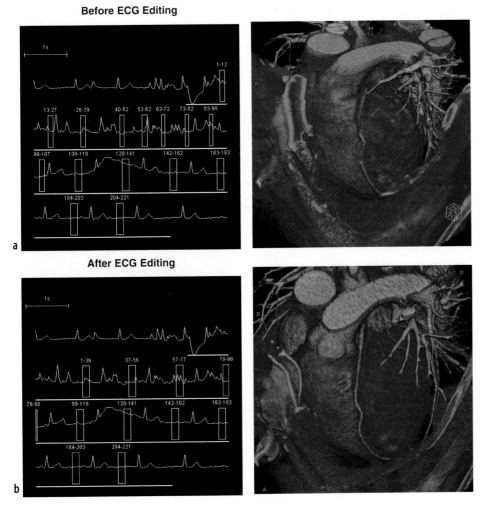

Fig. 14. ECG editing in a patient with suboptimal gating. The *top right* image demonstrates artifact that is explained by the locations (*rectangles* in the *top left image*) in the ECG where reconstruction was performed. Analysis of ECG tracing reveals that for some RR intervals, noise in the ECG is of great enough amplitude the the reconstruction algorithm mistook noise for an R wave. Thus, the different axial levels of the reconstruction reflect different phases of the cardiac cycle, rendering the study nondiagnostic. The *bottom left* image represents the ECG after editing; the location of the reconstruction has been manually placed to correspond with a relatively quiescent period in diastole. The subsequent ECG edited reconstruction (*bottom right image*) showed normal coronary arteries, using the high negative predictive value of coronary CT angiography (CTA) to eliminate coronary artery disease as a source of this patient's chest pain. Image post-processing courtesy of Melissa Ende, Siemens Medical Solutions

Summary

Imaging protocols for cardiac CT have been revolutionized by recent advances in technology. In addition to the widespread availability of ECG gating, CT equipment with submillimeter resolution, 64 slices per rotation, and gantry rotation times less than one-half second are available from all major vendors. Cardiac imaging protocols are more complicated than CT scanning of other body parts. Strict adherence to the protocol is required to maintain image quality. However, for the clinician familiar with CT, superior diagnostic images can be obtained routinely.

Acknowledgments

The authors gratefully acknowledge useful discussions with Bernhard Schmidt Ph.D., particularly with respect to the section of CT radiation dose.

References

1. International Electrotechnical Commission. Medical electrical equipment. Part 2-44: Particular requirements for the safety of X-ray equipment for computed tomography. IEC publication 60601-2-44 (2002). International Electrotechnical Commission (IEC) Central Office: Geneva. Accessed 17 Jan 2006

2. European Guidelines on Quality Computed Tomography. EUR16262 (2002). http://www.drs.dk/guidelines/CT/quality/index.htm. Accessed 17 Jan 2006

3. Morin R, Gerber T, McCollough C (2003) Radiation dose in computed tomography of the heart. Circulation 107:917–922

4. International Council on Radiation Protection (1991) 1990 recommendations of the International Commission on Radiological Protection. Publication 60. Annals of the ICRP. Pergamon, Oxford

5. Schmidt B, Kalender WA (2002) A fast voxel-based Monte Carlo method for scanner- and patient-specific dose calculations in computed tomography. Physica Medica XVIII(2):43–53

6. Zankl M, Panzer W, Drexler G (1991) The calculation of dose from external photon exposure using reference human phantoms and Monte Carlo methods. Part IV: Organ doses from tomographic examinations. GSF report 30/91. GSF, Neuherberg

7. Kalender WA, Schmidt B, Zankl M, Schmidt M (1999) A PC program for estimating organ dose and effective dose values in computed tomography. Eur Radiol 9:555–562

8. Stamm G, Nagel HD (2002) CT-Expo – ein neuartiges Programm zur Dosisevaluierung in der CT. Fortschr Röntgenstr 174:1570–1576

III.2

MDCT Angiography of the Thoracic Aorta

Geoffrey D. Rubin and Mannudeep K. Kalra

Introduction

Multidetector computed tomography angiography (MDCTA) is a noninvasive and accurate technique for assessment of many thoracic aortic abnormalities. It offers several advantages over conventional aortography for evaluation of the thoracic aorta. State-of-the-art MDCT scanners, with improved temporal and isotropic resolution, enable volumetric acquisition that provides clear anatomic delineation of thoracic aorta, its tortuous branches, and adjacent aneurysms and pseudo aneurysms. In contrast with the projectional technique of conventional aortography, these frequently overlapping structures can affect visualization and delineation of anatomic relationships. In addition, MDCTA allows simultaneous delineation of true and false luminal flow channels in thoracic aortic dissections, intramural hematomas communicating with the aortic lumen, slow perigraft blood flow around aortic stent grafts, as well as direct visualization of the aortic wall and noncommunicating intramural hematomas. This chapter reviews techniques for acquisition and interpretation of thoracic aortic MDCTA and describes abnormalities in which MDCTA provides valuable information.

Scanning Techniques

Scan Coverage

MDCTA scanning protocol for evaluation of thoracic aorta must extend, at the minimum, from the base of the neck (to assess proximal common carotid and vertebral arteries) to the origin of the celiac axis. Such scan coverage allows evaluation of the supraaortic arterial branches for possible extension of aortic lesions, such as aneurysm and aortic dissection, into these branches. MDCTA of thoracic aorta is often performed to diagnose and localize

aortic disease for planning endovascular and open repair, so inclusion of celiac origin aids in precise localization of lesions affecting distal thoracic aorta. However, in certain abnormalities, such as acute aortic dissection, additional scan coverage may be essential. In dissections, MDCTA is extended to cover the abdomen and pelvis to assess possible diminution of blood flow to the abdominal viscera or lower extremity. In other instances, upper-extremity arterial circulation (to evaluate for sources of embolization to the hands) or entire carotid arterial circulation (for assessing aortic dissection associated with symptoms of cerebral ischemia and large-vessel arteritis) may be included (Fig. 1).

Unenhanced Images

Generally, unenhanced CT images are acquired prior to MDCTA in the setting of suspected bleeding in the chest or aortic wall. These unenhanced images allow visualization of hyperattenuation of the mural crescent corresponding to intramural hematoma in patients with acute chest pain and possible intramural hematoma (Fig. 2). In addition, these images also aid in mapping the location of calcifications around the stent graft, which can simulate an endoleak following contrast administration. We typically use low radiation dose for acquiring these initial images (120 kV, 100 mA, 0.5 s rotation time, 1.3–1.7:1 pitch).

Contrast Media Considerations

For MDCTA of the thoracic aorta, we prefer contrast injection rate of at least 5 mL/s for an injection duration of less than 20 s. Generally, we do not perform MDCTA of thoracic aorta if flow rate is less than 4 mL/s. As a rule, the bolus duration must be equivalent to image acquisition duration plus

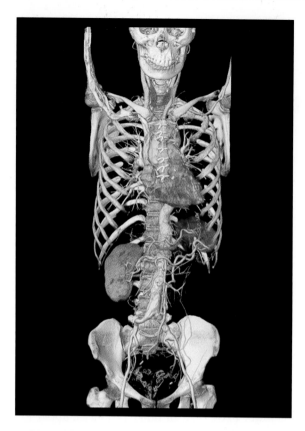

Fig. 1. A 16×1.25-mm multidetector computed tomography (MDCT) scan acquired in 15 s in a woman with Takayasu arteritis. All arterials beds that might be affected by the disease are imaged from the carotid arteries through the femoral arteries within a single breath hold

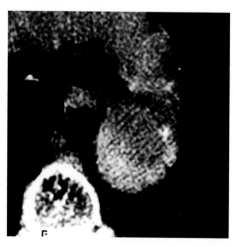

Fig. 2. Unenhanced transverse computed tomography (CT) section demonstrates a hyperattenuated crescent within the aortic wall diagnostic of an intramural hematoma

any delays by bolus monitoring algorithms. Our experience suggests that an iodinated contrast medium (370 mg of iodine/mL) volume of at least 80 mL is required for reliable opacification. As high CT attenuation values of undiluted contrast

medium in the veins can affect visualization of adjacent structures, we always administer contrast medium via a right antecubital venous source to avoid opacification of the left brachiocephalic, vein which can obscure the origins of the brachiocephalic, left common carotid, and left subclavian arteries.

To obtain optimum enhancement, it is necessary to use appropriate scan delay for contrast administration. We use an automated scan triggering technique for initiating image acquisition of the contrast-enhanced phase of MDCTA. As our MDCT scanners require about 8 s from the time that threshold enhancement is recognized in the descending aorta to the initiation of CTA acquisition, our injection duration is equal to scan duration plus 8 s. We have found that this is the most reliable technique for achieving consistently high-quality MDCTA studies.

Scanning Protocol

MDCTA of the thoracic aorta should be performed with ≤3 mm nominal section thickness and preferably with ≤1.5 mm thickness. The fastest possible gantry rotation time must be used to minimize scan duration and contrast dose. However, a slower gantry rotation time may improve image quality in larger patients by enabling a higher tube current-time product. Alternatively, some MDCT scanners allow use of higher tube current (up to 800 mA). Most MDCTA studies are performed with 120 kVp. We frequently use cardiac gating of MDCTA for evaluation of the ascending aorta and, in particular, coronary arteries [1, 2].

Scanning protocols for MDCTA must allow image acquisition in a single breath hold. If mechanical ventilation or extreme dyspnea does not permit single breath-hold scanning, then one should allow the patient to breathe quietly during image acquisition.

For most MDCTA studies, only arterial phase acquisition is required. However, for evaluation of stent-graft repair of aortic aneurysm, delayed images can be critical for detecting endoleak. These images are acquired about 70 s after initiation of arterial phase acquisition.

Reconstruction Considerations

We generally reconstruct MDCTA images with an interval that is 50% of the effective section thickness. These images are reconstructed with a smaller reconstructed field of view (25–30 cm) to only include the relevant arterial structures. Softer reconstruction algorithms are typically used to minimize noise in thin sections acquired with MDCTA.

Interpretation Techniques

Image Workstations

Soft copy reading of MDCTA image data sets at a postprocessing or picture archiving and communication system (PACS) workstation is recommended, as they allow scrolling through large number of source images, three-dimensional (3-D) postprocessing, and adjustment of window level and width. Due to variations in aortic enhancement, customization of window width and level settings is important to ensure that discrimination of luminal enhancement from mural calcifications is possible. In addition, very narrow windows are frequently necessary for assessing subtle endoleaks following stent-graft repair on delayed images.

Artifacts in MDCTA

Certain artifacts can affect assessment of patients with suspected aortic dissection. Perivenous streaks and arterial pulsations cause the most interpretative difficulties of MDCTA of thoracic aorta, typically on the visualization of the ascending aorta.

Perivenous streak artifacts result from both beam hardening and motion caused by transmitted pulsation in veins with undiluted contrast medium. Prior studies have recommended modification of scanning techniques to minimize these artifacts. These include the use of dilute contrast medium solutions [3, 4], caudal to cranial scan direction, and femoral venous access [5]. These methods have been abandoned due to the recent availability of dual-chamber contrast medium injectors, enabling the use of a saline chaser bolus to eliminate perivenous shunts (Fig. 3). In most instances, perivenous streaks are seldom misinterpreted as intimal dissection in the ascending aorta due to substantial variation in their orientation from image to image and extension beyond the confines of the aortic wall. However, the difficult area for perivenous streaks is the origin of the supraaortic branches adjacent to a contrast-opacified left brachiocephalic vein, where these artifacts can obscure extension of dissection to these branches as well as occlusive disease caused by atherosclerotic plaque at their origins. The best preventive strategy to avoid this artifact is to ensure peripheral venous access from the right upper extremity.

In addition to perivenous streaks, artifacts from arterial pulsation can also result in a false positive interpretation of aortic dissection. For example, pulsation in the ascending aorta can mimic an intimal flap. With faster acquisition speed and thin overlapping sections provided by MDCT scanners, this artifact may be eliminated. Use of

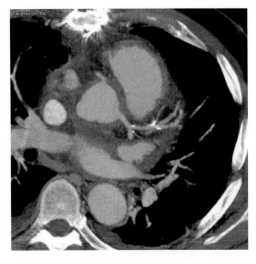

Fig. 3. Transverse multidetector computed tomography (MDCT) section obtained from a scan acquired with a 50-ml saline chaser bolus demonstrates mild superior vena cava opacification, allowing for artifact-free assessment of the aortic root

wider windows can also help in excluding "artifactual intimal flap" by documenting extension of artifacts beyond aortic walls. Segmented or partial reconstruction of helical scan data can also help in reducing motion artifacts observed on standard reconstructions [6] (Fig. 4). Aortic pulsation, which is particularly more pronounced in thinner patients, results in a serrated appearance to arteries that can simulate fibromuscular dysplasia in blood vessels such as renal arteries, but is rarely a limitation in the chest

Differential flow of contrast medium in the true and false lumina can simulate appearance of a thrombosed false lumen, particularly when scan delay is triggered on the basis of opacification of the true lumen of the aorta (Fig. 5). Thus, in patients with suspected aortic dissection, bolus tracking must be performed just caudal to the aortic arch, where transverse cross-sections of both the distal ascending as well as proximal descending aorta can be assessed. A region of interest must be placed in both the true and false lumen to obtain two time density curves. Delay time is selected to assure opacification of false lumen. Bolus duration is then increased by the time (seconds) between the true luminal peak and the selected delay time.

Reformation and Rendering

While axial source images remain the mainstay of MDCTA interpretation of the thoracic aorta, multiplanar reformation (MPR) and 3-D rendering techniques can aid in diagnosis. In addition, these techniques can provide an easier and more effec-

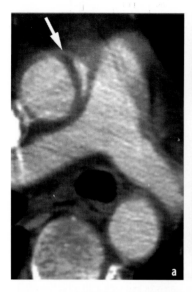
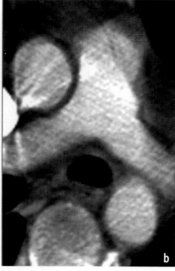

Fig. 4a, b. 3.75-mm transverse-section multidetector computed tomography (MDCT) sections obtained through the ascending aorta in a patient who had been run over by a tractor. Acquisition parameters are 3.75-mm detector width, pitch 1.5, table speed 22.5 mm per rotation, and 0.8 s per rotation. An apparent linear filling defect is present within the ascending aorta (*arrow*). (**a**) Identical image location from the same CT acquisition reconstructed with a half scan or segmented reconstruction algorithm. The segmented reconstruction requires approximately 220° of data, resulting in an effective temporal resolution of 0.5 s. By reconstructing the section using this algorithm, the apparent linear filling defects are revealed to be motion-related artifacts, and thus there is no suspicion for ascending aortic injury (**b**)

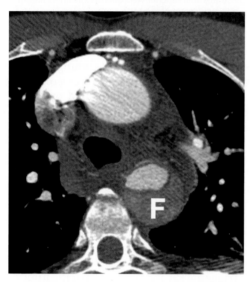

Fig. 5. Transverse section from multidetector computed tomography angiography (MDCTA) where the scan was triggered using a region of interest placed within the true aortic lumen results in an acquisition that is too early to allow the false lumen to fill, thus leading to the ambiguous appearance of a thrombosed versus a slowly filling false lumen (*F*)

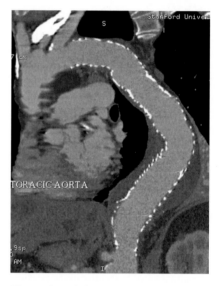

Fig. 6. Curved planar reformation (CPR) through the aortic arch and descending aorta allows clear delineation of the contrast-medium-enhanced aortic lumen, the stent graft, and the thrombosed portions of a descending thoracic aortic aneurysm outside of the stent graft

tive way of explaining critical anatomic relationships to clinicians. The most popular techniques include MPR, maximum-intensity projections (MIP), and volume rendering (VR). In our experience, curved planar reformations (CPR), and VR are the most useful 3-D techniques for assessing the thoracic aorta.

MPR, which also includes CPR and sagittal, coronal, and oblique tomograms, are typically single-voxel-thick tomographic images. The single-voxel-thick MPR, especially the CPR, is the most useful of the MPR techniques [7]. CPR is helpful for visualization of the luminal contents of the aorta or its branches in patients with aortic dissection

or aortic stent-graft deployment (Fig. 6). Combining information from adjacent voxels allows thicker MPR images, referred to as a thin-slab, or multiplanar volume rendered (MPVR) images [8]. Thin slabs require no pre-rendering segmentation or editing and help demonstrate vessel origins in different but adjacent planes, such as occurs with branches of the aortic arch.

MIP [9–11] has limited application in evaluation of thoracic aorta. As calcified atheroma is rarely of clinical significance, simultaneous display and distinction of the contrast-enhanced flow lumen and mural calcification with MIP images is not very useful in the thoracic aorta. Besides, in-

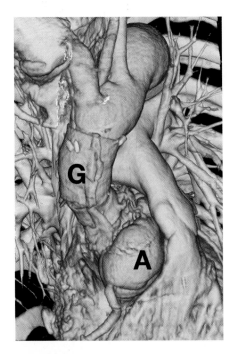

Fig. 7. Volume rendering (VR) allows clear depiction of the ascending aortic interposition graft (*G*) and a root aneurysm (*A*)

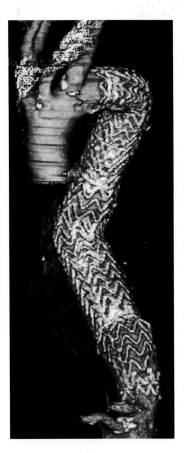

Fig. 8. Volume rendering (VR) demonstrates the metallic stent graft (*white*), the aortic lumen (*pink*), and the thrombosed aneurysm (*blue*) from the same patient as in Figure 6

ability of MIP to discern overlapping vascular anatomy is also a substantial disadvantage.

VR [12–16] is a volumetric 3-D technique that displays complex anatomic relationships, particularly in regions of vessel overlap (Figs. 7–9). With the exception of occlusive diseases, intramural hematomas and some thrombosed false lumina, VR provides the best information about lesion anatomy for surgical planning in most thoracic aortic diseases, such as aneurysms, congenital aberrant branching, and intimal dissection or intramural hematoma.

Clinical Applications of MDCTA of Thoracic Aorta

MDCTA of thoracic aorta provides useful information for congenital anomalies, aneurysms, dissection, aortic trauma, intramural hematoma, and open and endovascular interventions.

Congenital Anomalies

MDCTA of thoracic aorta allows noninvasive diagnosis and characterization of congenital anomalies of the thoracic aorta and aberrant branches of the descending aorta, such as vascular rings, aberrant supraaortic branching, coarctation (Fig. 10), and enlarged bronchial arteries or major arteriopul-

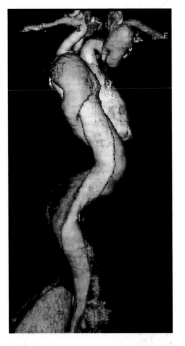

Fig. 9. The complex interrelationship between true and false lumina of the descending aorta are demonstrated with volume rendering (VR)

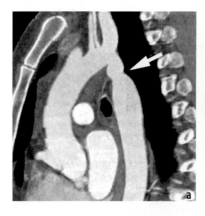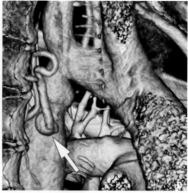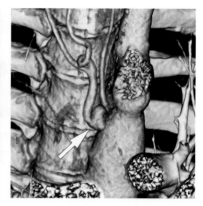

Fig. 10a-c. a Curved planar reformation (CPR) of computed tomography angiography (CTA) in a patient with aortic coarctation (*arrow*). **b** Volume rendering (VR) of the aortic arch and proximal descending aorta viewed from the right demonstrates an aneurysm (*arrow*) at the origin of an enlarged intercostal artery origin, which provides collateral circulation around the coarcted segment. **c** Frontal VR through the descending aorta demonstrates the intercostal artery aneurysm to better advantage (*arrow*)

monary communicating arteries [17, 18] In addition, thin section volumetric MDCTA studies provide information on lesions, such as pulmonary sequestration, as well as depict direct relationship between tracheobronchial narrowing and the presence of aberrant vessels.

Aortic Aneurysm

MDCTA allows accurate evaluation of thoracic aortic aneurysms, including presence of an aneurysm, its extent, size, complications, follow-up evaluation, and prediction of appropriate management [19]. Generally, diagnosis of aortic aneurysms is made from axial-source data, whereas CPR and VR are helpful in determining lesion extent (Figs. 11 and 12). As the thoracic aorta is a tortuous and curved structure, aneurysm size measurement is most accurate when double-oblique MPRs are generated in directions perpendicular to the aortic flow lumen (Fig. 13). This measurement technique for aneurysm sizing is also reproducible for evaluating the rate of aneurysm expansion on follow-up MDCTA studies. It is interesting to note that aneurysm volume allows the most complete measure of aneurysm size. Although volumetric MDCTA data should provide accurate aneurysm volume, the painstaking and time-consuming manual segmentation of patent, thrombosed, and atheromatous elements of the aorta from the adjacent structures is a substantial drawback of aneurysmal volume. To date, there is no data concerning the risk of aneurysm rupture and guidelines for intervention based on aneurysm volume expansion [20, 21].

Generally speaking, thoracic aortic aneurysms >5 cm in cross-sectional dimension have an increased risk for rupture. Surgical repair is often contemplated when thoracic aortic aneurysms

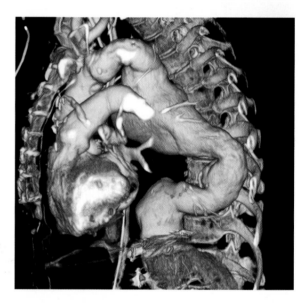

Fig. 11. Volume rendering (VR) of a large descending aortic aneurysm illustrates the tortuous course of the aorta distal the aneurysm

reach a diameter of 5–6 cm [20, 21]. For surgical planning, MDCTA provides a roadmap of aneurysms by depicting the precise anatomic extent of the aneurysm as well as the involvement of aortic branches. A recent study reported 94% accuracy, 95% positive predicative value, and 93% negative predictive value for successful prediction of the need for hypothermic circulatory arrest with transverse and MPR images [19].

Aortic Dissection

Accurate identification and localization [ascending aorta – type A (Fig. 14) or not proximal to the brachiocephalic artery – type B (Fig. 15)] of the in-

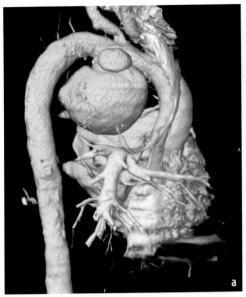
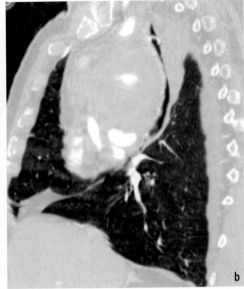

Fig. 12. a The lumen of a large pseudoaneurysm extending from the inferior aspect of the aortic arch is demonstrated with volume rendering (VR). The size of the mural thrombus (not visible) can be inferred from the compression on the superior vena cava. **b** Curved planar reformation (CPR) through the trachea demonstrates the marked compression of the airway by the large aneurysm

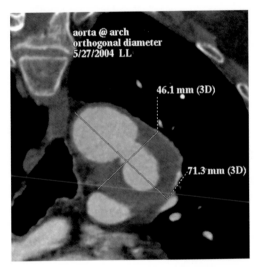
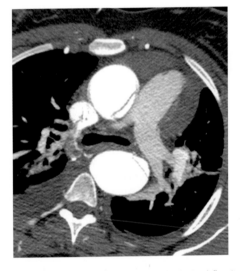

Fig. 13. Measurement of an aortic arch aneurysm using a double oblique view oriented perpendicular to the axis of the aneurysm

Fig. 14. Type A aortic dissection. An intimal flap is observed in both the ascending and descending aorta. Hemopericardium is demonstrated

timal flap is a prerequisite for application of any imaging technique in patients with suspected aortic dissection. Four imaging techniques, conventional angiography, CT scanning, MRI, and transesophageal echocardiography (TEE), can provide this information about aortic dissection and thus aid in decision making for emergent repair.

Although relative accuracy of these imaging modalities is controversial, technologic advances in CT, MRI and TEE have outpaced the ability of most researchers to compare these techniques in rigorous prospective trials. However, current opinion regards MRI or TEE as the most sensitive tests for aortic dissection [22] although this opinion is based on comparison of state-of-the-art MRI or TEE with relatively primitive conventional CT [23, 24]. Although radiation dose and iodinated contrast medium toxicity are relevant concerns with CT, to the best of our knowledge, no studies have compared state-of-the-art MDCT to either MRI or TEE. Although high-quality TEE offers several advantages over MDCT (on-site performance of TEE in emergency department and identification

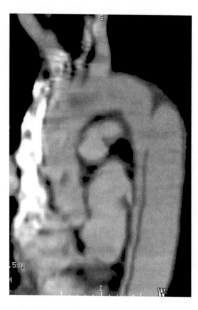

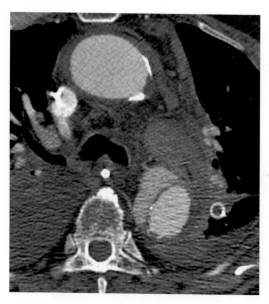

Fig. 15. Type B aortic dissection. The intimal flap originates distal to the brachiocephalic artery

Fig. 16. Rupturing type B aortic dissection. High attenuation blood is present in the mediastinum adjacent to the irregularly enlarged descending aortic false lumen

of aortic valvular insufficiency that requires immediate replacement), when TEE is unavailable, MDCTA will be the most accessible and staffed options to handle potentially hemodynamically unstable patients in most hospitals (Fig. 16).

The primary indication for diagnostic conventional angiography in patients with acute thoracic aortic dissection is in the setting of cardiac arrhythmia or electrocardiographic abnormalities, which suggest possible involvement of coronary artery and myocardial ischemia. However, in expert hands, it is most likely that the accuracy of TEE, MDCTA, and MRI will be nearly identical for diagnosis of aortic dissection.

Certain imaging modalities may be more useful in providing an alternative diagnosis when primary diagnosis is not present. For instance, unlike TEE, MDCTA may provide evidence of other vascular disease (such as coronary artery disease) mimicking aortic dissection. In addition, in patients with chronic or acute aortic dissection that do not require immediate surgical intervention, TEE does not provide sufficient information, such as extension of the intimal flap into aortic branches, true luminal compression by the false lumen that limits blood flow into the abdomen or pelvis, and presence of fenestrations that allow communication between the true and false lumen. However, MDCTA can provide information about extension of intimal flaps into aortic branches. Also, when catheter-based interventions are considered, preinterventional MDCTA can help identification of the best route for achieving access to aortic

branches as well as simultaneous visualization of all aortic lumina to avoid confusion in the angiography suite that results from opacification of only one of three or more lumina in a complex dissection. However, evaluation of thoracic aortic dissection with MDCTA does have pitfalls.

When considering reformation and rendering techniques, CPR is useful for depicting the flap within the center of the vessel (Fig. 17a). VR images demonstrate the interface of the intimal flap with the aortic wall (Fig. 17b). Usefulness of MIP images is limited, as they do not display the intimal flap unless it is oriented perpendicular to the plane of the MIP.

Intramural Hematoma

Several mechanisms have been proposed to explain formation of intramural hematoma, which include spontaneous rupture of the vasa vasorum, intimal fracture at the site of an atherosclerotic plaque, and intramural propagation of hemorrhage adjacent to a penetrating atherosclerotic ulcer. Patients with intramural hematomas exhibit symptoms, physical signs, and risk profiles that are almost identical to typical aortic dissection [25].

Prior studies on CT evaluation of intramural hematomas from penetrating atherosclerotic ulcers have reported that MDCTA aids in visualization of ulcers and intramural hematomas with confirmation of its subintimal location by the observation of displaced intimal calcifications [19, 26, 27] (Fig. 18).

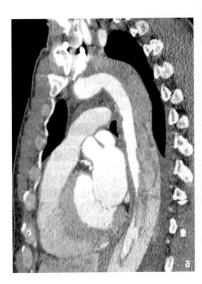

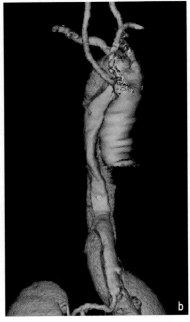

Fig. 17a, b. a Curved planar reformation (CPR) and **b** volume rendering (VR) of a type B aortic dissection. CPR depicts the interior of the lumen while VR demonstrates the interface of the lumen with the aortic wall

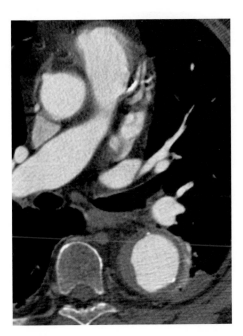

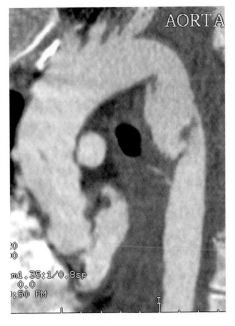

Fig. 18. Transverse section from a multidetector computed tomography angiography (MDCTA) demonstrates an intramural hematoma in the descending aorta. Intimal calcium along the posterior aspect of the aorta is displaced to the luminal surface supporting the conclusion that the mural collection is blood in the wall rather than atheroma within the lumen

Fig. 19. Curved planar reformation (CPR) through the aorta demonstrates a traumatic pseudoaneurysm at the aortic isthmus following high-speed deceleration in a motor vehicle collision

In patients with intramural hematoma, noncontrast images typically reveal a high-attenuation intramural crescent (Fig. 2). In addition, an intense contrast enhancement and thickening of the aortic wall external to the hematoma may be seen on contrast-enhanced images. These findings may represent adventitial inflammatory process.

Aortic Trauma

CT offers an accurate, rapid, and less expensive alternative to conventional aortography for evaluation of patients with suspected thoracic aortic trauma [28]. In such patients, MDCTA allows direct visualization of the aortic tear (Fig. 19). Prior

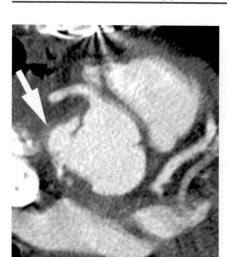

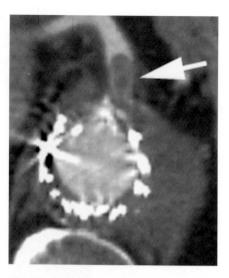

Fig. 20. Anastomotic dehiscence with resulting pseudoaneurysm (*arrow*) at the proximal anastomosis of an ascending aortic interposition graft

Fig. 21. Thrombotic occlusion of the celiac axis (*arrow*) following inadvertent extension of a thoracic aortic stent graft over the ostium of the celiac axis

studies have shown that helical CTA is a very sensitive technique for detection of aortic injury [29–31]. These studies have also reported that MPR and 3-D reformation do not contribute substantial information to axial source data for identification and characterization of aortic injury [31].

Evaluation of Aortic Interventions

MDCTA can be used for evaluation for assessment of open and endovascular aortic interventions. As vascular clips, sternal wires, and graft materials cause relatively little artifacts on MDCT images, MDCTA allows evaluation of perianastomotic complications following thoracic aortic or coronary artery bypass graft placement (Fig. 20) and complications following placement of access cannulas for cardiopulmonary bypass surgery.

MDCTA has been found useful for the evaluation of endoluminal thoracic aortic stent grafts [32]. It can demonstrate complications of stent grafting such as aortic-branch occlusions (Fig. 21), retroperitoneal hematoma, and iliac artery dissection or occlusion. As regards to imaging evaluation of aortic intervention, it is important to note that complete exclusion of aneurysm following stent-graft deployment determines the success of aneurysm treatment. In absence of complete exclusion of aneurysm, perigraft flow results, which can be very slow and therefore remains undetectable with flush aortography (Fig. 22). As MDCTA depends on intravenous injection of contrast medium for generalized arterial opacification, opacification of perigraft channels are often detected on postdeployment MDCTA, even when conventional aortography suggested complete ex-

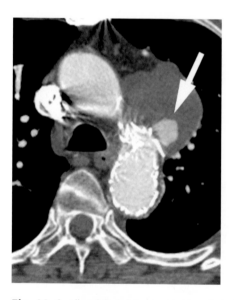

Fig. 22. Small endoleak following stent-graft deployment over an aortic arch aneurysm. The endoleak was not detected with flush aortography

clusion of such flow. MDCTA also helps in depicting the relationship of the aortic stent graft and the brachiocephalic arterial origins.

Conclusion

MDCTA offers a rapid, noninvasive, and accurate "one-stop" technique for evaluation of several thoracic aortic abnormalities [11, 33]. To optimize workflow and interpretation, efficient image postprocessing workstations and software are critical for large MDCTA image datasets [16]. In addition, it is important to update the scanning technique for optimum image acquisition and radiation dose as MDCT scanners evolve from 4-, 16-, 32-, and 40- to 64-slice configurations.

References

1. Lembcke A, Dohmen P, Rodenwaldt J et al (2003) Images in cardiovascular medicine. Recoarctation of the aorta associated with ascending aortic aneurysm demonstrated by ECG-gated multislice CT. Circulation. 107:e80–81

2. Marten K, Funke M, Rummeny EJ, Engelke C (2005) Electrocardiographic assistance in multidetector CT of thoracic disorders. Clin Radiol 60:8–21

3. Remy-Jardin M, Remy J, Wattinne L, Giraud F (1992) Central pulmonary thromboembolism: Diagnosis with spiral volumetric CT with the single-breath-hold technique - Comparison with pulmonary angiography. Radiology 185:381–387

4. Rubin GD, Lane MJ, Bloch DA (1996) Optimization of contrast enhanced thoracic spiral CT. Radiology 201:785–791

5. Prokop M, Schaefer CM, Leppert AGA, Galanski M (1993) Spiral CT Angiography of Thoracic Aorta: Femoral or Antecubital Injection Site for Intravenous Administration of Contrast Material? Radiology 189(P):111

6. Posniak HV, Olson MC, Demos TC (1993) Aortic motion artifact simulating dissection on CT scans: elimination with reconstructive segmented images. AJR Am J Roentgenol 161:557–558

7. Rubin GD, Dake MD, Semba CB (1995) Current status of three-dimensional spiral CT scanning for imaging the vasculature. Radiologic Clinics of North America 33:51–70

8. Napel S, Rubin GD, Jeffrey RB Jr (1993) STS-MIP: A new reconstruction technique for CT of the chest. J Comput Assist Tomogr 17:832–838

9. Rubin GD, Dake MD, Napel S et al (1994) Spiral CT of renal artery stenosis: comparison of three-dimensional rendering techniques. Radiology 190:181–189

10. Keller PJ, Drayer BP, Fram EK et al (1989) MR angiography with two-dimensional acquisition and three-dimensional display. Radiology 173:527–532

11. Napel S, Marks MP, Rubin GD et al (1992) CT angiography with spiral CT and maximum intensity projection. Radiology 185:607–610

12. Drebin RA, Carpenter L, Hanrahan P (1988) Volume rendering. Comput Graphics 22:65–74

13. Levoy M (1991) Methods for improving the efficiency and versatility of volume rendering. Prog Clin Biol Res 363:473–488

14. Rusinek H, Mourino MR, Firooznia H et al (1989) Volumetric rendering of MR images. Radiology 171:269–272

15. Fishman EK, Drebin B, Magid D et al (1987) Volumetric rendering techniques: applications for three-dimensional imaging of the hip. Radiology 163:737–738

16. Rubin GD, Beaulieu CF, Argiro V et al (1996) Perspective volume rendering of CT and MR images: applications for endoscopic imaging. Radiology 199:321–330

17. Katz M, Konen E, Rozsenman J et al (1995) Spiral CT and 3D image reconstruction of vascular ring and associated tracheobronchial anomalies. J Comput Assist Tomogr 19:564–568

18. Hopkins KL, Patrick LE, Simoneaux SF, Bank ER et al (1996) Pediatric great vessel anomalies: initial clinical experience with spiral CT angiography. Radiology 200:811–815

19. Quint LE, Francis IR, Williams DM et al (1996) Evaluation of thoracic aortic disease with the use of helical CT and multiplanar reconstructions: comparison with surgical findings. Radiology 201:37–41

20. Masuda Y, Takanashi K, Takasu J (1992) Expansion rate of thoracic aortic aneurysms and influencing factors. Chest 102:461–466

21. Dapunt L, Galla JD, Sadeghi AM et al (1994) The natural history of thoracic aortic aneurysms. J Thorac Cardiovasc Surg 107:1323–1333

22. Cigarroa JE, Isselbacher EM, DeSanctis RW, Eagle KA (1993) Medical progress. diagnostic imaging in the evaluation of suspected aortic dissection: old standards and new directions. AJR Am J Roentgenol 161:485–493

23. Erbel R, Daniel W, Visser C et al (1989) Echocardiography in diagnosis of aortic dissection. Lancet March 4:457–461

24. Nienaber CA, Kodolitsch Yv, Nicolas V et al (1993) The diagnosis of thoracic aortic dissection by non-invasive imaging procedures. NEJM 328:1–9

25. Nienaber CA, Kodolitsch Yv, Petersen B et al (1995) Intramural hemorrhage of the thoracic aorta: diagnostic and therapeutic implications. Circulation 92:1465–1472

26. Kazerooni EA, Bree RL, Williams DM (1992) Penetrating atherosclerotic ulcers of the descending thoracic aorta: evaluation with CT and distinction from aortic dissection. Radiology 183:759–765

27. Gore I (1952) Pathogenesis of dissecting aneurysm of the aorta. Arch Pathol Lab Med 53:142–153

28. Mirvis SE, Shanmuganathan K, Miller BH et al (1996) Traumatic aortic injury: diagnosis with contrast-enhanced thoracic CT - five year experience at a major trauma center. Radiology 200:413–422

29. Gavant ML, Manke PG, Fabian T et al (1995) Blunt traumatic aortic rupture: detection with helical CT of the chest. Radiology 197:125–133

30. Parker MS, Matheson TL, Rao AV et al (2001) Making the transition: the role of helical CT in the evaluation of potentially acute thoracic aortic injuries. AJR Am J Roentgenol 176:1267–1272

31. Dyer DS, Moore EE, Mestek MF et al (1999) Can chest CT be used to exclude aortic injury? Radiology 213:195–202

32. Armerding MD, Rubin GD, Beaulieu CF et al (2000) Aortic aneurysmal disease: assessment of stent-graft treatment-CT versus conventional angiography. Radiology 215:138–146

33. Rubin GD, Dake MD, Napel SA et al (1993) Abdominal spiral CT angiography: Initial clinical experience. Radiology 186:147–152

III.3

Pulmonary Embolism Imaging with MDCT

Joseph J. Kavanagh, Douglas R. Lake and Philip Costello

Introduction

The timely and accurate diagnosis of acute pulmonary embolism (PE) is crucial to providing appropriate patient care. Acute PE is a treatable condition with a 3-month mortality rate greater than 15% [1]. Potential complications include cardiogenic shock, hypotension, and myocardial infarction. PE is a relatively common condition, with an estimated overall incidence of about 1 per 1,000 patients within the United States [2]. Of approximately 1,000 computed tomography (CT) studies recently performed to assess for PE at our institution, roughly 10% were found to have PE. Unfortunately, the presenting symptoms of acute PE are relatively nonspecific and may be challenging for the clinician. Symptoms include dyspnea, cough, chest pain, and infrequently, hemoptysis. Chest radiography, electrocardiography (ECG), arterial blood gas measurements, and D-dimer assays all have the potential to suggest PE, but they are nonspecific [3–9]. Radiological imaging plays a crucial role in definitive diagnosis. Many modalities, including pulmonary angiography, ventilation-perfusion scintigraphy (V/Q), compression Doppler sonography, and CT have played important roles in the diagnosis of acute PE.

Over the last 5 years, multidetector CT (MDCT) pulmonary angiography has become the initial diagnostic test of choice in many institutions. Meanwhile, conventional angiography, V/Q scan, and Doppler sonography have been relegated to adjunctive roles [10–12]. Many retrospective and some prospective studies have been completed to prove the accuracy of MDCT for detecting and excluding patients suspected of acute PE. Through this research, there has been a transition from the "gold standard" of pulmonary angiography and V/Q scintigraphy to MDCT as the modality of choice for excluding PE.

Advantages of MDCT

CT has many advantages when compared with other available modalities in the detection of PE. MDCT pulmonary angiography is a rapid test, which can be obtained in a single 10-s breath hold with a 16-slice CT system. CT also has the ability to readily detect other abnormalities that may be contributing to the patient's clinical presentation, including congestive heart failure, pneumonia, interstitial lung disease, aortic dissection, malignancy (Fig. 1), and pleural disease [13, 14].

Due to the relative frequency of PE, its high mortality rate if not treated, and our ability to adequately treat it, the diagnosis of acute PE using CT has been the subject of much research. Multiple studies comparing MDCT with selective pulmonary angiography have shown a negative pre-

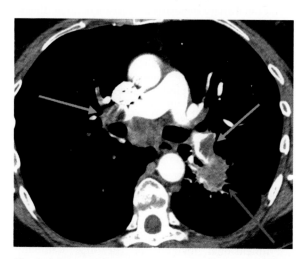

Fig. 1. A 53-year-old woman presented to the emergency department with acute shortness of breath and left-lower-extremity swelling. Multidetector computed tomography (MDCT) pulmonary angiogram axial image demonstrated large pulmonary emboli (*green arrows*) within the left and right main pulmonary arteries as well as an incidentally found left perihilar lung cancer (*purple arrow*)

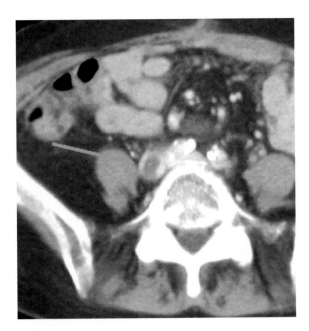

Fig. 2. A computed tomography venography (CTV) exam was performed simultaneously with a CT pulmonary angiogram in a 68-year-old woman with a history of ovarian cancer presenting with dyspnea. Axial CTV image demonstrates a filling defect (*arrow*) within the right common iliac artery consistent with thrombus. Images through the chest failed to demonstrate pulmonary embolism

dictive value greater than 96% for both single-slice [15–21] and MDCT [22, 14, 23–27] in PE detection. A large prospective study by Perrier et al. [28] showed that patients with a negative D-dimer and a negative MDCT pulmonary angiogram had test less than a 1% chance of having a lower-extremity deep venous thrombosis and a 3-month follow-up thromboembolic risk of only about 1.5%. A meta-analysis of 3,500 patients with a negative CT study who did not receive anticoagulation showed a neg-

ative predictive value (NPV) of 99%, which compares favorably with NPVs of conventional pulmonary angiography and greatly exceeds that of V/Q scintigraphy (76–88%) [15, 29–32]. These studies suggest that a negative MDCT pulmonary angiogram does not require any additional radiologic tests to help exclude the presence of acute PE. Because of its high sensitivity and specificity, MDCT can be both a screening and confirmatory study. Use of CT would help decrease additional and unnecessary imaging tests and limit the time between clinical presentation and effective treatment. More recently, the greater spatial resolution of MDCT has permitted the detection of small subsegmental emboli in sixth- and seventh-order arterial branches with a high degree of interobserver agreement [33–35]. Selective pulmonary angiography has low interobserver agreement rates, ranging from 45–66% [36, 37]. Similarly, V/Q scintigraphy has not only poor interobserver agreement rates but also poor specificity of low probability studies (10%). Additionally, up to 73% of V/Q scans are reported as intermediate probability [15, 30].

In addition to imaging the pulmonary arterial system, CT venography (CTV) may be performed to assess for venous thrombosis within the pelvis and lower extremities. Delayed venous-phase images from the pelvis through the knees are obtained 180 s following intravenous contrast injection. CTV is able to detect venous thrombosis in the pelvis veins, which is typically not possible during Doppler sonography due to overlying bowel gas (Fig. 2). Acute deep venous thrombosis (DVT) on CTV is detected as a filling defect within the vein (Fig. 3). Other signs include perivenous stranding, mural enhancement, and vein enlargement [38]. A study by Cosmic et al. [39] showed that up to 11% of patients with a negative chest CT

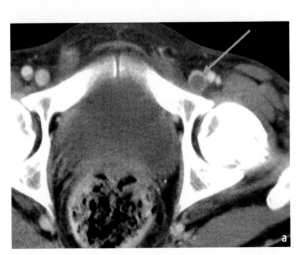
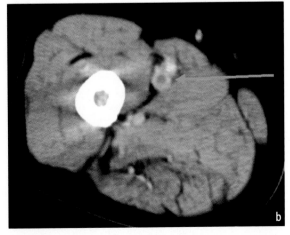

Fig. 3a, b. Axial computed tomography venography (CTV) images in two different patients presenting for CT pulmonary angiography demonstrate filling defects surrounded by intravenous contrast consistent with deep venous thrombosis (DVT) (*arrows*) in both the left common femoral vein (**a**) and right superficial femoral vein (**b**)

demonstrated venous thrombosis on CTV. Although this study did not take into account D-dimer levels, it proved the efficacy of imaging both the pelvis and lower-extremity venous structures following CT of the pulmonary arteries.

PE Findings Using MDCT

Most commonly, PE presents on CT as a filling defect within a pulmonary artery surrounded by a thin rim of contrast. These emboli often lodge at bifurcation points, extending into peripheral arteries (Fig. 4). When viewed in the transverse plane, the emboli may be described as having a "polo-mint" or "lifesaver" appearance (Fig. 5). When seen longitudinally, these filling defects may present as a "railway-track" sign, with the clot surrounded by contrast material within the vessel lumen (Fig. 6).

Occasionally, an abrupt arterial cutoff may be encountered, with complete obstruction of the pulmonary artery [40–43].

Secondary signs of acute PE are often present and may clue the radiologist to the presence of an embolus. On lung windows, small, wedge-shaped and peripheral areas of consolidation or ground glass opacity are seen in approximately 25% of patients [44]. These opacities mostly represent areas of pulmonary hemorrhage that clear within 4–7 days, but some represent pulmonary infarcts (Fig. 7). Pulmonary infarcts on CT appear as wedge-shaped peripheral opacities often characterized as a "Hampton hump" (Fig. 8). With larger emboli, there may be regions of localized oligemia and redistribution of blood flow (mosaic perfusion) in the involved portions of lung (Fig. 9). Frequent but nonspecific signs of PE include subsegmental atelectasis and small pleural effusions.

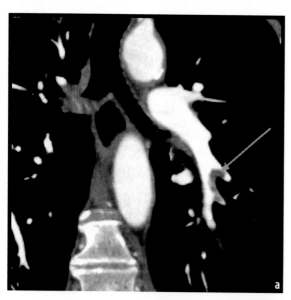

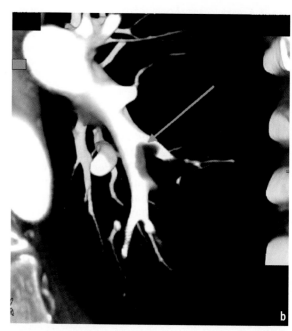

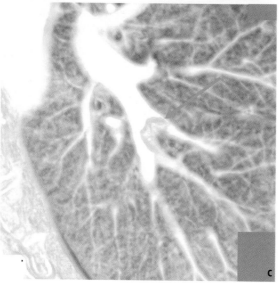

Fig. 4a-c. Sagittal multiplanar reformation (MPR) images (**a**) from a multidetector computed tomography (MDCT) pulmonary angiogram obtained in a patient with metastatic pancreatic cancer and shortness of breath demonstrate a filling defect at a branching point within the left lower lobe pulmonary artery, with extension into the segmental arterial branches (*arrow*). Three-dimensional (3-D) volume-rendered displays (**b, c**) help demonstrate the full extent of this embolus (*arrows*)

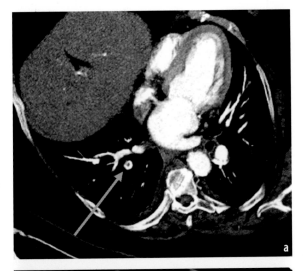

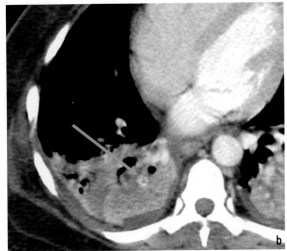

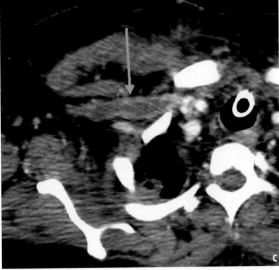

Fig. 5a-c. Multidetector computed tomography (MDCT) images of the "lifesaver" or "polo-mint" sign indicating pulmonary emboli visualized in the transverse plane. Oblique multiplanar reformation (MPR) images from an MDCT data set (**a**) demonstrate a filling defect within a right lower lobe segmental pulmonary artery (*arrow*). Axial MDCT images from a different patient, a 44-year-old woman with tachypnea and tachycardia following a motor vehicle collision (**b**), demonstrate a small subsegmental right lower lobe pulmonary artery filling defect surrounded by atelectatic lung (*arrow*). Axial images from higher in her chest (**c**) incidentally discovered thrombus in the right subclavian vein (*arrow*)

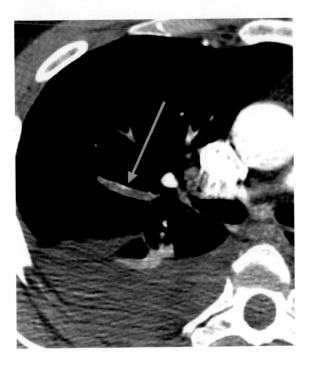

Fig. 6. Multidetector computed tomography (MDCT) images from CT pulmonary angiography in the axial plane demonstrate thrombus tracking longitudinally through a right middle lobe pulmonary artery feeding the lateral segment (*arrow*) with a characteristic "railway-track" appearance

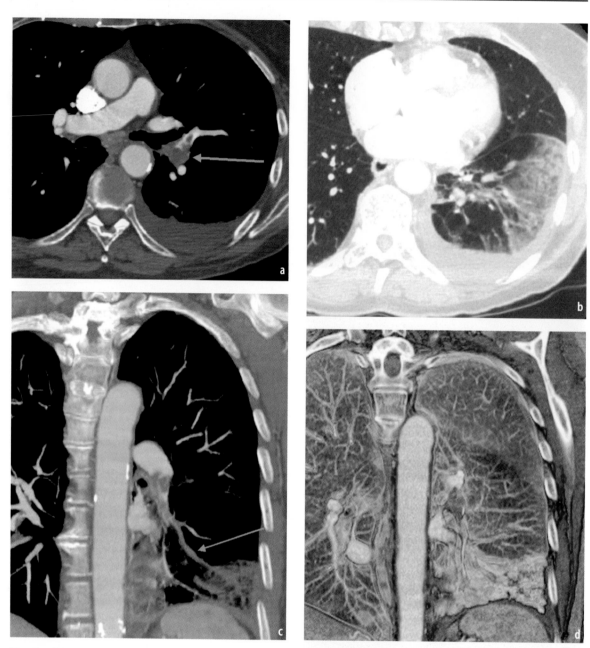

Fig. 7a-d. An 80-year-old woman presented with chest pain on the left with deep inspiration. Single-axial contrast-enhanced image (**a**) demonstrates a large embolus within the left main pulmonary artery extending into the left lower lobe pulmonary artery (*arrow*). Axial slice examined using lung windows (**b**) demonstrates a wedge-shaped region of ground-glass opacity in the periphery of the left lower lobe consistent with hemorrhage. Coronal multiplanar reconstruction (MPR) image (**c**) shows thrombus extending into the area of hemorrhage (*arrow*). Coronal three-dimensional (3-D) volume rendering (**d**) again demonstrates the large embolus and area of hemorrhage

Prognostic Value of CT in PE Patients

In addition to diagnosing emboli and other potential etiologies of dyspnea and chest pain, CT may provide some insight into the prognosis of patients with PE. There are cardiac findings on CT that may portend a worse clinical prognosis or warrant more emergent care in an intensive care unit and possible catheter intervention, thrombolysis, or surgical embolectomy, in addition to anticoagulation. Poor prognostic factors relate to the degree of right ventricular dysfunction and include the degree of right ventricular enlargement (Fig. 10), pulmonary artery thrombus load, enlargement of the main pulmonary artery, reflux of contrast into the hepatic veins (Fig. 11), and bowing of the ventricular septum toward the left ventricle.

Patients with a right ventricular diameter to

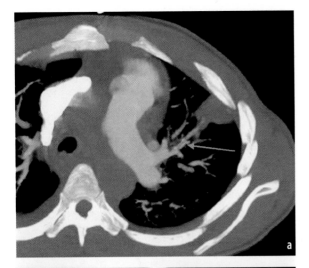

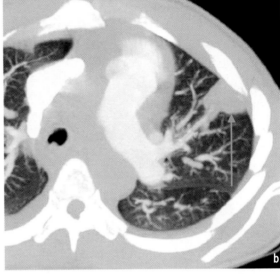

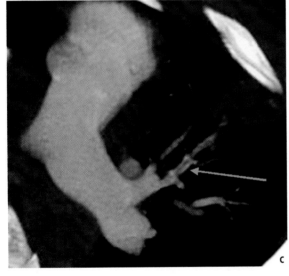

Fig. 8a-c. Axial image (**a**) from a computed tomographic (CT) pulmonary angiogram demonstrates a segmental embolus within the left upper lobe extending to a peripheral area of dense consolidation (CT Hampton hump) (*arrow*). Axial image obtained using lung windows (**b**) clearly defines the wedge-shaped region of infarcted lung (*arrow*). Magnified axial view of the embolus (**c**) demonstrates the "railway-track" appearance of the thrombus in the longitudinal plane (*arrow*)

left ventricular diameter (RVD/LVD) ratio of greater than 0.9 have a significant increase in mortality and a much greater likelihood of major complications [45–47]. One study showed a positive predictive value for PE-related mortality of 10.1% within the first 3 months after the diagnosis of PE with right ventricular enlargement (RVD/LVD ratio greater than 1.0). Perhaps more significantly, in those patients with a RVD/LVD ratio less than 1.0, there was a negative predictive value of 100% for an uneventful course [48]. Therefore, those patients without right ventricular enlargement are less unlikely to have an adverse outcome and are more likely to survive. Therefore, signs of right heart strain should be mentioned in the report and discussed with the referring physician, as they represent important prognostic factors that could assist in treatment planning and patient placement.

Studies have also shown a relationship between the percentage of pulmonary vascular bed obstruction and 3-month mortality. A scoring system based upon the number and degree of vascular obstructions was utilized. The highest possible score of 40 indicates complete obstruction of the pulmonary trunk [49]. Patients with a degree of vascular obstruction of greater than 40% have an 11% increased risk of dying from PE within the first 3 months. The negative predictive value in patients with a less than 40% degree of obstruction was 99%; indicating a very low rate of PE-related mortality [48, 50].

PE Protocol Using MDCT

Protocols employed for the detection of PE have evolved with rapid advances in CT technology. Current MDCT scanners are capable of providing

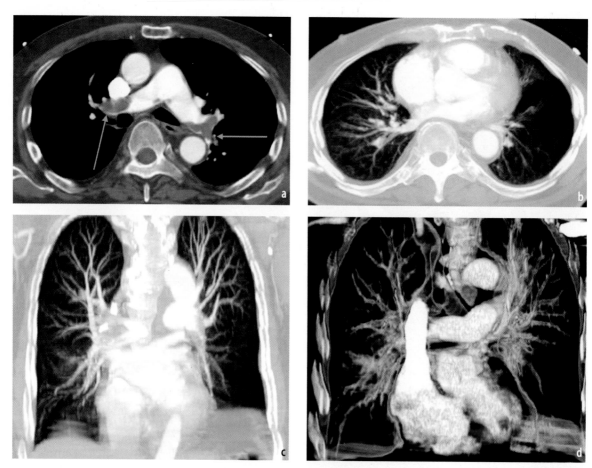

Fig. 9a-d. Axial image from a multidetector computed tomography (MDCT) pulmonary angiogram (**a**) demonstrates bilateral pulmonary emboli in a patient with acute shortness of breath and right lower extremity swelling (*arrows*). Axial image through the lower lobes using lung windows (**b**) demonstrates oligemia in the left lower lobe (CT Westermark sign). Coronal multiplanar reconstruction (MPR) image (**c**) again demonstrates the asymmetric hypovascularity in the left lower lobe. Three-dimensional (3-D) volume rendering in the coronal plane (**d**) more clearly defines the region of oligemia

image resolution of less than 1 mm. Patient respiratory motion artifacts have decreased dramatically over the last few years as acquisition of the entire thorax can be obtained in under 10 s using a 16-slice scanner and in less than 5 s with 64-slice units.

The quality of enhancement of the pulmonary arteries relies on several parameters: the amount and concentration of contrast agent used, the injection rate, and the delay between injection and scanning. To ensure adequate opacification of the pulmonary arteries, images are obtained 20 s following intravenous administration or, preferably, by using bolus tracking software to determine peak contrast delivery to the pulmonary arteries (Table 1).

Scan delay is obtained by injecting 15 ml of contrast material and placing a region of interest over the main pulmonary artery. Using a high con-centration contrast agent, such as Isovue-370, and a rapid flow rate of up to 4 ml/s ensures ideal vascular opacification. Injection of contrast media is typically via an 18- or 20-gauge peripheral intravenous line, preferably through the antecubital vein. A saline chaser may be used to decrease the amount of beam-hardening artifact caused by dense opacification of the superior vena cava and to decrease the amount of iodinated contrast needed to adequately opacify the pulmonary arteries [51–53]. While shorter scan times decrease respiratory motion and associated artifacts, timing the delivery of contrast becomes very critical with 16- and 64-slice protocols (Table 1).

In patients who are physically larger than average, 2.0–2.5 mm acquisitions can be used to decrease quantum mottle [43]. ECG gating has been recently implemented in some institutions to eliminate cardiac pulsation artifacts seen in small ves-

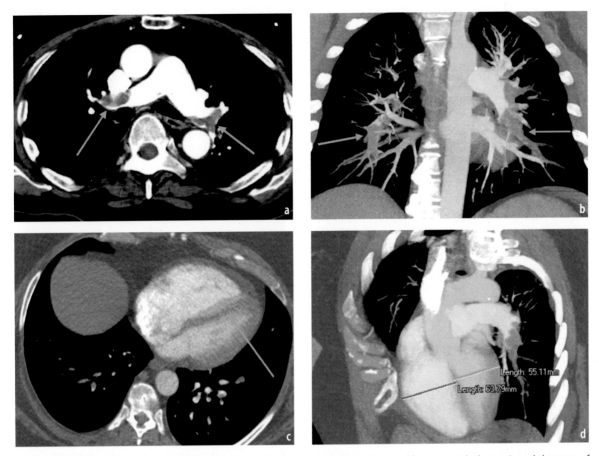

Fig. 10a-d. Computed tomographic (CT) pulmonary angiogram performed in a 49-year-old woman with chest pain and shortness of breath. Axial image through the pulmonary arteries (**a**) demonstrates large emboli within the left and right pulmonary arteries (*arrows*). Coronal multiplanar reconstruction (MPR) image (**b**) more clearly demonstrates the extent of the emboli (*arrows*). Axial image through the ventricular septum (**c**) reveals straightening of the septum and dilation of the right ventricle (*arrow*). Further evaluation with oblique MPR (**d**) clearly shows a right ventricular diameter (*red line*) that is larger than the left ventricular (*green line*) diameter (RVD/LVD ratio >1) consistent with right ventricular dysfunction

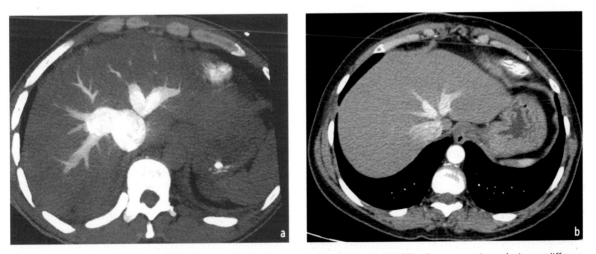

Fig. 11a, b. Axial images (**a, b**) obtained during multidetector computed tomography (MDCT) pulmonary angiography in two different patients show reflux of intravenous contrast into the hepatic veins, which is a sign of right ventricular dysfunction. The first image (**a**) also demonstrates distention of the hepatic veins. Both patients had large pulmonary emboli

Table 1. Computed tomography (CT) protocols: CT pulmonary angiography

Scanner type	4 slice	16 slice	64 slice
Collimation		16 × 0.75	64 × 0.6
Reconstruction (mm)	1.25	1.00	0.75
Rotation time (s)	0.8	0.5	0.33
Contrast volume (370 mgI/mL)	100 ml	100 ml	75–100 ml
Saline flush		50 ml	50 ml

sels adjacent to the heart; however, this technique requires a longer breath hold and increased radiation exposure. When viewing the pulmonary arterial system, window and level settings should be placed around 700 and 1,000 Hounsfield units (HU), respectively [43, 54].

Currently employed MDCT yields very large numbers of axial images – up to 1,000 with some newer systems. This can result in difficulties for the interpreting radiologist due to the sheer number of images to review. Two potential solutions include display tools and computer-aided diagnosis (CAD), which allow for rapid production of maximum intensity projection (MIP) images, multiplanar reconstructions (MPR), and three-dimensional (3-D) reformations. These reformations and reconstructions of the source images allow improved visualization of distal subsegmental pulmonary arterial branches with reconstruction of fewer overall images, without sacrificing PE detection sensitivity. CAD tools are under development and may be used as a second reader, potentially reducing study reading times. Preliminary experience in a small study population showed CAD tools can detect segmental emboli but are currently inaccurate for subsegmental emboli [55].

Disadvantages to MDCT

Approximately 3% of the CT scans completed for PE at our institution are inadequate for accurate interpretation [56]. Most problems relate to technical factors, including poor bolus timing and poor venous access. Correctly applied bolus tracking with density measurements over the pulmonary artery provides scan-precise delay times and optimal enhancement of the pulmonary arteries. Beam-hardening artifacts from dense contrast bolus within the superior vena cava may obscure small emboli in adjacent vessels (Fig. 12), particularly in the right main and right upper lobe pulmonary arteries [43]. Saline bolus chasing following initial contrast injection with a dual-head in-

jector can eliminate these artifacts completely. Abrupt loss of pulmonary artery opacification caused by the mixing of unopacified blood from the inferior vena cava may occur. This pulmonary artery flow artifact, also known as a "stripe sign," occurs during inspiration and results in loss of the contrast column in the pulmonary arteries; thus mimicking emboli [57, 58].

Patient factors that may hinder PE interpretation most often involve a large patient body habitus, leading to increased quantum mottle or an inability to breath hold for the desired length of time, resulting in motion artifact. Additional diagnostic pitfalls include partial volume averaging from hilar lymph nodes and mucous-filled bronchi. By utilizing a combination of workstation analysis, MIP, and MPR, both lymph nodes and mucous-filled bronchi can be distinguished from adjacent pulmonary arteries [59].

Radiation dose considerations with CT require careful evaluation when developing protocols. During a typical CT pulmonary angiogram, the effective patient dose ranges from 4-8 mSv, with an absorbed breast dose of 21 mGy [60]. As a comparison, the absorbed breast dose during a screening mammogram is only 2.5 mGy [60]. However, the risk-to-benefit ratio of using CT for diagnosing PE typically weighs heavily in favor of performing the study. CT pulmonary angiography using a single-slice scanner utilizes a radiation dose five times less than that of conventional angiography [61]. Performing CT examinations in young or pregnant women requires special considerations. In a young woman with a negative chest radiograph and low-to-moderate clinical suspicion, a V/Q scan might be considered as a more appropriate option. However, many patients undergo a subsequent CT study, so additional radiation burden to the female breast should be carefully evaluated. In pregnant patients with suspected PE, CT is recommended over V/Q scintigraphy, as the absorbed radiation dose to the fetus is 1–2 mGy for V/Q scans versus 0.1-0.2 mGy for CT [62, 63].

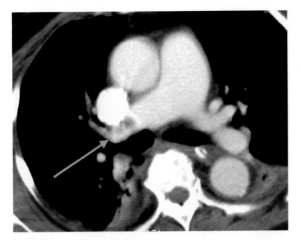 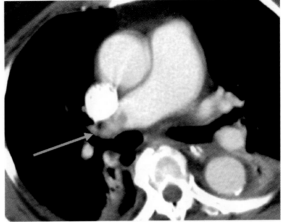

Fig. 12a, b. A 76-year-old woman who was postoperatively day 1 from a bilateral salpingoooophorectomy presented with decreased breath sounds in the right lung base, decreased oxygen saturation, and increased A-a gradient. Subsequent axial images from a contrast-enhanced multidetector computed tomography (MDCT) study (**a, b**) demonstrate beam-hardening artifact almost completely obscuring a large thrombus within the right main pulmonary artery (*arrows*). A saline chaser following injection of the iodinated contrast would have eliminated this artifact

Role of D-Dimer

D-dimer enzyme-linked immunosorbent assays (ELISA) play an important role in the workup for possible PE. D-dimer is a highly sensitive test (97%) with a negative predictive value of 99.6% [4]. This inexpensive measurement is an effective screening test in the outpatient setting for suspected PE. As a result, further diagnostic tests would be unnecessary in patients with a negative D-dimer assay, as there would be a very low likelihood of PE [64,65]. Taking this one step further, Perrier et al. [28] showed that patients have a very low likelihood of having any adverse affects related to PE when there is a negative CT angiogram and a negative D-dimer assay. Therefore, these patients are not only unlikely to have a PE, but they are also unlikely to suffer any adverse events secondary to venous thromboembolism within 3 months of the negative diagnostic tests. Unfortunately, the D-dimer assay is highly nonspecific and is of limited value within the inpatient setting. Other etiologies resulting in elevated D-dimer assays include cancer, myocardial infarction, pneumonia, sepsis, and pregnancy.

Future of MDCT

With continued technological improvements, MDCT pulmonary angiography will continue to be the test of choice for the diagnosis of PE. It is likely that these advances will center not only on hardware but also on the software used to reformat the large amount of acquired data during the CT examination. With slice thickness under 1.00 mm, there may be up to 1,000 axial images for the radiologist to evaluate. Unfortunately, small pulmonary emboli may be "overlooked" by having to individually examine each acquired image. In retrospect, these "perceptual errors" may be readily detectable: 60% of missed diagnoses occur because the embolus was simply not seen on first examination [66,67]. CAD for PE has shown potential for limiting these perceptual errors [68,69].

Advancements in the software used to create 2-D and 3-D reformations of the axial CT data will continue to improve our ability to detect emboli in obliquely oriented pulmonary arteries (Fig. 13) [70]. One promising technique involves performing "paddle wheel" reformations of the pulmonary arteries. A horizontal axis centered at the lung hila is used as a pivot point to image the pulmonary arteries. This type of multiplanar volume reformation helps prevent the "slicing" of pulmonary arteries into small fragments that are seen on coronal and sagittal reformations. Presumably, this will not only improve visualization of the pulmonary arterial tree but also decrease the overall number of images for the radiologist to review to accurately diagnose PE [71,72].

Studies are also underway to assess the possibility of using a single, contrast-enhanced, ECG-gated CT scan to assess patients with chest pain for coronary artery disease, pulmonary disease, and aortic disease [73]. Results of PIOPED II, which prospectively compared V/Q scanning, Doppler sonography for DVT, digital subtraction pulmonary angiography, and contrast venography with MDCT for the detection of venous thromboembolism [41], may provide practice guidelines.

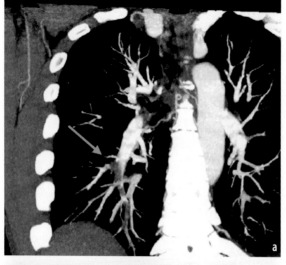

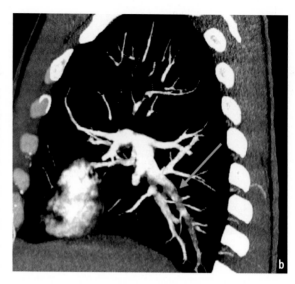

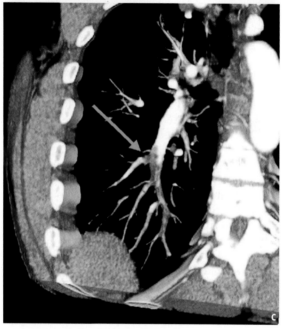

Fig. 13a-c. Computed tomographic (CT) pulmonary angiogram was obtained in a 42-year-old man presenting with chest pain and shortness of breath. Coronal (**a**) and sagittal (**b**) oblique multiplanar reproduction (MPR) images through the right lower lobe pulmonary artery demonstrate extensive thrombus extending almost the entire length of the artery (*arrows*). A three-dimensional (3-D) volume rendering of the multidetector computed tomography (MDCT) data set (**c**) more clearly demonstrates the mass-like nature and extent of the embolus (*arrow*)

Conclusion

CT pulmonary angiography has become the imaging modality of choice for the detection of acute PE. MDCT has proven sensitivity and specificity for detecting small pulmonary emboli in distal subsegmental pulmonary arteries with high interobserver agreement and cost effectiveness. Additionally, CT allows for the detection of other etiologies that may or may not be contributing to the patient's clinical presentation. When combined with CT venography, MDCT now provides a standalone test for excluding venous thromboembolism. High-risk patients with right ventricular dysfunction are also readily identifiable with CT pulmonary angiography, allowing for more appropriate management. Furthermore, continued im-

provements in postacquisition reformations and CAD will continue to enhance the ability to detect pulmonary emboli with an accuracy far exceeding that of other modalities.

References

1. Carson JL, Kelley MA, Duff A et al (1992) The clinical course of pulmonary embolism. N Engl J Med 326(19):1240–1245
2. Goldhaber SZ, Elliott CG (2003) Acute pulmonary embolism: part I: epidemiology, pathophysiology, and diagnosis. Circulation 108(22):2726–2729
3. Daniel KR, Courtney DM, Kline JA (2001) Assessment of cardiac stress from massive pulmonary embolism with 12-lead ECG. Chest 120:474–481
4. Dunn KL, Wolf JP, Dorfman DM et al (2002) Normal D-dimer levels in emergency department pa-

tients suspected of acute pulmonary embolism. J Am Coll Cardiol 40:1475–1478

5. Elliott CG, Goldhaber SZ, Visani L et al (2000) Chest radiographs in acute pulmonary embolism. Results from the international cooperative pulmonary embolism registry. Chest 118:33–38

6. Ferrari E, Imbert A, Chevalier T et al (1997) The ECG in pulmonary embolism: predictive value of negative T waves in precordial leads: 80 case reports. Chest 111:537–543

7. Kucher N, Walpoth N, Wustmann K et al (2003) QR in V1: an ECG sign associated with right ventricular strain and adverse clinical outcome in pulmonary embolism. Eur Heart J 24:1113–1119

8. Stein PD, Goldhaber SZ, Henry JW (1995) Alveolar-arterial oxygen gradient in the assessment of acute pulmonary embolism. Chest 107:139–143

9. Stein PD, Goldhaber SZ, Henry JW et al (1996) Arterial blood gas analysis in the assessment of suspected acute pulmonary embolism. Chest 109:78–81

10. Prologo JD, Glauser J (2002) Variable diagnostic approach to suspected pulmonary embolism in the ED of a major academic tertiary care center. Am J Emerg Med 20:5–9

11. Prologo JD, Gilkeson RC, Diaz M et al (2004) CT Pulmonary angiography: A comparative analysis of the utilization patterns in emergency department and hospitalized patients between 1998 and 2003. AJR Am J Roentgenol 183:1093–1096

12. Stein PD, Kayali F, Olson RE (2004) Trends in the use of diagnostic imaging in patients hospitalized with acute pulmonary embolism. Am J Cardiol 93:1316–1317

13. Kim KI, Muller NL, Mayo JR (1999) Clinically suspected pulmonary embolism: utility of spiral CT. Radiology 210:693–697

14. Kavanagh EC, O'Hare A, Hargaden G (2004) Risk of pulmonary embolism after negative MDCT pulmonary angiography findings. AJR Am J Roentgenol 182:499–504

15. Blachere H, Latrabe V, Montaudon M et al (2000) Pulmonary embolism revealed on helical CT angiography: comparison with ventilation-perfusion radionuclide lung scanning. AJR Am J Roentgenol 174:1041–1047

16. Bourriot K, Couffinhal T, Bernard V et al (2003) Clinical outcome after a negative spiral CT pulmonary angiographic finding in an inpatient setting from cardiology and pneumology wards. Chest 123:359–365

17. Garg K, Sieler H, Welsh CH et al (1999) Clinical validity of helical CT being interpreted as negative for pulmonary embolism: implications for patient treatment. AJR Am J Roentgenol 172:1627–1631

18. Goodman LR, Lipchik RJ, Kuzo RS et al (2000) Subsequent pulmonary embolism: risk after a negative helical CT pulmonary angiogram – prospective comparison with scintigraphy. Radiology 215: 535–542

19. Lomis NN, Yoon HC, Moran AG et al (1999) Clinical outcomes of patients after a negative spiral CT pulmonary arteriogram in the evaluation of acute pulmonary embolism. J Vasc Interv Radiol 10:707–712

20. Ost D, Rozenshtein A, Saffran L et al (2001) The negative predictive value of spiral computed tomography for the diagnosis of pulmonary embolism in patients with nondiagnostic ventilation-perfusion scans. Am J Med 110:16–21

21. Tillie-Leblond I, Mastora I, Radenne F et al (2002) Risk of pulmonary embolism after a negative spiral CT angiogram in patients with pulmonary disease: 1-year clinical follow-up study. Radiology 223: 461–467

22. Gottsater A, Berg A, Certergard J et al (2001) Clinically suspected pulmonary embolism: is it safe to withhold anticoagulation after a negative spiral CT? Eur Radiol 11:65–72

23. Krestan CR, Klein N, Fleischmann et al (2004) Value of negative spiral CT angiography in patients with suspected acute PE: analysis of PE occurrence and outcome. Eur Radiol 14:93–98

24. Musset D, Parent F, Meyer G et al (2002) Diagnostic strategy for patients with suspected pulmonary embolism: a prospective multicentre outcome study. Lancet 360:1914–1920

25. Nilsson T, Olausson A, Johnsson H et al (2002) Negative spiral CT in acute pulmonary embolism. Acta Radiol 43:486–491

26. Qanadli SC, Hajjam ME, Mesurolle B et al (2000) Pulmonary embolism detection: prospective evaluation of dual-section helical CT versus selective pulmonary arteriography in 157 patients. Radiology 217:447–455

27. Swensen SJ, Sheedy PF II, Ryu JH et al (2002) Outcomes after withholding anticoagulation from patients with suspected acute pulmonary embolism and negative computed tomographic findings: a cohort study. Mayo Clin Proc 77:130–138

28. Perrier A, Pierre-Marie R, Sanchez O et al (2005) Multidetector-row computed tomography in suspected pulmonary embolism. N Engl J Med 352:1760–1768

29. Henry JW, Stein PD, Gottschalk A et al (1996) Scintigraphic lung scans and clinical assessment in critically ill patients with suspected acute pulmonary embolism. Chest 109:462–466

30. PIOPED Investigators (1990) Value of the ventilation/perfusion scan in acute pulmonary embolism JAMA 95:498–502

31. Quiroz R, Kucher N, Zou KH et al (2005) Clinical validity of a negative computed tomography scan in patients with suspected pulmonary embolism – a systematic review. JAMA 293:2012–2017

32. van Beek EJ, Reekers JA, Batcherlor DA et al (1995) Feasibility, safety and clinical utility of angiography in patients with normal pulmonary angiograms. Chest 107:1375–1378

33. Ghaye B, Szapiro D, Mastora I et al (2001) Peripheral pulmonary arteries: how far in the lung does multi-detector row spiral CT allow analysis? Radiology 219:629–636

34. Patel S, Kazerooni EA, Cascade PN (2003) Pulmonary embolism: optimization of small pulmonary artery visualization at multi-detector row CT. Radiology 227:455–460

35. Schoepf UJ, Holzknecht N, Helmberger TK et al (2002) Subsegmental pulmonary emboli: improved detection with thin-collimation multi-detector row spiral CT. Radiology 222:483–490

36. Diffin DC, Leyendecker JR, Johnson SP et al (1998) Effect of anatomic distribution of pulmonary emboli on interobserver agreement in the interpretation of pulmonary angiography. AJR Am J

Roentgenol 171:1085–1089

37. Stein PD, Henry JW, Gottschalk A (1999) Reassessment of pulmonary angiography for the diagnosis of pulmonary embolism: relation of interpreter agreement to the order of the involved pulmonary arterial branch. Radiology 210:689–691

38. Washington L (2005) Venous thromboembolism: epidemiologic, clinical, and imaging perspectives. Cardiopulmonary imaging, categorical course syllabus. American Roentgen Ray Society 41–51

39. Cosmic MS, Goodman LR, Lipchik RJ et al (2002) Detection of deep venous thrombosis with combined helical CT scan of the chest and CT venography in unselected cases of suspected pulmonary embolism. Am J Respir Crit Care Med 165:A329

40. Ghaye B, Remy J, Remy-Jardin M et al (2002) Nontraumatic thoracic emergencies: CT diagnosis of acute pulmonary embolism-the first 10 years. Eur Radiol 12:1886–1905

41. Gottschalk A, Stein PD, Goodman LR et al (2002) Overview of prospective investigation of pulmonary embolism diagnosis II. Semin Nucl Med 32:173–182

42. Washington L, Goodman LR, Gonyo MB (2002) CT for thromboembolic disease. Radiol Clin North Am 40:751–771

43. Wittram C, Maher MM, Yoo AJ et al (2004) CT angiography of pulmonary embolism: diagnostic criteria and causes of misdiagnosis. Radiographics 24:1219–1238

44. Shah AA, Davis SD, Gamsu G et al (1999) Parenchymal and pleural findings in patients with and patients without acute pulmonary embolism detected at spiral CT. Radiology 211:147–153

45. Quiroz R, Kucher N, Schoepf UJ et al (2004) Right ventricular enlargement on chest computed tomography: prognostic role in acute pulmonary embolism, Circulation 109:2401–2404

46. Reid JH, Murchison JT (1998) Acute right ventricular dilation: a new helical CT sign of massive pulmonary embolism. Clin Radiol 53:694–698

47. Schoepf UJ, Kucher N, Kipfmueller F et al (2004) Right ventricular enlargement on chest computed tomography: a predictor of early death in acute pulmonary embolism. Circulation 110:3276–3280

48. Van der Meer RW, Pattynama PM, van Strijen MJ et al (2005) Right ventricular dysfunction and pulmonary obstruction index at helical CT: prediction of clinical outcome during 3-month follow-up in patients with acute pulmonary embolism. Radiology 235:798–803

49. Qanadli SD, El Hajjam M, Vieillard-Baron A et al (2001) New CT index to quantify arterial obstruction in pulmonary embolism: comparison with angiographic index and echocardiography. AJR Am J Roentenol 176(6):1415–1420

50. Wu AS, Pezzullo JA, Cronan JJ et al (2004) CT pulmonary angiography: quantification of pulmonary embolus as a predictor of patient outcome – initial experience. Radiology 230:831–835

51. Cademartiri F, Mollet N, van der Lugt A et al (2004) Non-invasive 16–row multislice CT coronary angiography: usefulness of saline chaser. Eur Radiol 14:178–183

52. Dorio PJ, Lee FT, Henseler KP et al (2003) Using a saline chaser to decrease contrast media in abdominal CT. AJR Am J Roentgenol 180:929–934

53. Haage P, Schmitz-Rode T, Hubner D et al (2000) Reduction of contrast material dose and artifacts by a saline flush using a double power injector in helical CT of the thorax. AJR Am J Roentgenol 174:1049–1053

54. Storto ML, Di Credico A, Guido F et al (2005) Incidental detection of pulmonary emboli on routine MDCT of the chest AJR Am J Roentgenol 184:264–267

55. Schoepf UJ, Schneider AC, Das M et al (2005) Pulmonary embolism: computer aided detection at multi-detector row spiral CT. Radiology (in press)

56. Schoepf UJ, Savino G, Lake DR et al (2005) The age of CT pulmonary angiography. J Thorac Imaging 20(4):273–279

57. Gosselin MV, Rassner UA, Thieszen SL et al (2004) Contrast dynamics during CT pulmonary angiogram: analysis of an inspiration associated artifact. J Thorac Imaging 19:1–7

58. Yoo AJ, Wittram C (2003) CTPA pulmonary artery flow artifact: pitfall in the diagnosis of pulmonary embolism Radiology 352(P):233

59. Gruden JF (2005) Pulmonary embolism: MDCT technique and interpretative pitfalls. Cardiopulmonary imaging, categorical course syllabus. American Roentgen Ray Society 53–60

60. Wiest PW, Locken JA, Heintz PH et al (2002) CT scanning: a major source of radiation exposure. Semin Ultrasound CT MR 23(5):402–410

61. Resten A, Mausoleo F, Valero M, Musset D (2003) Comparison of doses for pulmonary embolism detection with helical CT and pulmonary angiography. Eur Radiol 13:1515–1521

62. Huda W (2005) When a pregnant patient has a suspected pulmonary embolism, what are the typical embryo doses from a chest CT and a ventilation/perfusion study? Pediatr Radiol 25:25

63. Winer-Muram HT, Boone JM, Brown HL et al (2002) Pulmonary embolism in pregnant patients: fetal radiation dose with helical CT. Radiology 224(2):487–492

64. Abcarian PW, Sweet JD, Watabe JT et al (2004) Role of a quantitative D-dimer assay in determining the need for CT angiography of acute pulmonary embolism. AJR Am J Roentgenol 182:1377–1381

65. Kline JA, Wells PS (2003) Methodology for a rapid protocol to rule out pulmonary embolism in the emergency department. Ann Emerg Med 42: 266–275

66. Berlin L (1996) Malpractice issues in radiology. Perceptual errors. AJR Am J Roentgenol 167:587–590

67. Renfrew DL, Franken EA Jr, Berbaum KS et al (1992) Error in radiology: classification and lessons in 182 cases presented at a problem case conference. Radiology 183:145–150

68. Peldschus K, Herzog P, Wood SA et al (2005) Computer-aided diagnosis as a second reader: Spectrum of findings in computed tomography studies of the chest interpreted as normal. Chest 128:1517–1523

69. Wittram C, Meehan MJ, Halpern EF et al (2004) Trends in thoracic radiology over a decade at a large academic medical center. J Thorac Imaging 19: 164–170

70. Remy-Jardin M, Remy J, Cauvain O et al (1995): Diagnosis of central pulmonary embolism with helical CT: role of two-dimensional multiplanar reformations. AJR Am J Roentgenol 165:1131–1138

71. Chiang EE, Boiselle PM, Raptopoulos V et al (2003) Detection of pulmonary embolism: comparison of paddlewheel and coronal CT reformations – initial experience. Radiology 228:577–582

72. Simon M, Chiang EE, Boiselle PM (2001) Paddle-wheel multislice helical CT display of pulmonary vessels and other lung structures. Radiol Clin North Am 41:617–626

73. Schoepf UJ, Becker CR, Ohnesorge BM et al (2004) CT of coronary artery disease. Radiology 232:18–37

III.4

MDCT Angiography of Peripheral Arterial Disease

Geoffrey D. Rubin and Mannudeep K. Kalra

Introduction

Greater scan coverage and faster scanning with multidetector-row computed tomography (MDCT) has provided a unique opportunity for noninvasive and accurate imaging of vascular diseases of lower extremities [1]. This chapter describes scanning parameters, contrast medium administration features, image postprocessing techniques, and clinical applications of MDCT angiography (MDCTA).

Scanning Parameters

For an average-size patient, we use 120 kV and 300 mA for peripheral MDCTA. A lower tube current and/or tube potential can be used for smaller patients, greater current and potential can be used for obese patients. Alternatively, automatic exposure control techniques can also be used to adapt tube current to patient size. Using the greater trochanter as a bony landmark, a small to medium imaging field of view, is used for section reconstruction. For reconstruction of CT angiography (CTA) images, we use a soft or medium reconstruction kernel.

For peripheral CTA, the patient is placed supine and feet first on the CT table, with careful alignment of the patient's knees and feet positioned close to the gantry isocenter [2, 3]. The anatomic scan length for a typical lower-extremity CTA study is 110–130 cm and extends from the renal artery origins at T12 vertebra to the patient's feet. Compared with the 4- and 8-row MDCT scanners, 16- and 64-row MDCT scanners allow acquisition of thinner sections at faster speed. With these latter scanners, it is also possible to acquire submillimeter, isotropic images of the entire peripheral arterial tree. These "thinner" image data sets can improve visualization of small vessels (Fig. 1). This maximum spatial reso-

lution may translate into improved visualization and treatment planning of patients with advanced peripheral arterial occlusive disease. For most routine CTA of the entire peripheral arterial tree, we reconstruct images at 1.25- to 1.5-mm section thickness for 8- and 16-row scanners, and 1-mm section thickness with 64-row MDCT scanners while maintaining constant image quality with use of automatic exposure control techniques.

Contrast Medium

Oral contrast is not administered to patients undergoing peripheral CTA. Although the same principles for contrast medium injection for CTA (relationship of injection flow rate and injection duration with arterial enhancement) apply to peripheral CTA, the latter is more complex due to the need for acquiring optimum enhancement of the entire lower extremity arterial tree in a single CT acquisition.

For peripheral CTA studies, we inject 1–1.5 g of iodine per second for an average person (75 kg) and make patient-weight-based adjustment to the contrast volume and injection flow rate for heavier (>90 kg) or smaller (<60 kg) subjects. In peripheral CTA studies, attenuation values are usually lowest in the abdominal aorta and peak at the level of the infrageniculate popliteal artery [4]. This can be explained on the basis of continuous arterial enhancement with a continuous and prolonged intravenous injection of contrast media (e.g., 35 s) [5]. Thus, biphasic injections may result in more uniform enhancement over time, particularly for longer scan and injection times (>25–30 s) [6].

In addition to volume and injection for contrast media, an optimum scan delay for peripheral CTA is also critical. Contrast medium transit time (tCMT), the time interval between the beginning of an intravenous contrast medium injection and arrival of the bolus in the aorta, varies considerably between pa-

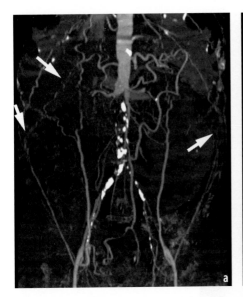
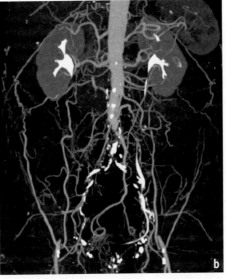

Fig. 1a, b. a Maximum intensity projection (MIP) from a multidetector computed tomography (MDCT) angiogram acquired with 4×2.5-mm-thick sections demonstrates an occlusion of the aorta and common iliac arteries. Collateral arteries connecting intercostal and lumbar arteries with deep lateral circumflex iliac arteries are not seen throughout their entire course and appear blurred (*arrows*). **b** MIP from an MDCT angiogram acquired in a different patient with 8×1.25-mm-thick sections demonstrates distal abdominal aortic and bilateral common and external iliac arterial occlusions. Similar collateral arteries are present, as in (**a**), but the thinner sections allow them to be visualized with less blurring

tients with coexisting cardiovascular diseases and may range from 12–40 s. Therefore, individualization of scanning delay (or determination of the individual's *t*CMT) is recommended in peripheral CTA with the help of either a small test-bolus injection or automated bolus triggering techniques. These techniques help the choice of scanning delays that may equal to the *t*CMT or exceed *t*CMT by being chosen at a predefined interval (e.g., "*t*CMT+5 s" implies that the scan starts 5 s after contrast medium has arrived in the aorta).

Contrast medium injection protocols in peripheral CTA are also complicated since arterial stenosis, occlusions, or aneurysms anywhere between the infrarenal abdominal aorta and the pedal arteries can substantially delay downstream arterial enhancement [7, 8] (Fig. 2). In fact, patients with peripheral arterial occlusive disease, transit times of intravenous (IV) contrast medium from the aorta to the popliteal arteries can range from 4 s (at transit speed of 177 mm/s) to 24 s (at a transit speed of 29 mm/s) [9]. This is particularly important with the use of faster acquisition speeds, as the scanner table may move faster than the intravascular contrast medium, and the scanner may thus outrun the bolus. It is important to note that this phenomenon of "outrunning" has only been reported at a table speed of 37 mm/s in one study on peripheral CTA [10], but it has not been reported at table speeds of 19-30 mm/s in other studies [10-14]. Thus, we categorize injection strategies for peripheral CTA into those for "slow" acquisitions (at a table speed of > 30 mm/s) and those for "fast" acquisitions (at a table speed of ≤ 30 mm/s).

For slow acquisitions, table speed usually translates into a scan time of approximately 40 s for the entire peripheral arterial tree. As data acquisition follows the bolus from the aorta to the feet, injection duration can be about 5 s shorter than the scan time (e.g., 40-s acquisition = 35-s injection duration). At a constant injection rate of 4 ml/s, this translates to 140 ml of contrast medium. If the beginning of data acquisition is timed closely to contrast arrival time in the aorta (using a test bolus or bolus triggering), biphasic injections achieve more favorable enhancement profiles with improved aortic enhancement.

In patients with peripheral arterial occlusive disease, fast acquisition protocols (>30 mm/s table speed) may be faster than contrast medium transit times through the peripheral arterial tree. In order to prevent CT acquisition from outrunning the bolus, the bolus should be given a "head start" by combining fixed injection duration of 35 s to fill the arterial tree and a delay of the start of CT acquisition relative to *t*CMT. The faster the acquisition, the longer "diagnostic delay" should be. We employ such a strategy with both a 16-row scanner with a 16×1.25-mm protocol, beam pitch 1.375:1, and 0.6-s gantry rotation period (table speed 45 mm/s) and a 64-row scanner with a 64×0.6-mm, beam pitch 1.0:1, and 0.5-s gantry rotation period, and table speed 45 mm/s. Our diagnostic delay is typically 15–20 s in these cases.

As there is a possibility of even more delayed arterial opacification than accounted for with the

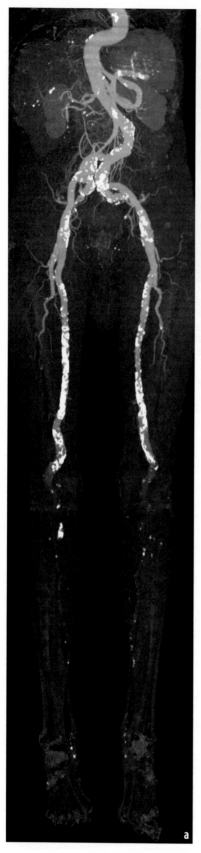

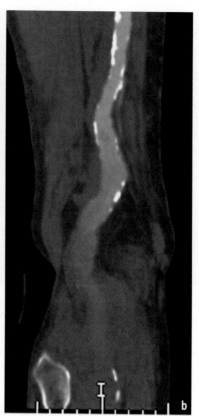

Fig. 2a, b. a Multidetector-row computed tomography angiogram (MDCTA) obtained with 32×1.0-mm-thick sections and a table speed of 80 mm/s immediately after arrival of contrast medium into the abdominal aorta. Arteriomegaly is present throughout but most notably in the iliofemoral arteries. Arterial opacification ceases in the popliteal artery, resulting in a nondiagnostic examination of the popliteal, crural, and pedal arteries. **b** A curved planar reformation through the proximal right popliteal artery demonstrates the presence of a popliteal artery aneurysm. The slow-flow characteristic of patients with large arteries results in a CT angiogram where the CT table is moving faster than the blood flow and the scanner thus overruns contrast medium bolus

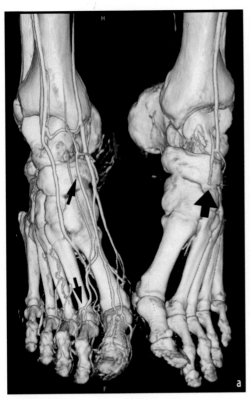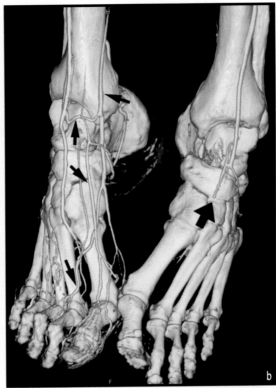

Fig. 3a,b. Two volume-rendered (VR) views of the feet in a patient with right-foot cellulitis. Extensive venous opacification (*narrow arrows*) complicates analysis of the right foot while arteries only are opacified in the left foot, allowing clear visualization of a dorsalis pedis arterial occlusion (*wide arrow*)

slow acquisition protocol [9], a second CTA acquisition (covering the popliteal and infrapopliteal vasculature) must be preprogrammed into the scanning protocol and can be initiated by CT technologists if they do not see any contrast medium opacification in the distal vessels. Opacification of deep and superficial veins cannot be completely avoided in some patients with rapid arteriovenous transit times [4, 15] and is more likely to occur with longer scan times and in patients with active inflammation, e.g., from infected or nonhealing ulcers (Fig. 3). However, stronger arterial enhancement with correct injection timing [4], along with adequate anatomic knowledge and postprocessing tools, can help to avoid diagnostic problems from venous enhancement.

Visualization Techniques

Despite the availability of state-of-the-art two- (2-D) and three- (3-D) dimensional image postprocessing techniques, transverse CT images are indispensable for assessment of nonvascular abdominal and/or pelvic abnormalities. These source images can also be used to analyze findings on 2-D or 3-D images that suggest artifactual lesions. For some vascular lesions, transverse images may provide an initial impression or may provide all the required information, for example, in patients with or without only minimal disease, trauma, or suspected acute occlusions. However, for most patients with peripheral vascular disease, review of large number of transverse images is time consuming and less accurate [11] than alternative 2-D and 3-D visualizations.

Three dimensional overview techniques with at least one 2-D technique are generally used for atherosclerotic peripheral vascular diseases. Our protocol for peripheral MDCTA comprises curved planar reformations (CPRs), thin-slab maximum intensity projections (MIPs) through the renal and visceral arteries, and interactive exploration of volume renderings (VRs) of the abdomen, pelvis, and each leg. These 2-D and 3-D techniques enable faster and easier interpretation of huge data sets of axial images. MIP and VR techniques facilitate assessment of vascular structures by providing "angiographic maps" of the arterial tree. Being closest to the angiographic map, MIP images are suitable for illustrating abnormalities to the requesting physicians and can serve as a vascular map for patient management in the catheter angiography suite or operating rooms (Fig. 4). However, need for time-consuming bone removal from image data, inadvertent removal of vascular structures adjacent

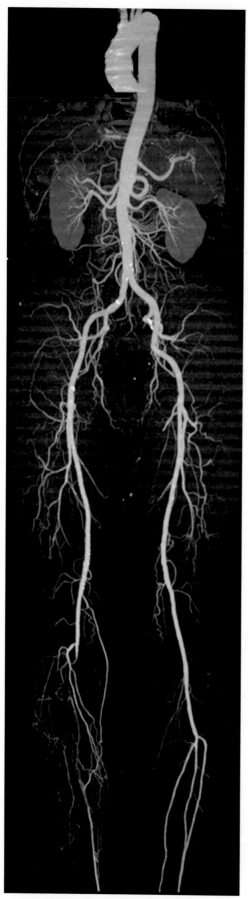

Fig. 4. Frontal maximum projection intensity (MIP) of computed tomography angiography (CTA) comprising the entirety of the aorta, iliac arteries, and runoff performed to assess for a source of distal embolization. This full-volume MIP requires preliminary removal of the bones to allow visualization of the arterial anatomy. There is an occlusion of the proximal right popliteal artery with robust collateralization reconstituting the posterior tibial artery

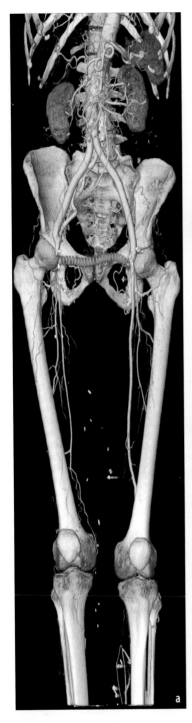
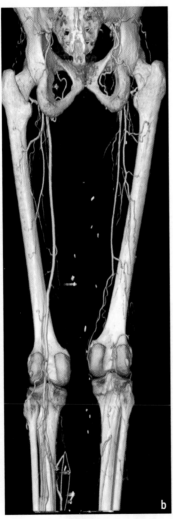

Fig. 5a, b. Anteroposterior **a** and posteroanterior volume renderings (VRs) **b** in a patient with an aortobifemoral bypass graft and an occluded femorofemoral bypass graft. The right femoral artery and distal right superficial femoral arteries are occluded. VRs allow visualization of complex, overlapping arterial channels without the need for preliminary bone removal, providing an excellent overview of the complex anatomy

to bony structures, and lack of depth information are some of the limitations of the MIP technique. On the other hand, VR techniques maintain 3-D depth information, and bone removal is not essential (Fig. 5). VR is an ideal technique for rapid and interactive viewing and exploration of peripheral CTA data sets. The main limitation of both MIP and VR is that vessel calcifications and stents may completely obscure the vascular flow channel. This precludes its exclusive use in up to 60% of patients with peripheral arterial occlusive disease [16].

In the presence of calcified plaque, diffuse vessel-wall calcification, or endoluminal stents, cross-sectional views such as transverse source images, sagittal, coronal, or oblique multiplanar reformations in conjunction with VR are important for assessing luminal contrast flow. Alternatively, longitudinal cross-sections along a predefined vascular centerline (CPR) can be created with either manual or (semi) automated tracing of the vessel centerlines for the most comprehensive cross-sectional display of luminal pathology [17, 18] (Figs. 6 and 7). At least

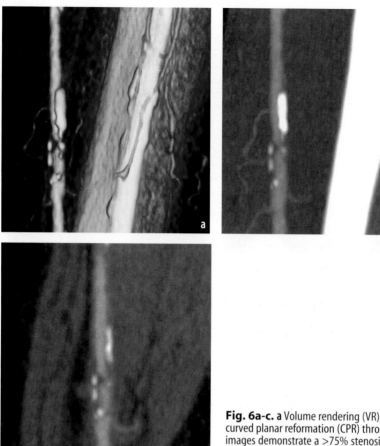

Fig. 6a-c. a Volume rendering (VR), **b** maximum intensity projection (MIP), and **c** curved planar reformation (CPR) through a mid superficial femoral artery lesion. All images demonstrate a >75% stenosis distal to a large calcified plaque. The lumen adjacent to the calcification is partially obscured on VR and MIP. The CPR (**c**) establishes that there is only minimal luminal narrowing as a result of this calcified plaque

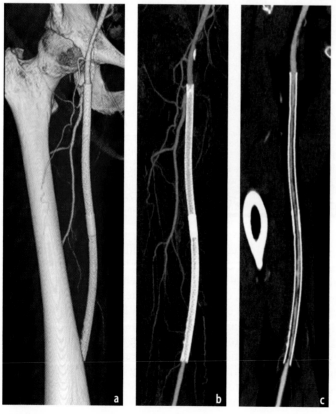

Fig. 7a-c. a Volume rendering (VR), **b** maximum intensity projection (MIP), and **c** curved planar reformation (CPR) through a stented segment of the superficial femoral artery. The lumen of the stent is obscured on both VR and the MIP. The CPR (**c**) demonstrates the lumen of the stent with irregular neointimal hyperplasia. (Images courtesy of Justus Roos, MD and Dominik Fleishmann MD, Department of Radiology, Stanford University School of Medicine, Stanford, CA, USA)

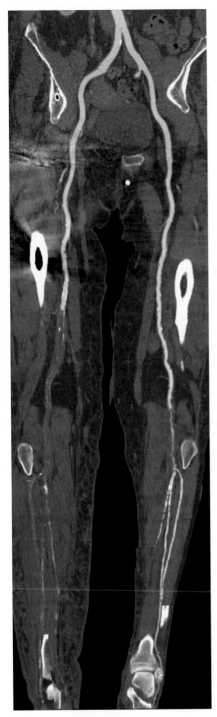

Fig. 8. Multipath curved planar reformation (CPR) demonstrates all iliac, femoral, and crural arteries bilaterally in a single image. Six traditional CPRs would be required to demonstrate all of the arterial lumina shown on this single view. There is extensive thrombus in the mid right superficial femoral artery (SFA) extending inferiorly to involve all three crural arteries. There is a high-grade stenosis of the left popliteal artery and occlusion of the mid left anterior tibial artery. (Reprinted with permission from Fleischmann D, Hallett RL, Rubin GD (2006) CT angiography of peripheral arterial disease. J Vasc Interv Radiol 17:3-26)

two orthogonal CPRs per vessel segment (e.g., sagittal and coronal views) are required for complete evaluation of eccentric disease. One problem of (single) CPRs in the context of visualizing the peripheral arterial tree is their limited spatial perception. Unless clear annotations are present, the anatomic context of a vascular lesion may be ambiguous. In this context, multipath CPRs provide simultaneous longitudinal cross-sectional views through the major blood vessels without obscuring

vascular calcifications and stents while maintaining spatial perception [18] (Fig. 8).

Despite remarkable improvements in 3-D image postprocessing, no algorithms allow fully automated detection of vessel centerlines, automated segmentation of bony structures, and detection (and subtraction) of vessel-wall calcification for peripheral CTA studies. Although it is reasonable to expect further improvements in computer-assisted segmentation and visualization in the not too distant future, it appears unlikely that expert user interaction (radiologist or 3-D technologist) can be completely avoided for creating clinically relevant and representative peripheral CTA images.

Clinical Applications

Several noninvasive imaging techniques, such as ultrasound, CTA, and magnetic resonance angiography (MRA) are available for evaluating clinical conditions involving the lower-extremity vascular structures. Peripheral CTA with state-of-the-art MDCT scanners has the advantages of high spatial resolution, relative freedom from operator dependence, and widespread (and increasing) availability. As a result, peripheral CTA is increasingly used in many imaging centers for a wide range of clinical indications. However, only sparse original data on its accuracy in patients with peripheral arterial occlusive disease, particularly for 16- or 64-row MDCTA, are available when compared with conventional angiography [4, 10–13]. Published studies suggest that peripheral CTA has a high diagnostic accuracy relative to conventional angiography [10–13]. Reported sensitivities and specificities range from 88% to 100%. In general, sensitivity and specificity are greater for arterial occlusions than for detection of stenoses. Accuracies and interobserver agreement are also higher for femoropopliteal and iliac vessels when compared with infrapopliteal arteries. Pedal arteries have not

been specifically analyzed in the literature. At least in patients with intermittent claudication, peripheral CTA has the potential to be cost effective [19].

Intermittent Claudication

Surgical or endovascular revascularization is performed when medical management of patients with claudication fails to improve the symptoms. Factors that influence choice of treatment include lesion morphology (degree of stenosis/occlusion and lesion length) [20], location, and, most importantly, status of runoff vessels, specifically the calf arteries, which can predict long-term patency rates after intervention [21]. Peripheral CTA provides complete delineation of both the femoropopliteal segment and inflow and outflow arteries, including lesion number, length, stenosis diameter and morphology, adjacent normal arterial caliber, degree of calcification, and status of distal runoff vessels. These findings help in planning the procedure with respect to route of access, balloon selection, and expected long-term patency after femoropopliteal intervention. Compared with catheter angiography, peripheral CTA provides better estimates of the effects of eccentric stenoses on luminal diameter reduction [22]. In addition, collateral vessels can be evaluated with MIP and VR images, and arterial segments distal to long-segment occlusions are well visualized (Fig. 9). It is also expected that peripheral CTA is more cost effective than digital subtraction angiog-

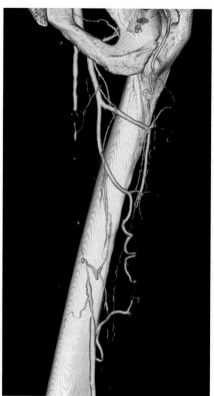

Fig. 9. Volume rendering (VR) of an occluded superficial femoral artery (SFA) in a patient with calf claudication. Computed tomography angiography (CTA) demonstrates the site of occlusion and associated collateral arteries that reconstitute the SFA via the profunda femoris

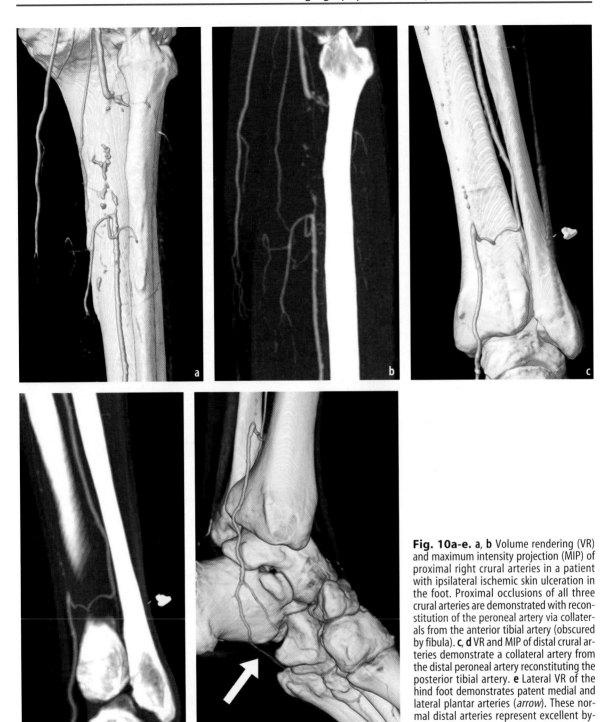

Fig. 10a-e. a, b Volume rendering (VR) and maximum intensity projection (MIP) of proximal right crural arteries in a patient with ipsilateral ischemic skin ulceration in the foot. Proximal occlusions of all three crural arteries are demonstrated with reconstitution of the peroneal artery via collaterals from the anterior tibial artery (obscured by fibula). **c, d** VR and MIP of distal crural arteries demonstrate a collateral artery from the distal peroneal artery reconstituting the posterior tibial artery. **e** Lateral VR of the hind foot demonstrates patent medial and lateral plantar arteries (*arrow*). These normal distal arteries represent excellent bypass graft candidates for pedal revascularization

raphy (DSA) for preprocedure evaluation of patients with claudication [23, 24].

Chronic Limb-Threatening Ischemia

In patients with chronic limb-threatening ischemia, the principal goal of treatment is prevention of tissue loss and need for amputation, assessment, and promotion of blood flow through the calf arteries. An accurate roadmap to lesions amenable to percutaneous transluminal angioplasty or other endovascular techniques and delineation of patent, acceptable target vessels for distal bypass are the challenges of vessel analysis in this advanced disease group (Fig. 10). In this respect, "isotropic" image data sets (<1 mm) and optimum contrast-medium delivery, especially with the state-of-the-art 64-row MDCT scanners, may provide improved visualization of small crural and pedal vessels in patients with chronic limb-threatening ischemia.

Acute Ischemia

For evaluation of acute lower-extremity ischemia, catheter angiography appears to be the most appropriate evaluation technique if urgent percutaneous (thrombolysis, etc.) or surgical intervention is planned [25]. However, in some situations, peripheral CTA may guide the choice of percutaneous or surgical intervention and help in preprocedural planning. For example, CTA can determine the extent and location of thrombosis and whether thrombus or emboli involves all trifurcation vessels, a previously patent bypass graft, or resides within a popliteal aneurysm, and whether thrombolytic therapy may be most efficacious [26] (Fig. 8). In addition, demonstration of thrombus in locations not accessible to embolectomy may direct treatment to catheter-based techniques. In the subacute ischemic population for whom surgical intervention may be best, peripheral CTA can provide a comprehensive map of the affected vascular territories for surgery planning. CTA may provide rapid and adequate evaluation for patients who refuse catherer angiography and/or thrombolysis. It is important to remember that in these settings, an additional CTA acquisition in a delayed phase immediately after the initial arterial phase is often helpful to differentiate patent but slowly flowing vessels from thrombus.

Aneurysms

Peripheral CTA is a noninvasive and cost-effective alternative to DSA for detection and characterization of lower-extremity aneurysms. It provides detailed information about aneurysm size, presence, and amount of thrombus, presence of distal embolic disease, associated significant proximal and distal steno-occlusive disease, and coexistent abdominal or iliac aneurysms. Three-dimensional volumetric analysis provides accurate measurement of aneurysm volume as well as luminal dimension.

Follow-Up and Surveillance After Percutaneous or Surgical Revascularization

Ultrasound is the first choice for routine bypass graft surveillance or serial follow-up evaluation after intervention (e.g., in research protocols) [27, 28]. However, peripheral CTA is an important problem-solving tool for the workup of patients with nondiagnostic (limited access due to skin lesions, wounds, draping, or obesity) or equivocal ultrasound studies. In these settings, CTA provides rapid, noninvasive, and accurate evaluation of peripheral arterial bypass grafts and stents and detects related complications, including stenosis, aneurysmal changes, and arteriovenous fistulae [29] (Fig. 7). CTA can also demonstrate the results of percutaneous interventions and reveal residual disease and both vascular and extravascular complications. Peripheral CTA has replaced catheter DSA completely at our institution in these settings and is used to decide upon further management.

Vascular Trauma

CTA provides rapid and accurate demonstration of traumatic arterial injuries, relationship of arterial segments to adjacent fractures, bone fragments, and soft tissue injuries, hematoma, associated vascular compression, or pseudoaneurysm. CTA can be performed in combination with CT of other organ systems (abdomen, chest, etc.) for complete delineation of the distribution and severity of injuries in each individual organ system [30]. Transverse source images are usually sufficient for interpretation, although MPRs may improve rapidity of analysis. VR images can improve depiction of the anatomic relationship between arteries and adjacent bony/soft tissue injuries and foreign bodies (Fig. 11).

Vascular Mapping

Peripheral CTA data sets can be used to generate vascular maps for subsequent surgical intervention. Prior to MDCTA, catheter angiography was used to generate these vascular maps. Peripheral CTA in the trauma setting is useful if subsequent surgical reconstruction is planned. Likewise, preoperative knowledge of vascular anatomy is also important for plastic surgery reconstruction for various diseases. Fibular free-flap procurement requires preoperative assessment of the limb to prevent ischemic complications and flap failure and to exclude variant peroneal artery anatomy and occlusive disease, which could alter the surgical procedure [31]. CTA allows high-resolution 3-D evaluation of arteries, veins, and soft tissues [32–34] with less risk and at lower cost than catheter angiography [34]. Vascular mapping with CTA is also useful for character evaluation and vascular supply of musculoskeletal tumors [30] and evaluation of suitability of the thoracodorsal and internal mammary arteries prior to trans-

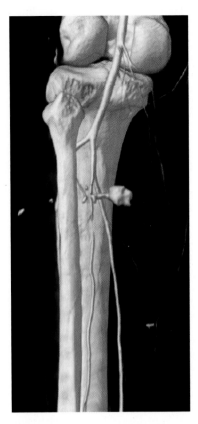

Fig. 11. Volume rendering (VR) of a 16-year-old male following a gunshot wound to the left calf demonstrates a pseudoaneurysm of the peroneal artery with distal occlusion due to peroneal arterial spasm

verse rectus abdominis muscle flap reconstruction.

Miscellaneous Applications

Peripheral CTA can provide important information about many other vascular conditions affecting the lower extremity, such as vascular malformations, arterial compression by adjacent masses, vasculitides, inflammatory/infective processes of soft tissue and bone affecting adjacent vessels, adventitial cystic disease, and popliteal entrapment syndrome [30, 35]. Image acquisition at rest and with provocative maneuvers (e.g., active plantar-flexion against resistance) in patients with popliteal entrapment syndrome allows anatomic delineation of the medial head of the gastrocnemius as well as the dynamic degree of arterial obstruction.

Pitfalls

It is important to review peripheral CTA studies in the context of a patient's symptoms, disease stage, and available therapeutic options. This can help overcome the learning curve and avoiding interpretation pitfalls associated with visual perception and interpretation of vascular abnormalities in a new and different format (such as VR or CPR images).

Commonly, pitfalls related to interpretation of peripheral CTA studies can occur with use of narrow viewing-window settings in the presence of arterial wall calcifications or stents. Blooming artifacts related to these high-attenuation structures leads to overestimation of a vascular stenosis or suggest spurious total occlusion, even at relatively wide window settings. Thus, we use a much higher window width of at least 1,500 HU for evaluating luminal patency at the site of a calcified lesion or a stent. Some vendors (Siemens Medical Solutions) recommend use of special higher spatial resolution reconstruction kernels in the presence of stents. Despite these measures, peripheral CTA studies may not resolve luminal diameter in presence of extensive atherosclerotic or media calcification within small crural or pedal arteries, such as those found in diabetic patients and in patients with end-stage renal disease.

Pitfalls related to image interpretation can also result from misinterpretation of editing artifacts (inadvertent removal of vascular structures in MIP images) and pseudostenosis and/or occlusions due to inaccurate centerline definition (in CPR images). These pitfalls underscore the importance of reviewing source images, additional views, or complimentary imaging modalities.

Conclusion

In conclusion, state-of-the-art MDCT scanners with 16 and 64 detector rows enable acquisition of high spatial resolution peripheral CTA, which helps in noninvasive imaging and treatment planning of peripheral arterial disease.

References

1. Rubin GD, Schmidt AJ, Logan LJ et al (1999) Multi-detector row CT angiography of lower extremity occlusive disease: a new application for CT scanning. Radiology 210(2):588
2. Fleischmann D, Hallett RL, Rubin GD (2006) CT angiography of peripheral arterial disease. J Vasc Interv Radiol 17(1):3–26
3. Fleischmann D, Rubin GD, Paik DS et al (2000) Stair-step artifacts with single versus multiple detector-row helical CT. Radiology 216(1):185–196
4. Rubin GD, Schmidt AJ, Logan LJ, Sofilos MC (2001) Multi-detector row CT angiography of lower extremity arterial inflow and runoff: initial experience. Radiology 221(1):146–158
5. Fleischmann D, Hittmair K (1999) Mathematical analysis of arterial enhancement and optimization

of bolus geometry for CT angiography using the discrete fourier transform. J Comput Assist Tomogr 23(3):474–784

6. Fleischmann D, Rubin GD, Bankier AA, Hittmair K (2000). Improved uniformity of aortic enhancement with customized contrast medium injection protocols at CT angiography. Radiology 214(2):363–371

7. Bron KM (1983) Femoral arteriography. In: Abrams HL (ed) Abrams angiography: vascular and interventional radiology, 3d edn. Little, Brown, Boston. pp 1835–1875

8. Versteylen RJ, Lampmann LE (1989) Knee time in femoral arteriography. AJR Am J Roentgenol 152(1):203

9. Fleischmann D, Rubin GD (2005) Quantification of intravenously administered contrast medium transit through the peripheral arteries: implications for CT angiography. Radiology 236(3):1076–1082

10. Martin ML, Tay KH, Flak B et al (2003) Multidetector CT angiography of the aortoiliac system and lower extremities: a prospective comparison with digital subtraction angiography. AJR Am J Roentgenol 180(4):1085–1091

11. Ofer A, Nitecki SS, Linn S et al (2003) Multidetector CT angiography of peripheral vascular disease: a prospective comparison with intraarterial digital subtraction angiography. AJR Am J Roentgenol 180(3):719–724

12. Ota H, Takase K, Igarashi K et al (2004) MSCT compared with digital subtraction angiography for assessment of lower extremity arterial occlusive disease: importance of reviewing cross-sectional images. AJR Am J Roentgenol 182(1):201–209

13. Catalano C, Fraioli F, Laghi A et al (2004) Infrarenal aortic and lower-extremity arterial disease: diagnostic performance of multi-detector row CT angiography. Radiology 231(2):555–563

14. Portugaller HR, Schoellnast H, Hausegger KA et al (2004) Multislice spiral CT angiography in peripheral arterial occlusive disease: a valuable tool in detecting significant arterial lumen narrowing? Eur Radiol 14(9):1681–1687

15. Milne EN (1967) The significance of early venous filling during femoral arteriography. Radiology 88(3):513–518

16. Koechl A, Kanitsar A, Lomoschitz E et al (2003) Comprehensive assessment of peripheral arteries using multi-path curved planar reformation of CTA datasets. In: European Congress of Radiology, p 268

17. Kanitsar A, Fleischmann D, Wegenkittl R et al (2002) Curved planar reformation. In: Moorehead R, Gross M, Joy KI (eds) Proceedings of the 13th IEEE Visualization 2002 Conference, Boston, 27 October–11 November 2002. IEEE Computer Society, Piscataway, pp 37–44

18. Raman R, Napel S, Beaulieu CF et al (2002) Automated generation of curved planar reformations from volume data: method and evaluation. Radiology 223(1):275–280

19. Visser K, Kock MCJM, Kuntz KM et al (2003) Cost-effectiveness targets for multi-detector row CT angiography in the work-up of patients with intermittent claudication. Radiology 227:647–656

20. Surowiec SM, Davies MG, Eberly SW et al (2005) Percutaneous angioplasty and stenting of the superficial femoral artery. J Vasc Surg 41(2):269–278

21. Clark TW, Groffsky JL, Soulen MC (2001) Predictors of long-term patency after femoropopliteal angioplasty: results from the STAR registry. J Vasc Interv Radiol 12(8):923–933

22. Hirai T, Korogi Y, Ono K et al (2001) Maximum stenosis of extracranial internal carotid artery: effect of luminal morphology on stenosis measurement by using CT angiography and conventional DSA. Radiology 221(3):802–809

23. Visser K, de Vries SO, Kitslaar PJ et al (2003) Cost-effectiveness of diagnostic imaging work-up and treatment for patients with intermittent claudication in The Netherlands. Eur J Vasc Endovasc Surg 25(3):213–223

24. Rubin GD, Armerding MD, Dake MD, Napel S (2000) Cost identification of abdominal aortic aneurysm imaging by using time and motion analyses. Radiology 215(1):63–70

25. Rutherford RB, Baker JD, Ernst C et al (1997) Recommended standards for reports dealing with lower extremity ischemia: revised version. J Vasc Surg 26(3):517–538

26. Costantini V, Lenti M (2002) Treatment of acute occlusion of peripheral arteries. Thromb Res 106(6):V285–V294

27. Mills JL, Harris EJ, Taylor LM Jr et al (1990) The importance of routine surveillance of distal bypass grafts with duplex scanning: a study of 379 reversed vein grafts. J Vasc Surg 12(4):379–386; discussion 387–389

28. Moody P, Gould DA, Harris PL (1990) Vein graft surveillance improves patency in femoropopliteal bypass. Eur J Vasc Surg 4(2):117–121

29. Willmann JK, Mayer D, Banyai M et al (2003) Evaluation of peripheral arterial bypass grafts with multidetector row CT angiography: comparison with duplex US and digital subtraction angiography. Radiology 229(2):465–474

30. Karcaaltincaba M, Akata D, Aydingoz U et al (2004) Three-dimensional MSCT angiography of the extremities: clinical applications with emphasis on musculoskeletal uses. AJR Am J Roentgenol 183(1):113–117

31. Whitley SP, Sandhu S, Cardozo A (2004) Preoperative vascular assessment of the lower limb for harvest of a fibular flap: the views of vascular surgeons in the United Kingdom. Br J Oral Maxillofac Surg 42(4):307–310

32. Karanas YL, Antony A, Rubin G, Chang J (2004) Preoperative CT angiography for free fibula transfer. Microsurgery 24(2):125–127

33. Chow L, Napoli A, Klein MB et al (2005) Vascular mapping with multidetector CT angiography prior to free-flap reconstruction. Radiology 237(1):353–360

34. Klein MB, Karanas YL, Chow LC et al (2003) Early experience with computed tomographic angiography in microsurgical reconstruction. Plast Reconstr Surg 112(2):498–503

35. Takase K, Imakita S, Kuribayashi S et al (1997) Popliteal artery entrapment syndrome: aberrant origin of gastrocnemius muscle shown by 3D CT. J Comput Assist Tomogr 21(4):523–528

SECTION IV

MDCT of Head and Neck

IV.1

CT Angiography of the Neck and Brain

David S. Enterline

Introduction

The evolution of multidetector computed tomography (MDCT) has allowed the development and advancement of CT angiography (CTA). While the concept of carotid artery evaluation by CT was introduced by Heinz and others in 1984 [1, 2], it has taken recent technological advances to bring the current methods into practice. CTA of the neck is used primarily to assess the carotid vessels. As CTA slice thickness and rendering methods have improved, so has the accuracy of stenosis determination. More recently, CTA of the neck has become the standard for traumatic injury. Routine utilization of CTA for the evaluation of carotid and vertebral arteries is now the norm. The technique also has been successfully applied to the intracranial vasculature. Detection of cerebral aneurysms and other vascular diseases are readily identified.

This chapter will discuss CT techniques and contrast optimization of MDCT for CTA of the neck and brain and discuss the interpretation of the diseases commonly evaluated by this technique.

CT Technique

Obtaining great quality CTA of the neck and brain requires optimizing CT technique and acquisition. Thin-slice CT attained while the contrast bolus is present is the fundamental doctrine. While some CT parameters are vendor specific, there are general principles that apply [3]. The scan for neck CTA is set up from the aortic arch to the skull base or to 1 cm above the top of the dorsum sella if additional information is desired about intracranial circulation. Alternatively, the scan can extend to the vertex of the skull. From a practical standpoint, this combined approach is most often used. For CTA of the brain, the scan starts at the C2 level and goes to 1 cm above the dorsum sella or to the vertex. In or-

der to evaluate a suspected vascular lesion more cephalad, such as in the case of an arteriovenous malformation (AVM), the volume covered needs to include this region, too. In most cases, a 20-cm field of view is used. This can be adjusted up or down as the situation warrants; however, use of a smaller field of view improves resolution. Patient chin position is adjusted to a neutral position since the scan is obtained at no gantry tilt, otherwise, the vasculature of the anterior head may be missed. Scanning from caudal to cephalad minimizes the contrast volume needed and venous opacification; however, it does risk producing a nondiagnostic scan if there is not sufficient contrast present.

Slice thickness directly determines resolution in the Z-axis. For neck CTA, use of slices in the 0.5- to 1.5-mm range provides adequate resolution and coverage. In general, for four- and eight-slice scanners, a thickness of 1 mm is used while in 16- and 64-slice scanners, the thinnest option is selected. This is due in large part to the overall detector configuration and length. Gantry rotation times have also decreased with newer scanner iterations. For neck CTA on a 4- or 8-slice scanner, a time of 0.7 s is typically used. For a 16-slice CT, 0.5 or 0.6 s is used while 0.4 s is used for 64-slice CT. This may be manufacturer specific. One interesting variant is a hybrid method. Since imaging a small vessel, such as the 3-mm in-plane middle cerebral artery (MCA), is different than the 5-mm transversely oriented proximal internal carotid artery (ICA), one can scan faster through the neck and then slow down for the circle of Willis where more resolution is needed. An example is to use 0.5-s scans through the neck with 1.0-s scans through the head. Pitch also has a significant impact on image quality. In general, keeping the pitch at about 1 provides a balance between coverage and resolution.

Historically, a tube voltage of 140 kVp was used for CT to minimize tube heating and maximize

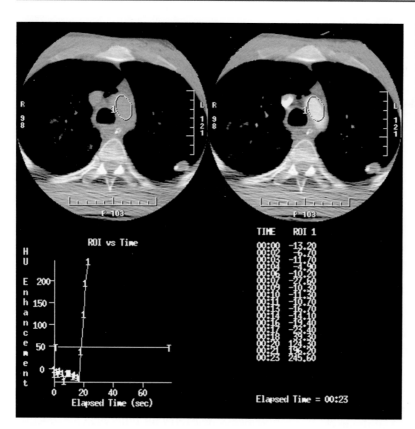

Fig. 1. Automatic triggering for CTA. The cursor is placed in the aorta, and sequential images are obtained during dynamic contrast injection. Scan commences when contrast density in Hounsfield units (HU) reaches a preset value of 50–100 or when the technologist visually sees sufficient opacity in the arteries. Note contrast enhancement versus time curve

tube life. However, one of the key advances of MDCT has been tube technology that improves heat unit dissipation and reliability. This has allowed the use of 120 kVp, which may improve relative opacification of contrast media. The tube load used depends on gantry speed, patient weight and size, and region scanned. In general, the milliampere second (mAs) used should be in the 220–260 range for an average adult patient. For a gantry rotation of 0.7 s, a 380-mA tube load is an acceptable starting point. The newer 16- and 64-slice scanners offer automatic mA adjustments based on in-plane and Z-axis attenuation. A range of mA is set, along with an image quality desired. For CTA of the brain, image quality needs to be set higher with lower noise. Neck studies permit a slightly higher noise setting.

In CT venography (CTV), the basic premise is that the contrast bolus needs to fill the major veins. CT parameters are adapted from CTA protocols. The field of view needs to include the entire head; 22 cm is suggested. For the 4-slice scanner, 2.5 mm slices may be used to provide coverage. Slice thickness of 1.25 mm is used in eight-slice scanners, which may be reduced to thinner slices on the 16- and 64-slice MDCT. Pitch may be increased to about 1.5. Less radiation is needed since the vessels are larger. Tube load and gantry rotation is adjusted for mAs of about 220, with gantry rotation of 0.7–0.8 s.

Contrast Optimization

Contrast timing is a key determinant of CTA image quality. Peak contrast opacification should occur at the time of the scan for each region evaluated. For the neck and brain, the use of high-concentration contrast optimizes visualization of small vessels and defines vessel boundaries for improved accuracy. It permits high iodine flux at an acceptable IV injection rate. Higher IV injection rates provide high iodine flux but at a greater risk of extravasation from the IV site. We typically use 4 ml/s in our patients. Ideally, the bolus of contrast only needs to be present for the length of time that is needed to scan the area of concern, offset by the time it takes to get to the artery of interest. In practice, it is difficult to always reliably time the contrast bolus. An arbitrary injection time of 15 s for the neck or 18 s for the brain might be in error due to poor cardiac output or arterial or venous stenosis. Anxious individuals or trauma patients may have a very rapid transit time due to increased cardiac output.

Bolus tracking and automatic triggering methods have improved with MDCT technology. For neck CTA, the aortic arch with a 500 HU trigger provides a good basis for beginning to scan (Fig. 1). Volume of contrast needed reflects the speed of the scanner, with 100 ml of contrast media needed for four- and eight-slice scanners and

75 ml needed for 16-slice scanners. For brain CTA, ideally, a 100 HU trigger at the distal cervical ICA is used. However, identification of this vessel can prove elusive in some patients, so the aortic arch trigger point can be used with an additional 2–3 s delay added. Contrast requirements for brain CTA is 50 ml for 16-slice and 75 ml for 4- and 8-slice scanners.

Image Processing

The acquired images are checked for adequacy at the scanner and then postprocessed. In the case of 16-slice scanners, the very thin slices are usually reconstructed at a thicker slice thickness of 1 mm. This reduces image noise and number of slices to review while permitting improved three-dimensional (3-D) images and reformation of the thinner slices due to isotropic pixel acquisition. There can be a substantial reduction in radiation exposure to the patient using this technique. The thin-slice data set is sent to the 3-D workstation while the reformatted axial images are sent to the picture archive and communication system (PACS).

The exception to automated processing is the acute stroke patient who is a candidate for thrombolysis intervention. This scenario makes evaluation of the ICA, the basilar artery, the proximal MCA, the anterior cerebral artery (ACA), and the posterior cerebral artery (PCA) immediately at the scanner imperative. This is easy to accomplish by reviewing the data dynamically. If these vessels are not opacified while the other head vessels are and the symptomatic patient is in the therapeutic time window, then immediate intervention is indicated. CT perfusion scans can add value; however, their processing time at this point precludes their routine clinical use.

The CTA data set is best evaluated at the workstation. This workstation may be from a third-party vendor or the scanner vendor. The data set is initially selected, and then a rendering technique selected. Each major vessel may be isolated for review using trimming of the data, isolation of the vessel by selecting an area of interest, or use of a curved multiplanar reconstruction (MPR) technique. In neck CTA, each carotid artery is traced entirely for completeness, with emphasis on the carotid bifurcation. Usually, this is done using both volume-rendered and maximal intensity projection (MIP) methods. For vessels that have little calcification, the 3-D views work best. However, with calcification, the reformatted MIP projections are more accurate. Vertebral arteries are also evaluated from their origins to the basilar artery. Attention to vertebral origins with MIP projections identifies well any areas of stenosis. The raw data set is also evaluated for incidental findings.

For brain CTA, often a different rendering setting is used that optimizes smaller vessel assessment. Again, systematic evaluation of the vessels is needed, as well as an overview of the images for ancillary findings. This may be done by averaging slices and adjusting window and level settings to see brain parenchyma or bone detail. In the case of the circle of Willis, the vital viewing regions include the vertebrobasilar area, the basilar tip, the PCAs, the ACA, the MCA, and their proximal trifurcation vessels; the supraclinoid and cavernous ICAs; and the pericallosal arteries. The 3-D surface-shaded volume-rendered views see these areas best. Reformatted MIP views provide additional and complementary information in the case of vessel calcification, vasculopathy, and aneurysms. Reformatted and source images are used primarily at the skull nase where the clinoids and adjacent bones obscure volume-rendered 3-D views. CTV coverage is of the entire head. Review of the axial data set is supplemented by reformatted MIP images. The 3-D-rendered images are less helpful. In all cases, selected images of important findings are captured and saved. These are then sent to be added to the PACS data set.

CTA of the Neck

Carotid Vascular Disease

Several multicenter trials have established the need to differentiate medical versus surgical therapy on the basis of degree of carotid stenosis. The North America Symptomatic Carotid Artery Trial (NASCET) established that carotid endarterectomy provides an improved outcome over medical therapy in cases where the stenosis measures greater than 70% [4]. Measurement is by diameter of the maximal stenosis divided by diameter of the more distal internal carotid artery beyond any poststenotic dilatation. At 2 years, the stroke risk was reduced from 26% to 9% in the surgical arm while major stroke risk was reduced from 13% to 2.5%. In the 50–69% stenosis group, a modest improvement in outcome was present at 5 years with surgery. Surgical skill was an important determinant in outcome, and the results were better in men than in women [5]. The European Carotid Surgery Trial (ECST) found significant improvement in the surgical endarterectomy group, reducing stroke from 21.9% to 12.3% in stenosis of 70–90% [6]. This trial measured stenosis as the diameter of the stenosis divided by the diameter of the expected vessel wall.

In the asymptomatic patient, there are a few large studies worthy of mention. The Carotid Artery Stenosis with Asymptomatic Narrowing Operation Versus Aspirin (CASANOVA) study and

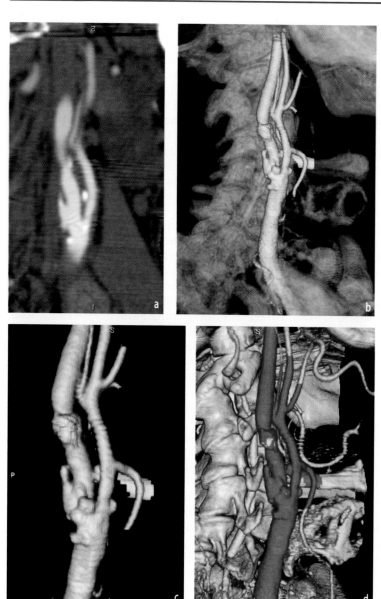

Fig. 2a-d. Carotid vascular disease on CTA. **a** Sagittal reformatted maximum intensity projection (MIP) demonstrates undermined, ulcerated plaque with moderate stenosis. **b** Volume-rendered surface-shaded three-dimensional (3-D) image of moderate stenosis and ulcerated plaque shows calcified plaque. **c** Magnified image with deleted background better exhibits carotid bifurcation region. The calcified plaque is lighter in this scheme, and the ulceration is well depicted posteriorly. **d** Automated vessel definition using a red color scheme example. Note the calcifications are not differentiated in this particular method

the Veterans Administration Asymptomatic Carotid Study (VAACS) are two of the earlier studies that have been overshadowed by the more recent Asymptomatic Carotid Atherosclerosis Study (ACAS) and Asymptomatic Carotid Surgery Trial (ACST) studies [7, 8]. The ACAS trial of 1,662 patients in 39 centers studied patients with greater than 60% stenosis. The 5-year stroke risk was 10.6% in the medical group versus 4.8% in the surgical group, resulting in an effective risk reduction of 1% per year with surgery. The benefit in women was much less with, relative risk reduction of 16% versus 69% in men [9]. The risk of surgery was less than 3%, and angiography constituted 1.2% of the total stroke risk. This often-cited statistic has helped to dramatically reduce the use of diagnostic angiography. The ACST study [10] involving 126 hospital trials in 30 countries followed 3,120 patients with greater than 70% stenosis. It demonstrated a 5-year stroke risk of 11.7% with medical therapy versus 6.4% with surgery. While there is criticism of the methods used in all of these trials, they all have clearly established the need for carotid artery evaluation.

Consequently, the most common indication for CTA of the neck is to assess vascular disease, most commonly carotid stenosis (Figs. 2–4). Its role in noninvasive testing is that of a secondary test along with magnetic resonance angiography (MRA). Ultrasound is a common noninvasive screening test for carotid assessment, and over two thirds of carotid cases are evaluated this way. If this test suggests only mild stenosis, then additional testing is not necessary. However, a moderate or severe degree of stenosis is worthy of further action. In many regions, ultrasound screening alone

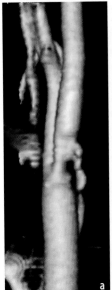
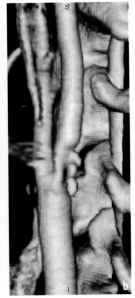
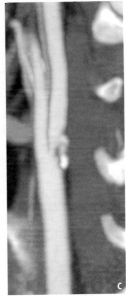

Fig. 3. Carotid vascular disease on CTA. **a** Coronal three-dimensional (3-D) image with eccentric plaque and approximately 70% stenosis. **b** Sagittal 3-D image with minimal calcification posteriorly. **c** Sagittal maximum intensity projection (MIP) reformatted image permits accurate viewing of severe stenosis and minimal calcification. Slice thickness and window/level settings affect visualized narrowing

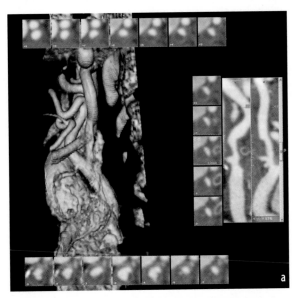
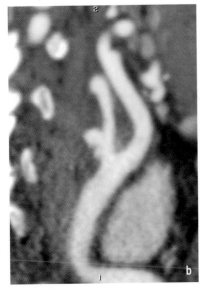

Fig. 4a, b. Carotid vascular disease on CTA. **a** Automated, curved, multiplanar reformation of carotid bifurcation. Multiple images are displayed perpendicular to the vessel long axis. Curved reformatted images to the *right* depict multiple ulcerations. The axial diameters are readily measured. **b** Manually trimmed sagittal maximum intensity projection (MIP) reformation also shows the multiple ulcerations with 50–55% stenosis

is seen as a clear surgical indication. However, the method does tend to exaggerate the degree of stenosis, so in cases of moderate or severe velocities, a correlative test may significantly improve accuracy and minimize false positives, thereby preventing unnecessary interventions. Also, this exam only evaluates a small window around the carotid bifurcation, not the entire vessel. The study by Johnston and Goldstein found a severe stenosis surgery misclassification rate of 28% on ultrasound results alone compared with conventional angiography [11]. While duplex ultrasound alone had a misclassification rate of 18%, the study illus-

trates the value of improved accuracy with multiple tests, reducing the miss rate to 7.9% with concordant exams. Consequently, if ultrasound is used as the screening modality, then MRA or CTA have value to confirm findings and provide additional information useful in patient assessment. This study has been confirmed by others.

MRA is also used widely for carotid evaluation. Most times, MRA is coupled with MR imaging (MRI) of the brain to evaluate the brain for stroke or other conditions and the vessels as a cause of the dysfunction. This "one-stop-shopping" method provides a useful clinical diagnostic procedure that is favored by neurologists. MRA can be obtained using time-of-flight (TOF) methods or with gadolinium enhancement [contrast-enhanced MRA (CEMRA)]. Improvements in MRI scanner gradient coils and slew rates have permitted more rapid data acquisition. Imaging methods such as elliptic-centric data ordering using 3-D fast-gradient-echo sequences or their equivalent allows the more important components of data to be captured when the contrast bolus is highest and for the scan time to be dramatically decreased. MRA is highly accurate. CEMRA tends to mildly overestimate degree of stenosis in the patient with severe stenosis. The two-dimensional (2-D) TOF method overestimates severe stenosis and may result in a "flow gap" due to intravoxel dephasing due to turbulent flow. Calcium is not evaluated since it does not have free hydrogen protons to give signal. The position of the carotid bifurcation is also difficult to assess. In cases of very severe stenosis, slow flow within a patent carotid may not be detected due to saturation effects inherent with MRA methods.

CTA of the neck provides many advantages and a few disadvantages compared with MRA and ultrasound. The entire vessel is evaluated, and the level of the bifurcation is clearly noted relative to the mandible. There is a small risk of allergic reaction due to iodinated contrast media. Radiation risk is difficult to quantify as to its significance but is of lesser importance in the typical older patient. Claustrophobia is certainly less of an issue than in MRI. The detection of calcification is a mixed advantage. This is an important feature to the surgeon and the interventionalist; however, it makes accurate stenosis analysis more difficult. While 3-D surface-shaded volume-rendered images are readily evaluated, in the case of calcification, the MIP reformatted images become the primary image of interpretation. In severe cases, the calcification must be windowed such that the calcium does not visually bloom and yet the vessel is well seen. Correlating the degree of stenosis in multiple planes improves the confidence level for an accurate reading.

Several papers have compared the accuracy of CTA, MRA, ultrasound, and conventional angiography [12, 13]. However, as the technology for each modality improves, the criteria by which they are judged is limited. One of the principal papers was written by Patel and colleagues in 2002 [12]. The sensitivity and specificity of ultrasound were 85% and 71%, of MRA 100% and 57%, and of CTA 65% and 100%, respectively. While the trend of MRA to overestimate and of CTA to underestimating stenosis but be more specific seems to hold, currently, MRA and CTA are considered to both be highly accurate with specificity and sensitivity in the 90–95% range. In our institution, neurologists favor MRA while vascular surgeons and interventionalists prefer CTA.

Stenosis alone does not fully predict who will present with neurologic events. The character of the carotid plaque is also important. Soft plaque and calcification are well depicted by CTA. Thrombus typically projects as a smooth intraluminal low-density image extending from an area of plaque. The detection of vulnerable plaque is more challenging to identify. The lipid-laden macrophages that are characteristic of vulnerable plaque are less focally defined than they are in the coronary circulation. Stratification of plaque by density is a potential way to suggest vulnerable plaque. Plaque with density below 60 HU is considered to be soft plaque that may be vulnerable while fibrous plaque may extend up to 150 HU. Ulceration is another plaque morphology that is hard to define, even by conventional angiography or direct inspection. A plaque that is undermined with a shelf-like appearance is suggestive of ulceration, but this is not definitive.

Carotid Occlusion

The diagnosis of carotid occlusion is clearly a forte of CTA (Fig. 5). The importance of this distinction lies in the potential for revascularization of a very severe stenosis, or "string sign" and the contraindication of surgery for occlusion. In actuality, it is important to distinguish between a small vessel with a focal severe narrowing that would be amenable to surgery and a diffusely irregular severely narrowed vessel that would preclude surgery. CTA is more of a volume technique than MRA, which is more flow sensitive. Consequently, CTA can provide this important information. With CTA, one can trace the lumen of the carotid artery and see if any contrast is visualized within it. If not, the diagnosis of occlusion is straightforward. Occlusion is also readily seen in the horizontal segment of the ICA. A pitfall is if imaging takes place too soon since slow flow may not be seen in this situation. Also of note is that collaterals from the external carotid artery can reconstitute the distal ICA, including the ophthalmic artery from ethmoidal internal maxillary artery branches, the artery of the foramen rotundum, and the Vidian artery.

Fibromuscular Disease

In addition to vascular stenosis, there are several other disorders that affect the carotid or vertebral arteries in the neck, including many of the collagen vascular disorders. One of these is fibromuscular dysplasia (FMD). This common disorder involves

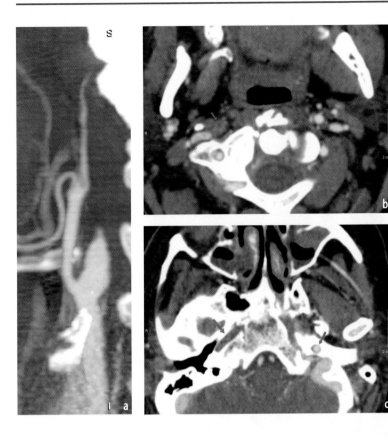

Fig. 5a-c. Carotid occlusion. **a** Sagittal reformatted maximum intensity projection (MIP) demonstrates carotid occlusion. **b** The occluded right internal carotid artery can be well seen on the axial image of the neck (*arrow*). No contrast is present within the lumen. **c** At the skull base, the right carotid occlusion is diagnosed by lack of contrast within the lumen

the mid- and distal cervical ICA and the distal vertebral artery. Involvement of the neck vessels is present in 30% of cases; there is a strong female predilection. Irregular beading with small outpouchings and multiple small septations is the characteristic appearance. Areas of more focal dilatations or smooth stenosis are also variants that may be seen. Dissection and pseudoaneurysms are common, and FMD should be considered when these entities present. Intracranial aneurysms are also associated with FMD.

CTA of FMD can be difficult to diagnose (Fig. 6). This is due to the relative smoothing that is inherent to the CTA method. Careful assessment of the mid- and distal ICA and the V3 and V4 vertebral artery segments can demonstrate small irregular undulations or a more irregular enlargement.

Dissection and Pseudoaneurysm

The diagnosis of dissection should be considered in any younger patient who presents with headache or acute neck pain in association with a neurologic complaint. Minimal trauma may be associated. Horner's syndrome of miotic pupil, ptosis, and anhydrosis are frequently seen. The intimal disruption of the vessel results in an expanded vessel and compromised, smoothly narrowed lumen.

Both CTA and MRA are useful in the diagnosis and treatment of dissection (Fig. 7). The expanded vessel can be seen compared with the contralateral vessel, and the intimal flap is typically depicted. If there is flow on both sides of the flap, this is well seen, particularly on the source images. If one lumen is occluded, then thrombus may be evident with flow in the other compromised lumen. By MRA, fat saturation T1 sequences may show methemoglobin in the vessel wall. CTA depicts well vessel expansion and compromised lumen of the vessel. The characteristic involvement of the distal cervical ICA is well seen.

Pseudoaneurysms are often associated with dissections. These represent the focal vessel wall expansion with flow. CTA and MRA are both useful, but CTA demonstrates the location relative to the skull base and the exact dimensions.

The diagnosis of dissection and pseudoaneurysm is readily made by CTA and MRA. These are treated by anticoagulation or antiplatelet therapy in most cases. Consequently, having a noninvasive test to follow therapy is also helpful. Both CTA and MRA can be used for this purpose.

Vertebral Artery Evaluation

The vertebral arteries are well seen by CTA (Fig. 8). However, the adjacent vertebral bodies may overlay the vessel, particularly on the 3-D images. The

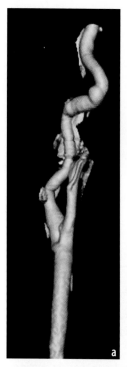
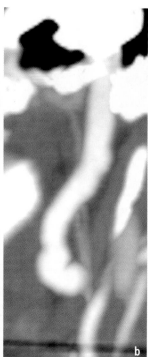
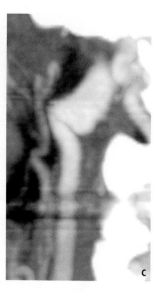

Fig. 6a-c. Fibromuscular dysplasia (FMD). **a** Irregular mid- and distal internal carotid artery (ICA) indicating FMD. **b** Maximum intensity projection (MIP) demonstrates the irregular vessel contour. **c** MIP on a different patient with FMD who also has pseudoaneurysm. Note the enlarged, tortuous vessel

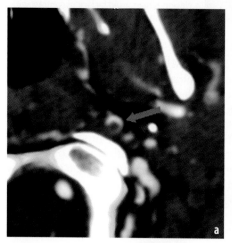
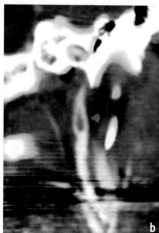

Fig. 7a, b. Carotid dissection. **a** Dissection of the left internal carotid artery (ICA) is diagnosed by enlarged vessel and compromised vessel lumen. Sometimes, a dissection flap is evident. Here, contrast is seen in the false lumen (*arrow*). **b** Reformatted image of dissection in a woman who was thrown from a horse. Note the dissection flap (*arrow*)

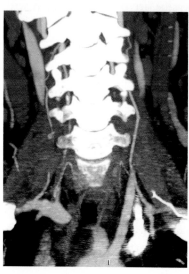

Fig. 8. Vertebral artery occlusion. Origins of the vertebral arteries can usually be well seen using thicker-slab maximum intensity projection (MIP) coronal images. Here, the left vertebral origin is occluded, and the ascending cervical artery reconstitutes the left vertebral artery in the transverse foramen at the C4 level. The right vertebral artery is hypoplastic

reformatted MIP images are useful to identify the vessel along with acquisition data. Normal variations of a dominant left vertebral artery or a vertebral artery ending in the posterior inferior cerebellar artery (PICA) are common. The origins of the vertebral arteries may be obscured by streak artifacts, superimposed contrast from the venous bolus, or calcification related to atherosclerotic disease. By magnifying the area of interest and adjusting the window/level of the image and adjusting the MIP slice thickness, one can usually resolve the vertebral artery well. In the case of atherosclerosis, measuring the maximal stenosis divided by the size of the normal vessel is used. Tortuosity of the vessel is often visualized in the mid-cervical spine region. Dissection of the vessel is more common distally.

Trauma

CTA has become the new standard in evaluating the patient with significant trauma to the neck or head [14]. The thin-slice CT technique provides evaluation of vessels in addition to surrounding soft tissue injury and evidence of fracture. Reformatted images also permit assessment of the cervical spine. Sensitivity for blunt cerebrovascular injury is quoted as 100%, with 94% specificity in a recent study by Berne [14]. Vertebral artery injury was more frequent than carotid injury, and there was a 21% mortality rate with vessel injury. Carotid canal fracture or transverse foramen fracture should alert one to the possibility of major vessel injury, specifically vessel dissection or occlusion (Fig. 9).

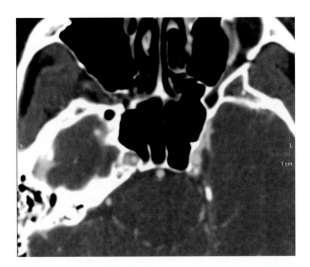

Fig. 9. Carotid traumatic dissection. CTA is used extensively to evaluate patients with significant trauma. Here, the right distal petrous internal carotid artery (ICA) is dissected in a patient post motor-vehicle collision. The compromised lumen is seen medial to the dissection laterally

CTA of the Brain

In the past, the evaluation of intracranial vasculature required conventional angiography. However, the development of MRA and CTA provides a noninvasive method of assessing these vessels. A major challenge is the small vessel size. The horizontal segment of the MCA (M1 branch) and the basilar artery are typically 3 mm and the distal ICA is about 4 mm. The more distal branches get progressively smaller. Consequently, voxel resolution is an issue. Small fields of view and thin slices combined with slow table speed and low pitch provide the ability to see most major vessels. Systematic evaluation of intracranial CTA minimizes omissions. While there are many ways to do this, one easy and quick way is outlined as follows:

- Trim the data set to see the back of the foramen magnum and above the top of the basilar artery. Also, trim from the sides to see the MCA branches, excluding most of the calvarium.
- Look at the 3-D view posteriorly to view the vertebral arteries and proximal basilar artery. Rotate along the basilar to see the basilar tip.
- Look from the top of the data set to see the circle of Willis, following the vessels with slight rotations. This will view the posterior and anterior communicating arteries.
- Look from anteriorly to see the ophthalmic artery origins and distal ICAs. The anterior communicating artery and MCAs are also seen from this view with some additional rotation of data.
- Trim data to see just between the ICAs to evaluate the ACA territory branches. Then shift to the right and then to the left to see the MCA territory branches.
- View the coronal and sagittal reformats using MIP, and vary the slab thickness to see vessels of interest, particularly in the cavernous sinus region.
- View the entire data set to look for incidental and related findings, such as stroke, tumor, or AVMs. This may be done by averaging data to 5-mm thickness. Also look at venous drainage for thrombosis.
- Document findings of images of interest.

Stenosis and Occlusion

The major intracranial vessels are usually well seen by CTA [15]. Stenosis represents an area of narrowing in the vessel caliber (Figs. 10, 11). This is calculated as the diameter of the narrowing relative to the normal vessel caliber. Due to the small size of these vessels, it can be difficult to measure this exactly; however, magnification of the image helps to improve accuracy.

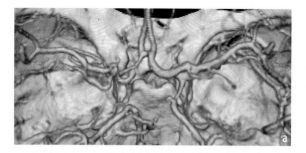

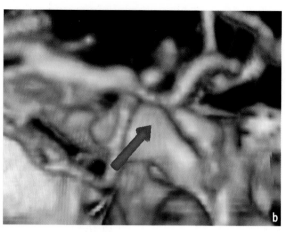

Fig. 10a, b. Intracranial stenosis. **a** Severe distal left internal carotid artery (ICA) and proximal middle cerebral artery (MCA) stenosis in this elderly patient with atherosclerotic disease causes reduced caliber of intracranial vessels. **b** By rotating and cropping the image, the severe stenosis at the ICA–MCA junction is well seen (*arrow*)

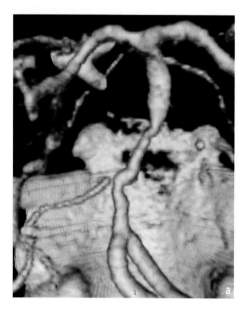

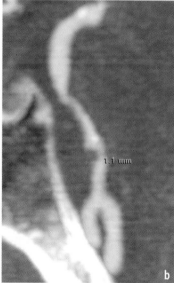

Fig. 11a, b. Intracranial stenosis. **a** Severe stenosis of the proximal and midbasilar artery due to atherosclerotic disease. **b** Sagittal maximum intensity projection (MIP) shows the irregularity of the basilar artery. Measurement of the vessel stenosis is demonstrated

Anomalies of the cerebral vasculature need to be considered as well. The left vertebral artery is equal or dominant in about 75% of patients, so asymmetry of the vertebral arteries is the rule. Frequently, a vertebral artery will diminish in size after the PICA origin. Also, hypoplastic P1 and A1 segments are frequently seen in about 25% of patients. These congenital narrowings should not be interpreted as acquired stenosis. The increased flow in the resultant compensatory feeding vessels makes aneurysms somewhat more likely, so these variations should be noted.

Stenosis of vessels is well seen on the 3-D images when the vessel is not calcified. However, in the setting of calcification, more reliance on MIP reformation is needed. The 3-D images will show a bump along the vessel wall, usually of a different color, but it can be complicated to differentiate the lumen from the calcified plaque. MIP reformation is more accurate to define the percentage stenosis.

In addition, CTA is very useful in the case of anticipated endovascular intervention. Measuring the vessel size, stenosis diameter and length, and landing zones of a stent permit more accurate and, presumptively, safer angioplasty and stent placement.

Occlusion of a branch vessel may be straightforward to detect if one knows the cerebral anatomy to realize that a vessel is missing (Figs. 12, 13). Often, there is a small tail of contrast at the origin or an abrupt caliber change that defines the occlusion site. One pitfall of occlusion in major vessels is due to collateral flow. This reconstitutes the more distal vessel but at a smaller caliber due to reduced pressure and flow. The diagnosis of occlusion is made by tracing the pathway of the vessel and noting that no flow is present in a segment. To be sure of this finding, the image level should be increased using a narrow window to eliminate the possibility of a high-grade stenosis rather than an occlusion.

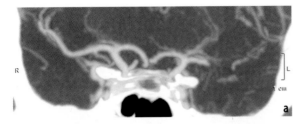

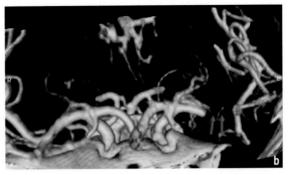

Fig. 12a, b. Acute thrombosis of the left middle cerebral artery (MCA). **a** Patient presents with acute right hemiplegia and aphasia. Thrombosis of the distal MCA is present, with occlusion of the distal M1 MCA segment and proximal M2 branches (*arrow*). **b** Three-dimensional (3-D) image of the acute thrombosis (*arrows*) demonstrates filling defect in contrasted vessels. Note reconstitution of distal collateral MCA branches

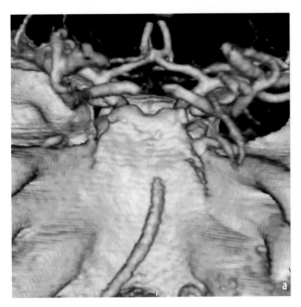

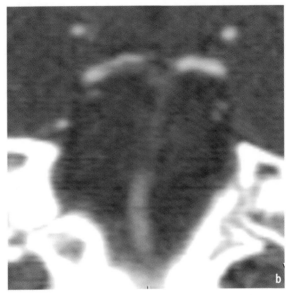

Fig. 13a, b. Acute basilar artery thrombosis. **a** Occlusion of the mid- and distal basilar artery is demonstrated in this patient who suddenly became comatose. **b** Coronal maximum intensity projection (MIP) image shows contrast opacification of the proximal basilar and posterior cerebral arteries with basilar artery thrombosis

Vasculopathy

Vasculopathy is a generalized term referring to any pathologic condition of the blood vessels. As such, it includes stenosis and occlusion and also includes vasospasm and vasculitis.

The detection of vasospasm by CTA has permitted a noninvasive method that complements transcranial Doppler [16]. Vasospasm typically arises in the 4–14 days following subarachnoid hemorrhage and is most common in the 7- to 10-day window. Standard clinical treatment includes "triple H" therapy consisting of hypertension, hypervolemia, and hemodilution in combination with the calcium channel blocker, nimodipine. This is effective in most patients, but in severe cases, endovascular angioplasty or arterial infusion is warranted. CT of the brain to evaluate for hydro-cephalus and infarction is performed prior to intervention. In this situation, CTA can be added to the evaluation although in many cases the decision to proceed to conventional angiography has already been made, negating the value of CTA. The appearance of vasospasm on CTA is that of regions of smooth narrowing of vessels, including the major intracranial vessels.

Vasculitis is an inflammatory infiltration of the blood-vessel wall (Fig. 14). There are many etiologies that can be grouped by the size of the vessel involved. Takayasu's arteritis has large-vessel involvement of the great vessels up to the carotid bifurcation. It shows smooth vessel narrowing and a thickened vessel wall. Giant-cell or temporal arteritis may involve the larger cerebral vessels, including the classic superficial temporal artery. Most of these cases show areas of smooth narrow-

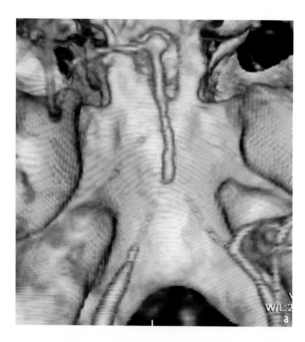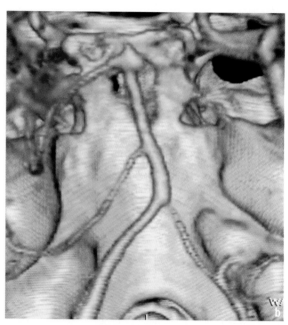

Fig. 14a, b. Vasculopathy. **a** Patient with sarcoid causing intracranial vasculopathy. Note narrowing of the basilar artery, distal vertebral arteries, and anterior inferior cerebellar artery. **b** Same patient after therapy demonstrates marked improvement in vessel caliber

ing of the vessel followed by a return to normal caliber – the so-called "beaded" appearance. There are also multiple autoimmune diseases and even primary CNS vasculitis with involvement of medium- to small-vessel beading. By CTA, involvement of the more proximal vessels is readily detected; however, medium- and small-vessel vasculitis is not able to be reliably found. Consequently, conventional angiography remains the standard diagnostic test.

Aneurysms

The detection of cerebral aneurysms by CTA has dramatically improved in the past few years. In many centers, it has moved to the forefront of evaluating patients with cerebral aneurysms [17–21]. There are two basic scenarios – the evaluation of the patient with subarachnoid hemorrhage (SAH) and the patient being screened or followed for cerebral aneurysm (Figs. 15–17).

SAH in the nontrauma patient without coagulopathy has a high likelihood of being due to a ruptured aneurysm. CT of the brain without contrast provides the diagnosis of SAH in most patients who present with the classical history of severe headache. Rarely, false negative cases may result from delayed presentation of the patient or from minimal amounts of blood in the spinal fluid. A compelling history warrants lumbar puncture (LP) for cerebral spinal fluid (CSF) analysis although the LP may also result in a traumatic tap. CTA pro-

vides a highly sensitive and specific method for detection and evaluation of cerebral aneurysms in all cases. A recent study by Karamessini and colleagues quotes a 93–100% sensitivity and 100% specificity for aneurysms 3 mm or larger. These values are comparable with conventional angiography [20]. In particular, anterior communicating artery aneurysms are seen equivalently or superiorly by CTA since both ACAs are visualized simultaneously.

MCA aneurysms, particularly complex aneurysms, are also seen equally as well or better by digital subtraction angiography (DSA). The basilar tip and artery and distal vertebral arteries are also evaluated equivalently or better by CTA. The posterior communicating artery is seen equivalently to DSA. Aneurysms that are seen better by DSA include those arising from the ICAs proximal to the ophthalmic arteries since adjacent bone can obscure the vessel on CTA. Also, mycotic aneurysms may be missed by CTA if they are not included in the imaging volume or involve small branches.

One advantage of CTA is that the aneurysm neck size and configuration can be accurately measured. Thus, the decision to surgically clip or endovascularly coil can be made in most situations. The need to reconstruct the parent vessel in the case of a broad-necked aneurysm is also suggested. CTA depicts calcified or partially thrombosed aneurysms. Calcification can be difficult to treat surgically. Thrombus within an aneurysm increases the risk of stroke or coil settling resulting

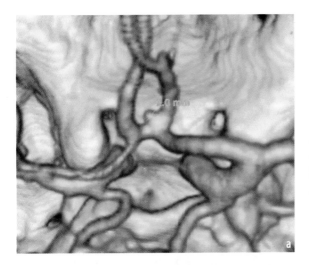

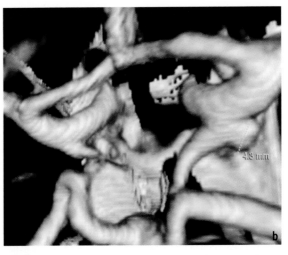

Fig. 15. Anterior communicating artery aneurysm. A small, 2-mm anterior communicating artery aneurysm is well visualized in this patient with prior subarachnoid hemorrhage (SAH) and "negative" cerebral angiography. By opacifying both anterior cerebral arteries simultaneously, the anterior communicating artery is typically seen better than by conventional angiography. Size and contours of the aneurysm are also well depicted

Fig. 16. Posterior communicating artery aneurysm. There is a 4-mm posterior communicating artery aneurysm in this patient who has a prominent associated posterior communicating artery. Note that the aneurysm neck is well seen, as is the contralateral infundibulum

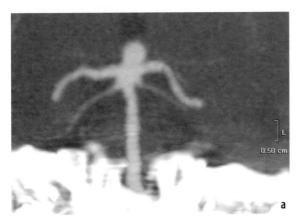

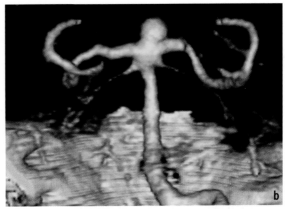

Fig. 17a, b. Basilar artery aneurysm. **a** Coronal maximum intensity projection (MIP) demonstrates the basilar tip aneurysm and relation to the posterior cerebral arteries with relatively broad neck configuration. **b** The three-dimensional (3-D) image gives better perspective of the aneurysm configuration

in incomplete treatment. Cases of endovascular stenting as an adjunct to coiling are also suggested.

An aneurysm may be detected incidentally in many cases where neuroimaging is performed. In the patient without SAH, finding an aneurysm presents a dilemma. Are the risks of rupture high enough to indicate treatment or should the aneurysm be followed medically? The International Study of Unruptured Intracranial Aneurysms (ISUIA) suggested that the risk of rupturing an aneurysm less than 10 mm is very low [22]. Many patients with incidental aneurysms are followed noninvasively to assess for interval change since a growing aneurysm is at higher risk for rupture.

CTA provides an accurate means to measure and compare sequential exams.

Arteriovenous malformations (AVM)

The detection of AVMs is usually made by means other than CTA. In the case of ruptured AVM, brain CT without contrast demonstrates SAH, usually with parenchymal hematoma around the AVM. If the AVM is not ruptured, increased density or calcification at the AVM site is common and may be seen on noncontrasted CT. MRI shows flow voids, mixed signal intensity, and possibly hemo-

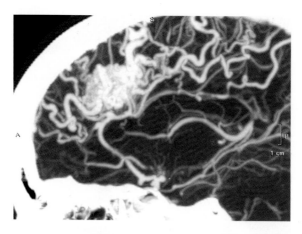

Fig. 18. Arteriovenous malformation (AVM). Sagittal maximum intensity projection (MIP) image demonstrates a 30cm AVM in the frontal lobe. Note the complex superficial venous drainage pattern. Aneurysms are also present in the distal internal carotid artery (ICA) posteriorly and the anterior communicating artery

siderin at the AVM. Conventional angiography is the procedure of choice for diagnosis since it demonstrates the relative flow in the feeding arteries, including dominant and lesser branches, and the nidus configuration. Most importantly, the venous drainage, including any venous constriction, is seen. CTA can be used to evaluate AVMs; however, the scan volume obviously needs to include the AVM and its feeding and draining vessels. The nidus is well depicted, which may be of benefit for radiosurgery planning. Associated flow-related aneurysms are well seen. However, it is difficult to see all the feeding arteries and to represent the relative flow in each branch (Fig. 18).

CT Venography of the Brain

CTV is a variation of CTA whereby the area of interest is the venous drainage rather than the arterial supply to the brain. As such, the timing reflects the transit time of blood to fill the venous system.

CTV Protocol

The entire head is included, using a 22-cm field of view with craniocaudal scanning using thin slices. For a 16-slice scanner, a pitch over 1 can be used with rotation time of 0.7 s. Tube load in the 320-mA range for 120 kVp with noise index of 5 provides excellent image quality. Image reconstruction at 2.5 mm or 1.25 mm is suggested. At the workstation, CTV is evaluated somewhat differently than CTA. The axial images provide the most information while reformatted data depicts the venous sinuses well. The 3-D images are sliced to

look at the vertex and then the posterior head as an adjunct to the 2-D images.

Congenital Variants

The right transverse and sigmoid sinus are dominant in 50–75% of patients. Consequently, seeing a small left-venous sinus is common. Typically, the transverse sinus is smaller, and the sigmoid is a little larger due to inflow from the vein of Labbe and posterior fossa veins. The true size of the sigmoid sinus is easy to determine since the bony defect of the vein coincides with the vein on the CT source images.

The ability of CTV to show a hypoplastic sinus is one of its principal advantages over MR venography (MRV). Frequently, small low-density defects are visualized in the major venous sinuses. These represent arachnoid granulations where CSF is resorbed. MRV may mistakenly portray these defects as nonobstructive thrombus.

The significance of sinus stenosis is uncertain. If the sinuses connect, then compromise of one sinus is not of consequence. However, sometimes the sagittal sinus or straight sinus drains via only one transverse sinus. In these circumstances, severe sinus stenosis could be symptomatic [23]. Restriction of venous outflow inherently increases intracranial pressure, but the degree and nature of compensation is unknown. It has been postulated that there is an association with pseudotumor cerebri; however, the nature of this link and the contribution of other factors, such as the demographic association of an obese woman of childbearing age, is unknown.

Venous Thrombosis

Contrast-filled venous sinuses are commonly seen in almost every CTA and contrast-enhanced brain CT. By adjusting the window and level to see the contrast-filled veins, the entire venous system can be readily traced. Thrombosis represents a filling defect within the sinus and is readily evaluated [24] (Fig. 19). As a consequence of the venous obstruction, collateral veins along the sinus may be seen. As the thrombosis matures, the clot becomes adherent and synechia are seen. While thrombosis is demonstrated superiorly by CTV over MRV, MRI is better than CT at looking at the sequelae of the thrombosis. This includes venous infarction and cerebral edema. Hemorrhage, which is common with venous infarction, can be seen with both modalities.

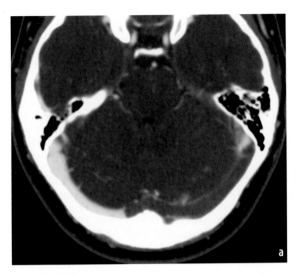
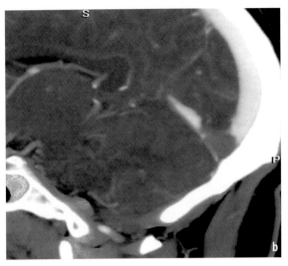

Fig. 19a, b. Venous thrombosis. **a** Axial image demonstrates a large filling defect of the left transverse sinus involving the torcula. This indicates acute thrombosis. **b** Sagittal maximum intensity projection (MIP) image demonstrates thrombus within the torcula. The posterior superior sagittal sinus and the straight sinus are widely patent and opacify with contrast

Summary

CTA provides an excellent method of evaluating the vasculature of the neck and brain. Technical improvements in MDCT and the improvement in workstation software provide for accurate diagnosis in a timely manner. In many cases, this currently replaces conventional angiography. The evaluation of carotid stenosis; trauma to the neck; and detection of cerebral stenosis, aneurysm, and thrombosis are but some of the growing indications for the routine utilization of CTA.

References

1. Heinz ER, Fuchs J, Osborne D et al (1984) Examination of the extracranial carotid bifurcation by thin-section dynamic CT: direct visualization of intimal atheroma in man (Part 2). AJNR Am J Neuroradiol 5(4):361-366
2. Heinz ER, Pizer SM, Fuchs H et al (1984) Examination of the extracranial carotid bifurcation by thin-section dynamic CT: direct visualization of intimal atheroma in man (Part 1). AJNR Am J Neuroradiol 5(4):355-359
3. Enterline D, Lowry CR, Tanenbaum LN (2005) Brain, and head and neck applications. In: Multidetector CT protocols developed for GE scanners. BDI, Princeton, pp E1-57
4. North American Symptomatic Carotid Endarterectomy Trial Collaborators (1991) Beneficial effect of carotid endarterectomy in symptomatic patients with high-grade carotid stenosis. N Engl J Med 325:445-453
5. Barnett HJ, Taylor DW, Eliasziw M et al for the North American Symptomatic Carotid Endarterectomy Trial Collaborators (1998) Benefit of carotid endarterectomy in patients with symptomatic moderate or severe stenosis. N Engl J Med 12:339(20):1415-1425
6. European Carotid Surgery Trialists' Collaborative Group (1991) MRC European carotid surgery trial: interim results for symptomatic patients with severe (70–99%) or with mild (0–29%) carotid stenosis. Lancet 337:1235-1243
7. Hobson RW 2nd, Weiss DG, Fields WS et al (1993) The Veterans Affairs Cooperative Study Group. Efficacy of carotid endarterectomy for asymptomatic carotid stenosis. N Engl J Med 28:328(4):221-227
8. CASANOVA Study Group (1991) Carotid surgery versus medical therapy in asymptomatic carotid stenosis. Stroke 22(10):1229-1235
9. Executive Committee for the Asymptomatic Carotid Atherosclerosis Study (1995) Endarterectomy for asymptomatic carotid artery stenosis. JAMA 273:1421-1428
10. Halliday A, Mansfield A, Marro J et al for the MRC asymptomatic carotid surgery trial (ACST) collaborative group (2004) Prevention of disabling and fatal strokes by successful carotid endarterectomy in patients without recent neurological symptoms: randomized controlled trial. Lancet 363:1491-1502
11. Johnston DCC, Goldstein LB (2001) Clinical carotid endarterectomy decision making: Noninvasive vascular imaging versus angiography. Neurology 56:1009-1015
12. Patel SG, Collie DA, Wardlaw JM et al (2002) Outcome, observer reliability, and patient preferences if CTA, MRA, or Doppler ultrasound were used, individually or together, instead of digital subtraction angiography before carotid endarterectomy. J Neurol Neurosurg Psychiatry 73(1):21-28
13. Randoux B, Marro B, Koskas F et al (2001) Carotid artery stenosis: prospective comparison of CT, three-dimensional gadolinium-enhanced MR, and conventional angiography. Radiology 220(1):179-185
14. Berne JD, Norwood SH, McAuley CE, Villareal DH (2004) Helical computed tomographic angiography: an excellent screening test for blunt cerebrovascular

injury. J Trauma 57(1):11-17

15. Bash S, Villablanca JP, Jahan R et al (2005) Intracranial vascular stenosis and occlusive disease: evaluation with CT angiography, MR angiography, and digital subtraction angiography. AJNR Am J Neuroradiol 26(5):1012-1021

16. Goldsher D, Shreiber R, Shik V (2004) Role of multisection CT angiography in the evaluation of vertebrobasilar vasospasm in patients with subarachnoid hemorrhage. AJNR Am J Neuroradiol 25(9):1493-1498

17. Dammert S, Krings T, Moller-Hartmann W (2004) Detection of intracranial aneurysms with multislice CT: comparison with conventional angiography. Neuroradiology 46(6):427-434

18. Hoh BL, Cheung AC, Rabinov JD (2004) Results of a prospective protocol of computed tomographic angiography in place of catheter angiography as the only diagnostic and pretreatment planning study for cerebral aneurysms by a combined neurovascular team. Neurosurgery 54(6):1329-1340

19. Kangasniemi M, Makela T, Koskinen S et al (2004) Detection of intracranial aneurysms with two-dimensional and three-dimensional multislice helical computed tomographic angiography. Neurosurgery 54(2):336-340

20. Karamessini MT, Kagadis GC, Petsas T et al (2004) CT angiography with three-dimensional techniques for the early diagnosis of intracranial aneurysms. Comparison with intra-arterial DSA and the surgical findings. Eur J Radiol 49(3):212-223

21. White PM, Teasdale EM, Wardlaw JM, Easton V (2001) Intracranial aneurysms: CT angiography and MR angiography for detection prospective blinded comparison in a large patient cohort. Radiology 219(3):739-749

22. International Study of Unruptured Intracranial Aneurysms Investigators (1998) Unruptured intracranial aneurysms: risk of rupture and risks of surgical intervention. N Engl J Med 339:1725–1733

23. Rajpal S, Niemann DB, Turk AS (2005) Transverse venous sinus stent placement as treatment for benign intracranial hypertension in a young male: case report and review of the literature. J Neurosurg 102 [Suppl 3]:342-346

24. Casey SO, Alberico RA, Patel M et al (1996) Cerebral CT venography. Radiology 198:163-170

IV.2

MDCT Perfusion in Acute Stroke

Sanjay K. Shetty and Michael H. Lev

Introduction

Acute cerebrovascular stroke ranks amongst the foremost causes of morbidity and mortality in the world [1]. In acute settings, the rapid evaluation of acute stroke is invaluable due to the ability to treat patients with thrombolytics. In addition to anatomic information about the acute stroke, state-of-the-art radiologic techniques can also provide critical information about capillary-level hemodynamics and the brain parenchyma. Computed tomography perfusion (CTP) provides this information and can help in understanding the pathophysiology of stroke [2–5]. CTP helps the physician to identify critically ischemic or irreversibly infarcted tissue ("core") and to identify severely ischemic but potentially salvageable tissue ("penumbra"). This information can guide triage and management in acute stroke.

Overall application of CT and magnetic resonance (MR) perfusion techniques and estimation of cerebral perfusion parameters such as cerebral blood flow (CBF), cerebral blood volume (CBV), and mean transit time (MTT) are similar for both MR imaging (MRI) and CT. However, faster imaging time, affordability, and wider availability of CT technology in the acute setting makes the combination of CT angiography (CTA) and CTP a potential surrogate marker of stroke severity, likely exceeding the National Institutes of Health Stroke Scale (NIHSS) or the Alberta Stroke Program Early CT Score (ASPECTS) as a predictor of outcome [6–14].

CTP: Scanning Technique

Scanning protocol for acute stroke must facilitate patient triage. At Massachusetts General Hospital, the scanning protocol for acute stroke has the following three parts: the noncontrast CT; CTA from aortic arch to vertex; and dynamic, first-pass, cine CTP (Table 1). The noncontrast CT excludes hemorrhage prior to thrombolysis [15] and can reveal a large territory infarction [such as a hypodensity occupying greater than one third of the middle cerebral artery (MCA) territory], which is also considered to be a contraindication to thrombolysis [16].

The CTA component of acute stroke protocol provides information about important vessels of the head and neck and generates source images (CTA-SI), which serve as relevant data for tissue level perfusion. According to theoretical perfusion models, the CTA-SI data are predominantly blood-volume rather than blood-flow weighted [17–19]. As this perfused blood volume technique requires the assumption of an approximately steady-state level of contrast media during the period of image acquisition [18], our CTA protocols use a biphasic contrast injection to attain a better approximation of the steady state [20, 21].

Finally, for dynamic, quantitative CTP, an additional bolus of contrast is administered (at a rate of 4–7 ml/s) during continuous cine imaging over a single region of the brain. In order to track the "first pass" of the contrast bolus through the intracranial vasculature without recirculation effects, images over 45–60 s are acquired. The coverage volume of each acquisition depends on the vendor and type of the multidetector CT (MDCT) scanner. We use two contrast boluses to acquire two slabs of CTP data at different locations to increase overall Z-axis coverage [22]. Appropriate scanning planes allow multiple vascular territories to be assessed [3, 23, 24]. It is important to include a major intracranial artery in at least one image slice in each acquisition for CTP map reconstruction (Fig. 1). In this respect, the previously acquired CTA data allows one to target the tissue of interest with the CTP, which is important given the relatively restricted Z-axis coverage obtained even

Table 1. Sample acute stroke computed tomography (CT) protocol employed at the authors' institution, incorporating CT angiography (CTA) and CT perfusion (CTP). The protocol is designed to answer the four basic questions necessary for stroke triage described. Note the alteration in the kilovolt peak (kVp) for perfusion acquisition. Parameters are presented for illustrative purposes and have been optimized for the scanner currently employed (General Electric Healthcare Lightspeed 16) in our emergency department. Parameters should be optimized for each scanner

Scan series	Unenhanced	CTA head	CTA neck	Cine perfusion ×2
Contrast		Biphasic contrast injection: 2.5 cc/s for 50 cc, then 1.0 cc/s for 20 cc		7 cc/sec for 40 cc for each CTP acquisition
Scan delay		Delay: 25 s (35 s if poor cardiac output, including atrial fibrillation)		Delay: 5 s (each series is a 60-s cine acquisition)
Range	C1 to vertex	C1 to vertex	Arch to C1	Two CTP slabs
Slice thickness	5 mm	2.5 mm	2.5 mm	5 mm
Image spacing	5mm	2.5 mm	2.5 mm	N/A
Table feed	5.62 mm	5.62 mm	5.62 mm	N/A
Detectors configuration (mm)	16×0.625	16×0.625	16×0.625	16×1.25
Pitch	0.562:1	0.562:1	0.562:1	N/A
Mode	Helical	Helical	Helical	Cine 4i
kVp	140	140	140	80
mA	220	200	250	200
Rotation time	0.5 s	0.5 s	0.5 s	1 s
Scan FOV	Head	Head	Large	Head
Retrospective slice thickness/interval	None	1.25/0.625 mm	1.25/1.0 mm	None

Standard reconstruction algorithm is used for all image reconstruction
CTA computed tomography angiography, *CTP* computed tomography perfusion, *kVp* kilovolt peak, *mA* milliampere, *FOV* field of view

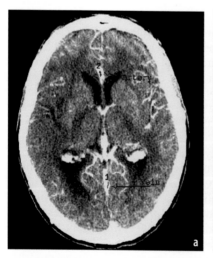
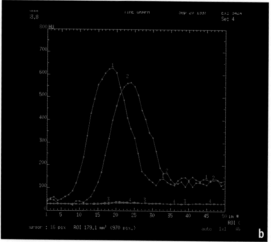

Fig. 1a, b. Computed tomography perfusion (CTP) postprocessing. Appropriate region of interest (ROI) placement on an artery (a major vessel running perpendicular to the plane of section to avoid volume averaging) and on a vein (also running perpendicular to the plane of section and placed to avoid the inner table of the skull) (**a**). The time density curves (TDC) generated from this artery (*A*) and vein (*V*) show the arrival, peak, and passage of the contrast bolus over time (**b**). These TDCs serve as the arterial input function (AIF) and the venous output for the subsequent deconvolution step with two CTP acquisitions. To keep the total iodine dose for acute stroke protocol within reasonable limits, the contrast bolus for the CTA is restricted to allow two 40-cc boluses for the CTP acquisition.

It is also important to bear in mind that there is considerable variability in CTP scanning protocols, as this technique has only recently gained acceptance as a clinical tool and because construction of perfusion maps depends on the particular mathematical model used to analyze the dynamic, contrast-enhanced data. Algorithm-dependent differences in contrast injection rates exist, and, regardless of injection rate, higher contrast concentrations are likely to produce maps with improved signal-to-noise ratios [25].

CTP: Comparison with Perfusion-Weighted MR (MR-PWI)

CTP has several advantages and disadvantages compared with perfusion-weighted MR (MR-PWI). Wider availability and easy, rapid scanning in seriously ill patients with monitors or ventilators make CTP a feasible option. Furthermore, in patients with absolute contraindication to MR, CT may be the only option. Although capillary-level hemodynamics can be assessed with both MR-PWI and CTP, there are several important distinctions between these two techniques (Table 2, Fig. 2). Dynamic susceptibility contrast MR-PWI techniques depend on induction of the indirect T2* effect in adjacent tissues by high concentrations of gadolinium. Thus, MR-PWI may have more "contamination" from large vascular structures and is also limited in certain regions of brain because of susceptibility effects from adjacent structures. On the other hand, CTP depends on direct visualization of the contrast medium. As there is a linear relationship between attenuation and contrast concentration in CT, CTP readily allows quantitation. This is not possible with MR-PWI.

Another advantage of CTP is that CT has greater spatial resolution than MRI. Thus, visual evaluation of core/penumbra mismatch may be more reliable with CTP than with MR-PWI [26, 27].

Conversely, there are notable disadvantages of CTP when compared with MR-PWI. These include limited Z-axis coverage and more labor-intensive postprocessing of CTA and CTP data sets. Another limitation of our CTP protocol is the use of a large amount of contrast material, which may be particularly problematic in older patients, who are most likely to be undergoing evaluation for acute stroke. Several studies have highlighted the issue of radiation risk inherent to CT [3, 28].

CTP: Fundamentals

CTP and MR-PWI evaluate capillary, tissue-level circulation, which is beyond the resolution of traditional anatomic imaging and provides valuable information about blood flow to the brain parenchyma [29]. Cerebral blood flow can be assessed using various parameters, which include CBF, CBV, and MTT. For accurate analysis of CTP maps, it is important to understand associations between these perfusion parameters, as cerebral perfusion pressure drops in acute stroke. CBV is the total blood volume in a given unit volume of the brain, which includes blood in the tissues and blood in the larger vessels such as arteries, arterioles, capillaries, venules, and veins. CBV is measured as units of milliliters of blood per 100 g of cerebral tissue (ml/100 g). CBF is the blood volume moving through a given unit volume of brain per unit time. CBF is measured in units of milliliters of blood per 100 g of brain tissue per minute. MTT is the mean of the transit time of blood through a given region of the brain, which depends on the distance traveled between arterial inflow and venous outflow. MTT is related to both CBV and CBF according to the central volume principle, which

Table 2. Advantages and disadvantages of computed tomography perfusion (CTP) relative to magnetic resonance (MR) perfusion-weighted imaging (PWI)

Advantages	Disadvantages
• Wider availability of CT with lower cost	• Associated radiation dose
• Improved resolution with quantitative perfusion information	• Risks and complications of iodine-based contrast
• Rapid acquisition	• Limited scan coverage
• Easier monitoring and intervention in critical patients	• More complex data postprocessing
• Possible in patients with pacemakers or other contraindications to MR or in patients who cannot be screened for MR safety	

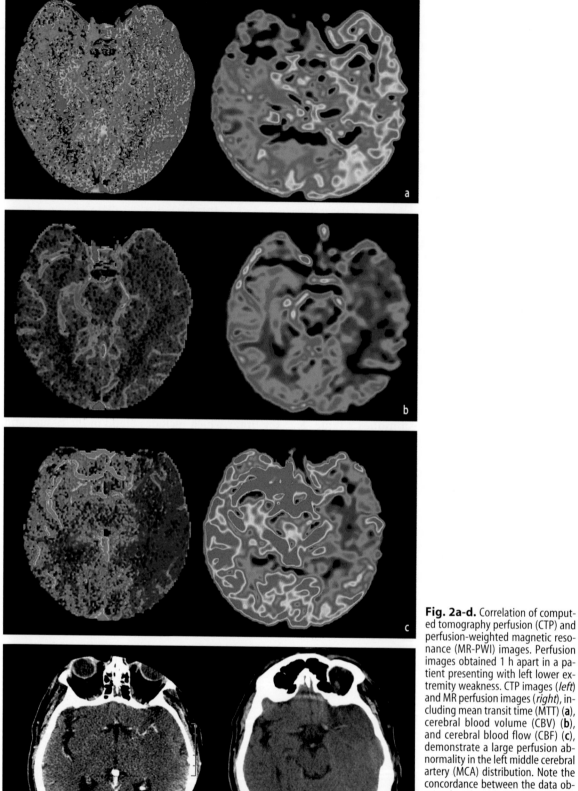

Fig. 2a-d. Correlation of computed tomography perfusion (CTP) and perfusion-weighted magnetic resonance (MR-PWI) images. Perfusion images obtained 1 h apart in a patient presenting with left lower extremity weakness. CTP images (*left*) and MR perfusion images (*right*), including mean transit time (MTT) (**a**), cerebral blood volume (CBV) (**b**), and cerebral blood flow (CBF) (**c**), demonstrate a large perfusion abnormality in the left middle cerebral artery (MCA) distribution. Note the concordance between the data obtained with each modality. Corresponding computed tomography angiography source images (CTA-SI) (*left*) and subsequent unenhanced CT are also shown, revealing an infarct in the left MCA distribution (**d**)

states that MTT=CBV/CBF [30, 31].

The CTP parameters of CBV, CBF, and MTT can be difficult to quantify in practice. The dynamic, first-pass, CTP approach is performed with the dynamic intravenous administration of contrast agent, which is tracked with serial scanning during its first-pass circulation through the capillary bed of brain tissue. Depending on the assumptions regarding the arterial inflow and the venous outflow of the contrast agent, CBV, CBF, and MTT can then be calculated. Dynamic, first-pass CTP models assume that the agent used for perfusion measurement is *nondiffusible* (neither absorbed nor metabolized) in the tissue bed through which it traverses. Therefore, "contrast leakage" outside of the intravascular space in cases of blood brain barrier breakdown associated with tumor, infection, or inflammation, requires a more complex model for calculations. The two major mathematical models used for calculating CTP parameters include deconvolution based and nondeconvolution-based methods.

Nondeconvolution-based CTP models depend on the application of the *Fick principle* to a given region of interest (ROI) within the cerebral parenchyma. A time-density curve (TDC) is derived for each pixel, and CBF is calculated based on the concept of conservation of flow. This calculation is dependent on the assumptions made regarding blood inflow and outflow to the brain region. Although common models simplify the calculations by assuming that there is no venous outflow, these models necessitate high injection rates. CBV can be estimated as the area under the "fitted" tissue TDC divided by the area under the fitted arterial TDC [17]. This equation forms the basis for the quantitative estimation of CBV using the "whole-brain perfused blood volume" when it is assumed that there is a steady state of contrast concentration in the arteries and capillaries [18, 19]: CBV is a function of the density of tissue contrast, normalized by the density of arterial contrast, after soft tissue components have been removed by coregistration and subtraction of the noncontrast scan.

Deconvolution models to estimate CTP parameters have also been validated in a number of studies [32–40]. These methods allow direct computation of CBF, which is applicable for even relatively slow injection rates [41] and compensates for inability to deliver a complete, instantaneous contrast bolus into the artery supplying a given region of brain. Indeed, a contrast bolus (especially one that is given via a peripheral vein) does undergo delay and dispersion before arriving in the cerebral circulation. With the deconvolution model, correct CBV and CBF are estimated by calculating the *residue function*. CBF is calculated directly as proportional to the maximum *height* of the scaled residue function curve. CBV is represented as the *area* under the scaled residue function curve. Once CBF and CBV are estimated, MTT is calculated using the central volume principle.

Potential imaging pitfalls in the calculation of CBF with the deconvolution model include partial volume averaging as well as patient motion, which can lead to underestimation of the arterial input function (AIF). To minimize errors in CTP parameters due to these pitfalls, image coregistration software programs can be used to correct for patient motion and to carefully select ROIs for the AIF. Comparison with the contralateral (normal) side to establish a percentage change from normal can also be a useful adjunctive technique, particularly since the reliability of quantitative CTP parameters is in the range of 20–25%.

In general, nondeconvolution models are more sensitive to changes in underlying vascular anatomy than the deconvolution models. The reason is that nondeconvolution cerebral CTP models assume that a single feeding artery and a single draining vein supports blood circulation in a given area, and that the precise arterial, venous, and tissue TDC can be uniquely identified by imaging. This assumption is an oversimplification of cerebral circulation. In fact, a delay correction is present in most available CTP processing software, so that this oversimplification is less of a concern in CTP.

CTP: Data Postprocessing

In emergent cases, CTP can allow immediate detection of perfusion changes by direct visual inspection of the axial source images at the user interface. Review of CTP data set at an image workstation using a "movie" or cine mode can provide information about relative perfusion changes over time. However, detection of subtle perfusion changes requires advanced postprocessing and quantification. To accomplish this, source CTP images are usually networked to a freestanding workstation for computation of quantitative, first-pass, cine cerebral perfusion maps. Users are generally required to input some information for quantification purposes (Fig. 1), which include:

- *Arterial Input ROI*: A small ROI is placed over the central portion of a large intracranial artery (with maximal peak contrast intensity), preferably orthogonal to the image acquisition plane so that partial volume averaging can be minimized. It is critical to ensure that the image acquisition slab for CTP contains a major intracranial artery to generate the AIF. Some programs allow ROI selection in a semiautomated manner.
- *Venous Outflow ROI*: In addition to an arterial

ROI, a small venous ROI with similar attributes is also selected, most commonly at the superior sagittal sinus. For certain programs, appropriate venous ROI are crucial for accurate CTP maps [42].

Major variations in the aforementioned input values may cause variation in the image quality of CTP maps as well as variation in the CBF, CBV, and MTT.

CTP: Clinical Indications and Applications

Advanced "functional" imaging of acute stroke in the first 12 h can include the following [42]:

- Inclusion of cases most likely to benefit from thrombolysis
- Exclusion of cases most likely to hemorrhage
- Extension of the time window beyond 3 h for intravenous thrombolysis and 6 h for anterior circulation intra-arterial thrombolysis
- Triage to other available therapies, such as hypertension or hyperoxia
- Appropriate treatment of "wake-up" strokes, for which precise time of onset is unknown
- Management decisions regarding admission to neurological intensive care unit or discharge from emergency department

The Desmoteplase in Acute Ischemic Stroke (DIAS) trial suggests that intravenous desmoteplase can be used in an extended therapeutic window of 3–9 h postictus, with substantial improvements in reperfusion rates and clinical outcomes achieved in patients with a diffusion/perfusion mismatch on MRI [43]. On the basis of this study and other ongoing studies, some investigators have cautiously proposed the use of either MR-PWI or CTP for extending the traditional therapeutic time window [44, 45]. These authors cite evidence of a relevant volume of salvageable cerebral tissue present in the 3- to 6-h time frame in more than 80% of acute stroke patients [43, 46, 47].

CTP: Infarct Detection

Several studies have opined that CTA-SI, like diffusion-weighted MRI, can detect tissue destined to infarct despite successful recanalization [11, 48, 49]. In theory, if an approximately steady state of contrast in the cerebral arteries and parenchyma during image acquisition is assumed, CTA-SI are predominantly blood-volume rather than blood-flow weighted [17–19, 50]. An early report suggested that CTA-SI can be used to delineate minimal final infarct size and to identify "infarct core" in an acute stroke [48]. CTA-SI subtraction maps, ob-

tained by commercially available platforms for coregistration and subtraction of the noncontrast head CT from the CTA source images, can provide information about quantitative blood-volume maps of the entire brain [3, 18, 19]. As these maps cover the entire brain, they are especially appealing for clinical use. An exploratory study in patients with MCA stem occlusion who underwent intra-arterial thrombolysis after imaging revealed that CTA-SI and CTA-SI subtraction maps improve conspicuity of cerebral infarct when compared with nonenhanced CT in hyperacute stroke.

In another study, CTA-SI preceding diffusion-weighted MRI was performed in patients with clinically suspected acute stroke presenting within 12 h of symptom onset (42 patients were scanned within 6 h) [11]. The authors reported that CTA-SI and diffusion-weighted imaging (DWI) lesion volumes were independent predictors of final infarct volume, and overall sensitivity and specificity for parenchymal stroke detection were 76% and 90% for CTA-SI, and 100% and 100% for diffusion-weighted imaging, respectively. Although diffusion-weighted imaging is more sensitive than CTA-SI for detection of small lacunar and distal infarcts, both diffusion-weighted imaging techniques are highly accurate predictors of final infarct volume. It is important to remember that, like diffusion-weighted imaging, not every acute hypodense ischemic lesion seen with CTA-SI is destined to infarct [51, 52] (Fig. 3). In the presence of early complete recanalization, CTA-SI can show occasional dramatic sparing of regions with reduced blood pool.

CTP maps can also improve detection of acute infarct, improving both sensitivity (MTT maps) and specificity (relative CBF and relative CBV maps) for the detection of infarct relative to noncontrast CT images [53] (Fig. 4). These maps are also more accurate for determining the extent of infarct, especially for the percentage of MCA territory infarct [53]. A prior study has shown that the relative CBV (rCBV) map correlated better with final infarct volume than admission diffusion-weighted imaging [54].

CTP: Interpretation of Penumbra and Core

Advanced stroke imaging in acute settings must allow for evaluation of the viability of ischemic tissue that transcends an arbitrary "clock time" [55–57]. Two thresholds from prior experimental studies gave rise to the original theory of penumbra [58, 59]. One threshold defined a specific CBF value below which there was no cortical function, without extracellular potassium increment or pH

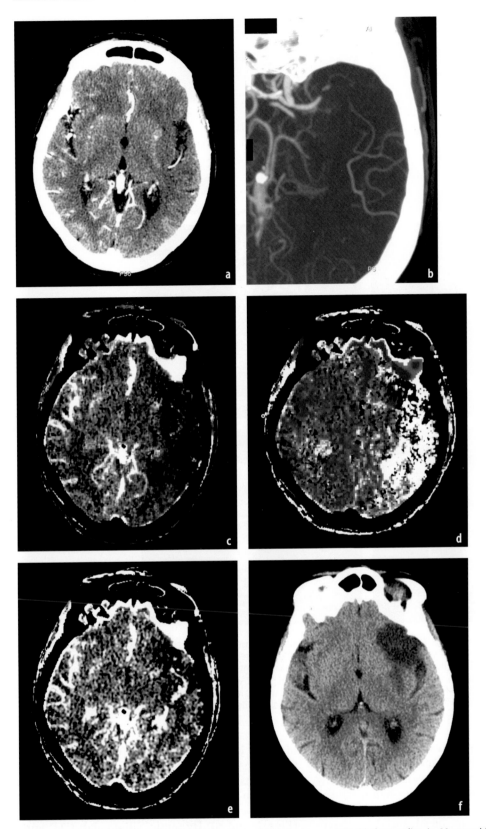

Fig. 3a-f. Reversal of computed tomography angiography source images (CTA-SI) abnormality. An 80-year-old woman presented with a devastating exam. CTA-SI initially demonstrated a large area of hypodensity in the left middle cerebral artery (MCA) distribution (**a**). CTA shows occlusion of the distal left internal carotid artery (ICA) and the entire left middle cerebral artery (MCA) (**b**). CT perfusion (CTP) images obtained at the same time, including cerebral blood flow (CBF) (**c**), mean transit time (MTT) (**d**), and cerebral blood volume (CBV) (**e**), show a large CBF/MTT abnormality involving nearly the entire left MCA territory while the CBV shows only a small area of abnormality anteriorly. After successful intra-arterial thrombolysis, subsequent unenhanced CT shows that the infarct is confined to the initial CBV abnormality (**f**). Although the CTA-SI abnormality characteristically predicts infarct, this case demonstrates the unusual possibility of a reversal of the CTA-SI abnormality. The final infarct volume was better predicted by the initial CBV map

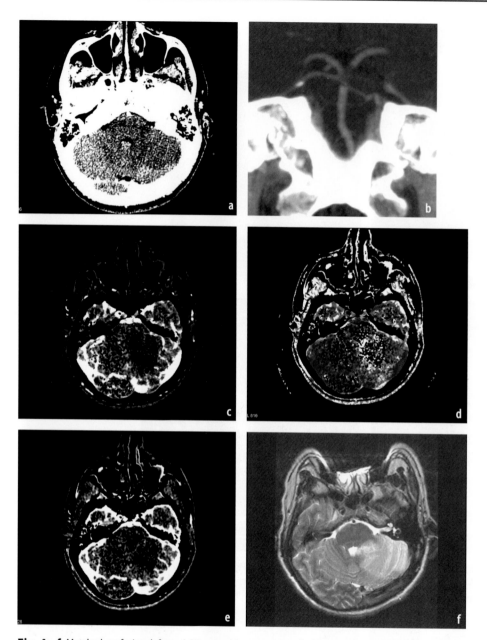

Fig. 4a-f. Matched-perfusion defects. A 36-year-old man presented with acute onset ataxia. Computed tomography angiography source images (CTA-SI) demonstrates an infarct in the left cerebellar hemisphere (**a**). CTA reformat shows thrombus at the basilar tip (**b**). Concurrent CT perfusion (CTP) images, including cerebral blood flow (CBF) (**c**), mean transit time (MTT) (**d**), and cerebral blood volume (CBV) (**e**), show no evidence of a perfusion mismatch to suggest additional territory at risk. T2-weighted magnetic resonance (MR) image obtained 5 days later show an infarct in the left superior cerebellar artery distribution, with no interval expansion of the infarct territory as predicted by the matched perfusion defect initially (**f**). Note that MR perfusion is typically limited in the posterior fossa due to susceptibility artifact

reduction. The second threshold defined a CBF value below which cellular integrity was disrupted. Subsequently, a clinically relevant "operationally defined penumbra," which defines hypoperfused but potentially salvageable tissue, has gained acceptance with emergence of advanced cross-sectional imaging techniques and modern stroke therapy protocols [55, 59–61].

"Ischemic penumbra" can be defined as ischemic but still viable tissue. The operationally defined penumbra may be described as the volume

of tissue in the region of CBF/CBV mismatch on CTP maps, where the region of CBV abnormality represents the infarct tissue core and the CBF/CBV mismatch identifies the surrounding region of hypoperfused tissue that is potentially salvageable (Figs. 5 and 6). Dynamic, single-slab CTP with quantitative maps of CBF, CBV, and MTT can describe regions of ischemic penumbra.

Prior human and animal studies with MRI, positron emission tomography (PET), single photon emission tomography (SPECT), and xenon,

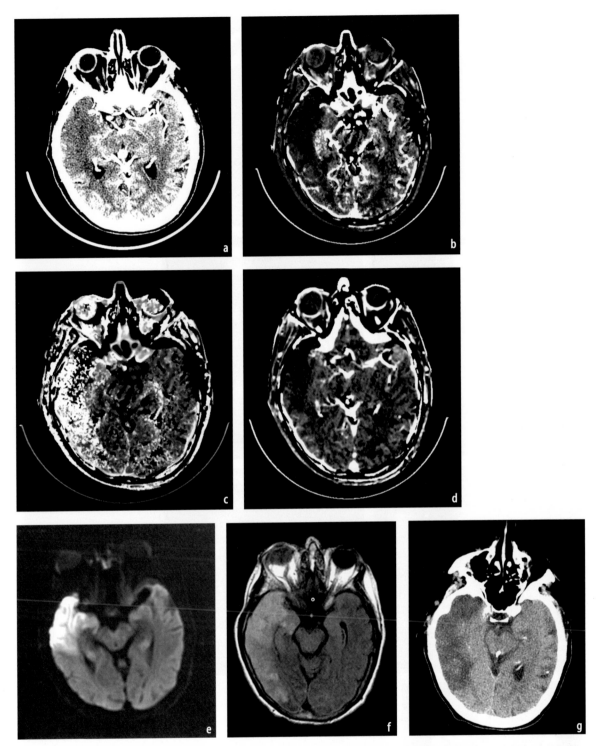

Fig. 5a-g. Expansion of infarct into territory at risk. A 77-year-old woman presented with acute left-sided weakness. Initial computed tomography angiography source images (CTA-SI) performed several hours postictus demonstrates an area of infarct in the anterior right temporal lobe (**a**). CT perfusion (CTP) images obtained concurrently, including cerebral blood flow (CBF) (**b**), mean transit time (MTT) (**c**), and cerebral blood volume (CBV) (**d**) show an area of mismatch posteriorly within the right temporal lobe. Note that the initial infarct corresponds to the CBV abnormality. Diffusion-weighted image (DWI) obtained 30 min later confirms that the infarct is limited to the area seen on CTA-SI and CBV (**e**). Therapy was withheld because of suspected hemorrhage in the cerebellum (not shown). Subsequent magnetic resonance MR (2 days later) (**f**) and CT (5 days later) (**g**) reveal expansion of the infarct into the region at risk as predicted on the initial CTP

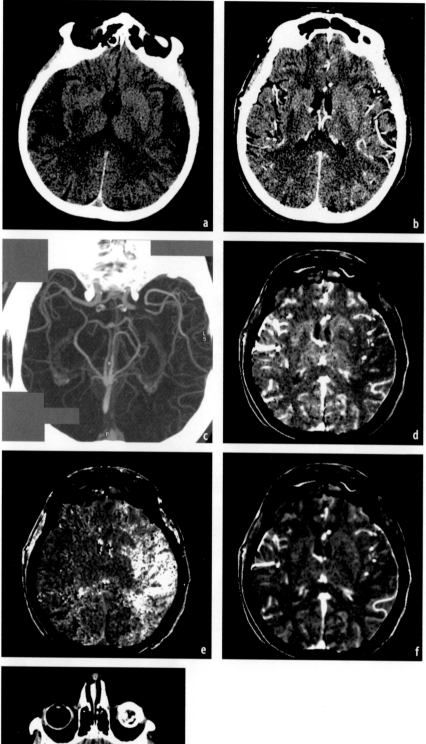

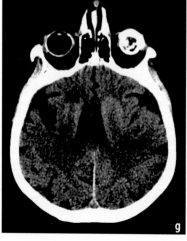

Fig. 6a-g. Successful therapy to preserve territory at risk. A 76-year-old woman presented with acute onset weakness and dysphasia. Computed tomography (CT) (**a**) and CT angiography source images (CTA-SI) (**b**) show no evidence of infarct while CTA reformat shows nonocclusive thrombus in the proximal M1 segment (**c**). Concurrent CT perfusion (CTP), including cerebral blood flow (CBF) (**d**), mean transit time (MTT) (**e**), and cerebral blood volume (CBV) (**f**) show a large area of CBF/CBV mismatch, suggesting territory at risk. The patient underwent intravenous (IV) thrombolysis and an attempt at intra-arterial (IA) mechanical thrombolysis. Unenhanced CT 2 day later shows only small areas of infarct in the posterior left temporal lobe and inferior parietal lobe, in a region much smaller than the territory at risk (**g**). The patient was unable to have a magnetic resonance (MR) image because of a pacemaker

Table 3. Normal values for perfusion parameters in brain tissue (adapted from [80])

CTP	CBF	CBV	MTT
Gray matter	60 ml/100 g per minute	4 ml/100 g	4 s
White matter	25 ml/100 g per minute	2 ml/100 g	4.8 s

CTP computed tomography perfusion, *CBF* cerebral blood flow, *CBV* cerebral blood volume, *MTT* mean transit time

Table 4. Summary of computed tomography perfusion (CTP) interpretation

Small CBV, larger CBF
- Ideal for therapy
- Perfusion mismatch identifies territory at risk
- Consider no treatment if prolonged time postictus

CBV/CBF match
- No territory at risk
- No therapy regardless of lesion size

Large CBV, larger CBF
- Possible therapy based on time postictus, size
- Perfusion mismatch suggests territory at risk
- Consider no therapy if CBV is greater than 100 ml

CBV cerebral blood volume, *CBF* cerebral blood flow

which investigated the role of CTP in acute stroke triage, have assumed predefined threshold values for infarct core and ischemic penumbra and determined the accuracy of these modalities in predicting stroke outcome [22]. An excellent correlation (r=0.946) was noted between diffusion-weighted imaging and CTP-CBF infarct core and the MR-MTT and CT-CBF ischemic penumbra with assumed cutoff values of ≥34% reduction from baseline CTP-CBF for ischemic penumbra and ≤2.5 ml/100 g CTP-CBV for infarct core [22] (refer to Table 3 for normal values).

The interpretation of CTP in acute stroke is summarized in Table 4. CTP-CBF/CBV mismatch correlates significantly with increase in lesion size. Acute stroke patients who are not treated or are unsuccessfully treated and have a large CBF/CBV mismatch exhibit substantial increase in lesion size on follow-up imaging (Fig. 5). However, in patients without substantial mismatch or with early, complete recanalization, progression of their initial CTA-SI lesion volume is not exhibited (Fig. 6). Hence, CBF/CBV mismatch might serve as a marker of salvageable tissue, which can be useful in triaging patients for thrombolysis [62].

Interpretation of CTP-CBV maps can benefit from a semiautomated thresholding approach to segmentation for a more precise definition of the infarct size [27]. More sophisticated probability maps, synthesizing information derived from different CTP parameters, as well as other imaging series may eventually provide a means to facilitate interpretation of CTP, particularly in the acute setting (Fig. 7).

Prior studies with MR perfusion have shown that CBF maps are superior to MTT maps for distinguishing viable from nonviable penumbra, as MTT maps depict circulatory derangements that are not necessarily ischemic changes (such as large-vessel occlusions with compensatory collateralization and reperfusion hyperemia following revascularization) [63–65].

There have been several improvements in the traditional penumbra model. As not all tissue within the operationally defined penumbra is destined to infarct, the operationally defined penumbra is an oversimplified term. Indeed, there is an area of "benign oligemia" in the region of the CTP-CBV/CBF mismatch that is not expected to infarct even in the absence of reperfusion. Thus, refinement of the traditional penumbra model is important from a clinical standpoint, as therapies based on an overestimated "at-risk" tissue volume can be overaggressive and result in higher risks and complications of treatment for tissue that may not have progressed to infarct even without these therapies. Very few studies have addressed this problem using CTP. Prior studies have reported a significant difference between the MR-CBF thresholds for ischemic penumbra likely to infarct and penumbra likely to remain viable [63, 65]. They also suggested a good correlation between MR perfusion and CTP parameters [50, 66–69]. We reported that normalized, or relative, CBF (rCBF) is the most robust

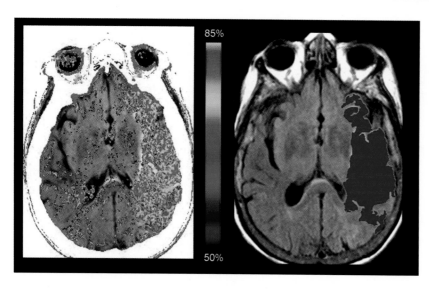

85%

50%

Fig. 7. Probability maps. Scans from a patient who presented to the emergency department with acute stroke symptoms of aphasia and right hemiparesis. The image on the *left* is a probability map constructed from the admission computed tomography angiography source images (CTA-SI) and CT perfusion (CTP) data, with brain regions likely to be irreversibly injured despite successful treatment shown in color. On the *right* is a follow-up magnetic resonance (MR) scan, with the region of the final stroke shown in red. This portends improved methods for visualizing perfusion defects and synthesizing several imaging parameters into a single set of images, facilitating interpretation. (Figure courtesy of Ona Wu, Ph.D.)

CTP parameter for differentiating viable from nonviable penumbra. In general, CTP-CBF penumbra with less than 50% reduction from baseline values has a high probability of survival. Conversely, CTP-CBF penumbra with a greater than two-thirds reduction from baseline values has a high probability of infarction. Furthermore, no region with an average rCBV less than 0.68, absolute CBF less than 12.7 ml/100 g per minute, or absolute CBV less than 2.2 ml/100 g survived. Due to differences in CBV and CBF between gray matter (GM) and white matter (WM) (Table 3), it is important that the contralateral ROI used for normalization have the same GM/WM ratio as the ipsilateral ischemic area under study.

CTP: Relationship with Clinical Outcome

As stated in the prior section, estimation of the penumbra is technically challenging. Depending on the applied techniques, there is substantial variation in CBF thresholds for various states of tissue perfusion among different studies [70]. However, several studies, evaluating heterogeneous cohorts of patients receiving different therapies, have consistently reported that there is a strong correlation between clinical outcome and initial infarct core lesion volume, regardless of the technique used for measuring it (DWI, CT-CBV, subthreshold xenon CT-CBF, or noncontrast CT) [71–75]. One of these studies reported that clinical outcome was influenced by two factors: recanalization at 24 h ($p=0.0001$) and day-0 lesion volume on diffusion-weighted imaging ($p=0.03$) [76]. Likewise, a CTP study in patients with MCA stem occlusions and patients with admission whole-brain CTP lesions volumes greater than 100 ml (about a third of the

volume of the MCA territory) had poor clinical outcomes, irrespective of degree of recanalization [49]. Furthermore, final infarct volume was closely approximated by the lesion size of the initial whole-brain CTP in patients from the same cohort who had early complete MCA recanalization.

In addition to the prediction of clinical outcome from identification of infarct core, CTP, particularly the extent of early CBF reduction in patients with acute stroke, may also help in predicting risk of hemorrhage. Our initial studies indicate that severe hypoperfusion relative to normal cerebral tissue on whole-brain CTP images may also help to localize ischemic regions more likely to have hemorrhage after intra-arterial thrombolysis [77]. Our results are also supported by a recent SPECT study in patients with complete recanalization within 12 h of stoke onset [78]. This study demonstrated that patients with less than 35% of normal blood flow at infarct core had substantially higher risk for hemorrhage [79]. Supportive evidence suggests that cerebral parenchyma with severe ischemia with early reperfusion have the highest risk for hemorrhage [73, 78].

Conclusion

Technologic revolution in MDCT hardware and software has enhanced speed, coverage, and resolution of CTP. CTP has the potential to decrease morbidity of acute stroke. Incorporation of CTP as part of a "one-stop" acute stroke imaging examination is possible with the current MDCT scanners to rapidly and accurately answer the crucial questions related to acute stroke triage. As new treatments are developed for stroke, the potential clinical applications of CTP in the diagnosis, triage, and therapeutic monitoring of these diseases will increase.

References

1. Heart disease and stroke statistics – 2004 update (2003) American Heart Association, 2003, Dallas

2. Lev MH, Farkas J, Rodriguez VR et al (2001) CT angiography in the rapid triage of patients with hyperacute stroke to intraarterial thrombolysis: accuracy in the detection of large vessel thrombus. J Comput Assist Tomogr 25(4):520–528

3. Lev MH, Gonzalez RG (2002) CT Angiography and CT Perfusion Imaging. In: Toga AW, Mazziotta JC (eds) Brain mapping: the methods, 2nd edn. Academic Press, San Diego, pp 427–484

4. Wildermuth S, Knauth M, Brandt T et al (1998) Role of CT angiography in patient selection for thrombolytic therapy in acute hemispheric stroke. Stroke 29(5):935–938

5. Knauth M, vonKummer R, Jansen O et al (1997) Potential of CT angiography in acute ischemic stroke. AJNR Am J Neuroradiol18(6):1001–1010

6. Albers GW (1999) Expanding the window for thrombolytic therapy in acute stroke. The potential role of acute MRI for patient selection. Stroke 30(10):2230–2237

7. Barber PA, Demchuk AM, Zhang J, Buchan AM (2000) Validity and reliability of a quantitative computed tomography score in predicting outcome of hyperacute stroke before thrombolytic therapy. ASPECTS Study Group. Alberta Stroke Programme Early CT Score. Lancet 355(9216):1670–1674

8. Broderick JP, Lu M, Kothari R et al (2000) Finding the most powerful measures of the effectiveness of tissue plasminogen activator in the NINDS tPA stroke trial. Stroke 31(10):2335–2341

9. Schellinger PD, Jansen O, Fiebach JB et al (2000) Monitoring intravenous recombinant tissue plasminogen activator thrombolysis for acute ischemic stroke with diffusion and perfusion MRI. Stroke 31(6):1318–1328

10. Tong D, Yenari M, Albers G et al (1998) Correlation of perfusion- and diffusion-weighted MRI with NIHSS Score in acute (<6.5 hour) ischemic stroke. Neurology 50(4):864–870

11. Berzin T, Lev M, Goodman D et al (2001) CT perfusion imaging versus MR diffusion-weighted imaging: prediction of final infarct size in hyperacute stroke [abstract]. Stroke 32:317

12. Warach S (2001) New imaging strategies for patient selection for thrombolytic and neuroprotective therapies. Neurology 57 [Suppl 2]:48–52

13. Von Kummer R, Holle R, Grzyska U, Hofmann E et al (1996) Interobserver agreement in assessing early CT signs of middle cerebral artery infarction. AJNR Am J Neuroradiol 17:1743–1748

14. Grotta JC, Chiu D, Lu M et al (1999) Agreement and variability in the interpretation of early CT changes in stroke patients qualifying for intravenous rtPA therapy. Stroke 30(8):1528–1533

15. Von Kummer R, Allen KL, Holle R et al (1997) Acute stroke: usefulness of early CT findings before thrombolytic therapy. Radiology 205(2):327–333

16. Von Kummer R (2003) Early major ischemic changes on computed tomography should preclude use of tissue plasminogen activator. Stroke 34(3):820–821

17. Axel L (1980) Cerebral blood flow determination by rapid-sequence computed tomography. Radiology 137:679–686

18. Hunter GJ, Hamberg LM, Ponzo JA et al (1998) Assessment of cerebral perfusion and arterial anatomy in hyperacute stroke with three-dimensional functional CT: Early clinical results. AJNR Am J Neuroradiol 19:29–37

19. Hamberg LM, Hunter GJ, Kierstead D et al (1996) Measurement of cerebral blood volume with subtraction three-dimensional functional CT. AJNR Am J Neuroradiol 17(10):1861–1869

20. Bae KT, Tran HQ, Heiken JP (2000) Multiphasic injection method for uniform prolonged vascular enhancement at CT angiography: pharmacokinetic analysis and experimental porcine model. Radiology 216(3):872–880

21. Fleischmann D, Rubin GD, Bankier AA, Hittmair K (2000) Improved uniformity of aortic enhancement with customized contrast medium injection protocols at CT angiography. Radiology 214(2):363–371

22. Wintermark M, Reichhart M, Thiran JP et al (2002) Prognostic accuracy of cerebral blood flow measurement by perfusion computed tomography, at the time of emergency room admission, in acute stroke patients. Ann Neurol 51(4):417–432

23. Aksoy FG, Lev MH (2000) Dynamic contrast-enhanced brain perfusion imaging: technique and clinical applications. Semin Ultrasound CT MR 21(6):462–477

24. Eastwood JD, Lev MH, Provenzale JM (2003) Perfusion CT with iodinated contrast material. AJR Am J Roentgenol 180(1):3–12

25. Lev MH, Kulke SF, Weisskoff RM et al (1997) Dose dependence of signal to noise ratio in functional MRI of cerebral blood volume mapping with sprodiamide. J Magn Reson Imaging 7:523–527

26. Coutts SB, Simon JE, Tomanek AI et al (2003) Reliability of assessing percentage of diffusion-perfusion mismatch. Stroke 34(7):1681–1683

27. Roccatagliata L, Lev MH, Mehta N et al (2003) Estimating the size of ischemic regions on CT perfusion maps in acute stroke: is freehand visual segmentation sufficient? In: Proceedings of the 89th Scientific Assembly and Annual Meeting of the Radiological Society of North America, 2003, Chicago, p. 1292

28. Mullins ME, Lev MH, Bove P et al (2004) Comparison of image quality between conventional and low-dose nonenhanced head CT. AJNR Am J Neuroradiol 25(4):533–538

29. Villringer A, Rosen BR, Belliveau JW et al (1988) Dynamic imaging with lanthanide chelates in normal brain: Contrast due to magnetic susceptibility effects. Magn Reson Med 6:164–174

30. Meier P, Zieler K (1954) On the theory of the indicator-dilution method for measurement of blood flow and volume. J Appl Physiol 6:731–744

31. Roberts G, Larson K (1973) The interpretation of mean transit time measurements for multi-phase tissue systems. J Theor Biol 39:447–475

32. Cenic A, Nabavi DG, Craen RA et al (1999) Dynamic CT measurement of cerebral blood flow: a validation study. AJNR Am J Neuroradiol 20(1):63–73

33. Cenic A, Nabavi DG, Craen RA et al (2000) A CT method to measure hemodynamics in brain tumors: validation and application of cerebral blood flow maps. AJNR Am J Neuroradiol 21(3):462–470

34. Nabavi DG, Cenic A, Dool J et al (1999) Quantitative assessment of cerebral hemodynamics using CT: stability, accuracy, and precision studies in dogs. J Comput Assist Tomogr 23(4):506–515

35. Nabavi DG, Cenic A, Craen RA et al (1999) CT assessment of cerebral perfusion: experimental validation and initial clinical experience. Radiology 213(1):141–149

36. Nabavi DG, Cenic A, Henderson S et al (2001) Perfusion mapping using computed tomography allows accurate prediction of cerebral infarction in experimental brain ischemia. Stroke 32(1):175–183

37. Ostergaard L, Weisskoff RM, Chesler DA et al (1996) High resolution of cerebral blood flow using intravascular tracer bolus passages. Part I: Mathematical Approach ad Statistical Analysis. Magnetic Resonance Imaging in Medicine 36(5):715–725

38. Ostergaard L, Chesler DA, Weisskoff RM et al (1999) Modeling cerebral blood flow and flow heterogeneity from magnetic resonance residue data. J Cereb Blood Flow Metab 19(6):690–699

39. Wintermark M, Thiran JP, Maeder P et al (2001) Simultaneous measurement of regional cerebral blood flow by perfusion CT and stable xenon CT: a validation study. AJNR Am J Neuroradiol 22(5):905–914

40. Wirestam R, Andersson L, Ostergaard L et al (2000) Assessment of regional cerebral blood flow by dynamic susceptibility contrast MRI using different deconvolution techniques. Magn Reson Med 43(5):691–700

41. Wintermark M, Maeder P, Thiran JP (2001) Quantitative assessment of regional cerebral blood flows by perfusion CT studies at low injection rates: a critical review of the underlying theoretical models. Eur Radiol 11(7):1220–1230

42. Sanelli PC, Lev MH, Eastwood JD et al (2004) The effect of varying user-selected input parameters on quantitative values in CT perfusion maps. Academic Radiology 11(10):1085–1092

43. Hacke W, Albers G, Al-Rawi Y et al (2005) The Desmoteplase in Acute Ischemic Stroke Trial (DIAS): a phase II MRI-based 9-hour window acute stroke thrombolysis trial with intravenous desmoteplase. Stroke 36(1):66–73

44. Schellinger PD, Fiebach JB, Hacke W (2003) Imaging-based decision making in thrombolytic therapy for ischemic stroke: present status. Stroke 34(2):575–583

45. Rother J (2003) Imaging-guided extension of the time window: ready for application in experienced stroke centers? Stroke 34(2):575–583

46. Rother J, Schellinger PD, Gass A et al (2002) Effect of intravenous thrombolysis on MRI parameters and functional outcome in acute stroke <6 hours. Stroke 33(10):2438–2445

47. Parsons MW, Barber PA, Chalk J et al (2002) Diffusion- and perfusion-weighted MRI response to thrombolysis in stroke. Ann Neurol 51(1):28–37

48. Lev MH, Segal AZ, Farkas J et al (2001) Utility of perfusion-weighted CT imaging in acute middle cerebral artery stroke treated with intra-arterial thrombolysis: prediction of final infarct volume and clinical outcome. Stroke 32(9):2021–2028

49. Schramm P, Schellinger PD, Fiebach JB et al (2002). Comparison of CT and CT angiography source images with diffusion-weighted imaging in patients with acute stroke within 6 hours after onset. Stroke 33(10):2426–2432

50. Schramm P, Schellinger PD, Klotz E et al (2004) Comparison of perfusion computed tomography and computed tomography angiography source images with perfusion-weighted imaging and diffusion-weighted imaging in patients with acute stroke of less than 6 hours' duration. Stroke 35:1652–1658

51. Kidwell CS, Saver JL, Mattiello J et al (2000) Thrombolytic reversal of acute human cerebral ischemic injury shown by diffusion/perfusion magnetic resonance imaging. Ann Neurol 47(4):462–469

52. Kidwell CS, Saver JL, Starkman S et al (2002) Late secondary ischemic injury in patients receiving intraarterial thrombolysis. Ann Neurol 52(6):698–703

53. Wintermark M, Fischbein NJ, Smith WS et al (2005) Accuracy of dynamic perfusion CT with deconvolution in detecting acute hemispheric stroke. AJNR Am J Neuroradiol 26(1):104–112

54. Bisdas S, Donnerstag F, Ahl B (2004) Comparison of perfusion computed tomography with diffusion-weighted magnetic resonance imaging in hyperacute ischemic stroke. J Comput Assist Tomogr 28(6):747–755

55. Warach S (2003) Measurement of the ischemic penumbra with MRI: it's about time. Stroke 34(10):2533–2534

56. Wu O, Koroshetz WJ, Ostergaard L et al (2001) Predicting tissue outcome in acute human cerebral ischemia using combined diffusion- and perfusion-weighted MR imaging. Stroke 32(4):933–942

57. Barber PA, Darby DG, Desmond PM et al (1998) Prediction of stroke outcome with echoplanar perfusion- and diffusion-weighted MRI. Neurology 51(2):418–426

58. Astrup J, Siesjo BK, Symon L (1981) Thresholds in cerebral ischemia – the ischemic penumbra. Stroke 12(6):723–725

59. Sorensen AG, Buonanno FS, Gonzalez RG et al (1996) Hyperacute stroke: evaluation with combined multisection diffusion- weighted and hemodynamically weighted echo-planar MR imaging. Radiology 199(2):391–401

60. Sunshine JL, Tarr RW, Lanzieri CF et al (1999) Hyperacute stroke: ultrafast MR imaging to triage patients prior to therapy. Radiology 212:325–332

61. Schlaug G, Benfield A, Baird AE et al (1999) The ischemic penumbra: operationally defined by diffusion and perfusion MRI. Neurology 53(7):1528–1537

62. Mehta N, Lev MH, Mullins ME et al (2003) Prediction of final infarct size in acute stroke using cerebral blood flow/cerebral blood volume mismatch: added value of quantitative first pass CT perfusion imaging in successfully treated versus unsuccessfully treated/untreated patients. In: Proceedings of the 41st Annual Meeting of the American Society of Neuroradiology, 2003, Washington

63. Rohl L, Ostergaard L, Simonsen CZ et al (2001) Viability thresholds of ischemic penumbra of hyperacute stroke defined by perfusion-weighted MRI and apparent diffusion coefficient. Stroke 32(5):1140–1146

64. Grandin CB, Duprez TP, Smith AM et al (2001) Usefulness of magnetic resonance-derived quantitative measurements of cerebral blood flow and volume in prediction of infarct growth in hyperacute stroke. Stroke 32(5):1147–1153

65. Schaefer PW, Ozsunar Y, He J et al (2003) Assessing tissue viability with MR diffusion and perfusion imaging. AJNR Am J Neuroradiol 24(3):436–443

66. Eastwood JD, Lev MH, Wintermark M et al (2003) Correlation of early dynamic CT perfusion imaging with whole-brain MR diffusion and perfusion imaging in acute hemispheric stroke. AJNR Am J Neuroradiol 24(9):1869–1875

67. Wintermark M, Reichhart M, Cuisenaire O et al (2002) Comparison of admission perfusion computed tomography and qualitative diffusion- and perfusion-weighted magnetic resonance imaging in acute stroke patients. Stroke 33(8):2025–2031

68. Lev MH, Hunter GJ, Hamberg LM et al (2002) CT versus MR imaging in acute stroke: comparison of perfusion abnormalities at the infarct core. In: Proceedings of the 40th Annual Meeting of the American Society of Neuroradiology, 2002, Vancouver

69. Lev MH (2003) CT versus MR for acute stroke imaging: is the "obvious" choice necessarily the correct one? AJNR Am J Neuroradiol 24(10):1930–1931

70. Heiss WD (2000) Ischemic penumbra: evidence from functional imaging in man. J Cereb Blood Flow Metab 20(9):1276–1293

71. Jovin TG, Yonas H, Gebel JM et al (2003) The cortical ischemic core and not the consistently present penumbra is a determinant of clinical outcome in acute middle cerebral artery occlusion. Stroke 34(10):2426–2433

72. Lev MH, Roccatagliata L, Murphy EK et al (2004) A CTA based, multivariable, "benefit of recanalization" model for acute stroke triage: core infarct size on CTA source images independently predicts outcome. In: Proceedings of the 42nd Annual Meeting of the American Society of Neuroradiology, 2004, Seattle

73. Suarez J, Sunshine J, Tarr R et al (1999) Predictors of clinical improvement, angiographic recanalization, and intracranial hemorrhage after intra-arterial thrombolysis for acute ischemic stroke. Stroke 30:2094–2100

74. Molina CA, Alexandrov AV, Demchuk AM et al (2004) Improving the predictive accuracy of recanalization on stroke outcome in patients treated with tissue plasminogen activator. Stroke 35(1):151–156

75. Baird AE, Dambrosia J, Janket S et al (2001) A three-item scale for the early prediction of stroke recovery. Lancet 357(9274):2095–2099

76. Nighoghossian N, Hermier M, Adeleine P et al (2003) Baseline magnetic resonance imaging parameters and stroke outcome in patients treated by intravenous tissue plasminogen activator. Stroke 34(2):458–463

77. Swap C, Lev M, McDonald C et al (2002) Degree of oligemia by perfusion-weighted CT and risk of hemorrhage after IA thrombolysis. In: Stroke – Proceedings of the 27th International Conference on Stroke and Cerebral Circulation, 2002, San Antonio

78. Ogasawara K, Ogawa A, Ezura M et al (2001) Brain single-photon emission CT studies using 99mTc-HMPAO and 99mTc-ECD early after recanalization by local intraarterial thrombolysis in patients with acute embolic middle cerebral artery occlusion. AJNR Am J Neuroradiol 22(1):48–53

79. Ueda T, Sakaki S, Yuh W (1999) Outcome in acute stroke with successful intra- arterial thrombolysis procedure and predictive value of initial single-photon emission-computed tomography. J Cereb Blood Flow Metab 19:99–108

80. Calamante F, Gadian DG, Connelly A (2000) Delay and dispersion effects in dynamic susceptibility contrast MRI: simulatinos using singular value decomposition. Magn Reson Med 44(3):466-473

SECTION V

MDCT of Trauma

V.1

MDCT of Abdominal Trauma

Robert A. Halvorsen

Introduction

Trauma is a significant public health problem, representing the third leading cause of death in the United States. Trauma is also the leading cause of mortality in Americans under the age of 40. With the widespread availability of multidetector-row computed tomography (MDCT) in trauma centers, the traditional workup of trauma patients has changed. Blunt chest injuries are now frequently studied with MDCT to evaluate the aorta, and workup of the blunt trauma victim with abdominal injury is evolving with MDCT. MDCT now allows not only the detection of injuries but provides new information on the severity of injuries with improved detection of vascular injury manifested by "active extravasation." Until recently, patients with a history of penetrating trauma went directly to the operating room for surgical therapy without preoperative imaging. Today, MDCT is often performed in patients with penetrating trauma in order to best identify vascular injuries prior to surgical intervention.

This chapter reviews the technique of MDCT and discusses major findings in abdominal MDCT in the trauma patient. The varied manifestations of bleeding are emphasized. Common mistakes and pitfalls in interpretation are described along with a step-by-step technique for interpretation.

MDCT Utilization in the Trauma Patient

Workup of the blunt trauma patient has evolved with the advent of MDCT. In the past, a large number of patients with deceleration injuries had abdominal CT in the search for solid-organ or hollow viscus injury, but few had a chest CT. With the installation of MDCT scanners in major trauma centers, the frequency of chest CT in the trauma pa-

tient has increased dramatically. MDCT provides the capability to perform high-definition multiplanar reconstruction (MPR) based upon thin sections reconstructed from MDCT raw data. Chest MDCT with MPR effectively produces CT angiograms, probably equal in quality to angiography (Fig. 1). A trauma surgeon can be provided definitive information concerning aortic injuries almost immediately with MDCT without the additional contrast load and invasiveness of traditional angiography. At many institutions, MDCT of the chest has almost completely replaced angiography in the initial workup of patients with possible aortic injuries. Angiography is often relegated to the role of a problem-solving tool. An MDCT of the chest not only provides diagnostic information concerning potential aortic injuries but also evaluates lungs, pleura, and bones. MPRs of the thorax

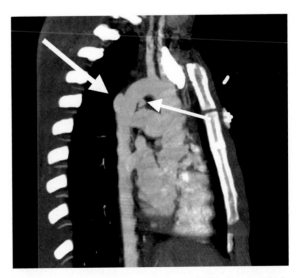

Fig. 1. Computed tomography angiogram (CTA) of motor vehicle accident victim demonstrating two pseudoaneurysms of the aorta (*arrows*), the smaller located on the anterior surface at the bottom of the aortic arch and the second located on the posterior proximal descending thoracic aorta

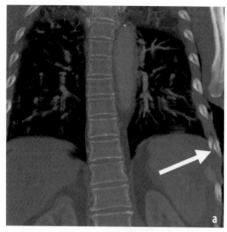
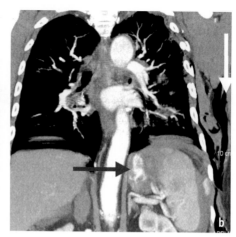
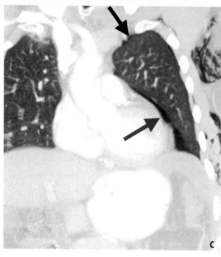

Fig. 2a-c. Computed tomography (CT) of high-speed motor vehicle accident victim. **a** Coronal CT with bone windows readily identifies rib fracture (*arrow*). **b** Soft tissue coronal view demonstrates large amount of subcutaneous emphysema (*white arrow*) and active extravasation in upper abdomen medial to spleen (*black arrow*). **c** Lung window in coronal projection demonstrates medial and small apical pneumothorax (*black arrows*)

facilitate detection of rib and spine fractures (Fig. 2a)

Alternative Strategies in MDCT Acquisitions

While the introduction of MDCT has dramatically changed the way many thoracic injuries are evaluated, it has had a lesser impact on evaluation of the abdomen and pelvis. Optimal use of MDCT below the diaphragm has not yet been established. Evaluation of the abdomen and pelvis with MDCT is currently performed differently in different institutions. Some centers, such as Massachusetts General Hospital, advocate the use of a "whole-body" CT in the trauma patient [1]. They utilize a continuous scanning technique through the areas to be scanned, such as cervical spine, chest, abdomen, and pelvis. Other centers, such as ours, continue to perform separate MDCT data acquisitions for each type of CT. For instance, a patient who has multiple types of CT studies in our Emergency Department will have them performed sequentially but not

continuously, facilitating the optimization of contrast enhancement timing and radiation dose. Sequential rather than continuous scanning makes possible the use of different types of reconstruction algorithms for different anatomical segments.

Alternative Means of MDCT Interpretation

Another variable is the availability of freestanding image processing workstations. Workstations linked to CT scanners allow the interpreting radiologist to take raw data at the workstation and make customized MPRs. Off-line reconstruction has the added benefit of allowing the technologist to move on to the next patient without waiting for the CT computers to perform the MPRs. Alternatively, technologists can produce routine MPRs using standard imaging planes, such as sagittal or coronal planes. Our technologists obtain routine coronal and sagittal MPRs in chest trauma patients and also reconstruct an oblique sagittal MPR along the plane of the aortic arch (Fig. 1). When obtaining MPRs using the 16-detector-row MDCT scanner computer, time costs are of interest. An MDCT of the chest requires a 20/second scan time. Initial reconstruction at 3 mm is performed, and axial images are sent to our PACS system for interpretation. This initial reconstruction requires 3 min 20 s. Then, to obtain MPRs, the raw data is reconstructed at thinner intervals and MPRs are constructed, requiring 7 min 10 s. Therefore, in order to prepare data obtained from an MDCT of the chest for interpretation, scan time (data acquisition) is only 20 s, but total reconstruction time is 10 min 30 s.

Changes in Interpretation Strategies with MDCT

Interpretation of MDCT in trauma patients requires attention to detail. The use of a rigorous routine in the interpretation of these studies significantly diminishes missed traumatic lesions [2]. We routinely review all trauma CTs with five settings:

- Lung window
- Soft tissue window
- Liver window
- Bone window
- MPR: sagittal and coronal multiplanar reconstructions

Interpretation: Routine Approach

Following is a detailed routine for interpretation of abdominal and pelvic MDCT in trauma patients:

Lung Windows
In our experience, the most frequently overlooked finding in trauma CT is a pneumothorax. We use lung windows to search for pneumothorax as well as pneumoperitoneum (Figs. 2c, 3, and 4). Not only the entire chest, but also the abdomen and pelvis are scanned from top to bottom using lung windows for the detection of free intraperitoneal air, intraperitoneal air adjacent to bowel loops, and retroperitoneal air.

Soft Tissue Windows
After scanning from top to bottom using lung windows, we switch to soft tissue windows and scroll from bottom back to top. This primary initial soft tissue survey is performed to search for free intraperitoneal fluid consistent with blood in a trauma patient (Fig. 5) Intraperitoneal fluid in a trauma patient is most likely due to either solid-organ or bowel injury and is a good indicator of injury severity. Careful attention is paid to the presence or absence of free fluid in the pelvis, where small amounts of fluid are easily overlooked. After the initial survey of the abdomen for blood, individual organs are scrutinized. When intraabdominal fluid is encountered on an MDCT of a trauma patient, an analysis of fluid density is extremely helpful. Clotted blood next to or adjacent to a bleeding site is called a sentinel clot [4] (Fig. 6). This clotted blood will be of higher density than the more serous blood further away from the site of bleeding. Identification of the sentinel clot is helpful in identifying the site of bleeding.

Spleen Survey
We evaluate the spleen twice. First, we look within the splenic parenchyma for areas of low or high density. Low density can represent splenic laceration or fracture. Fracture of a solid organ is defined as a laceration that extends from one capsular surface to the other. Splenic lacerations are usually identified because of the hematoma within the splenic parenchyma (Fig. 6). Whenever a

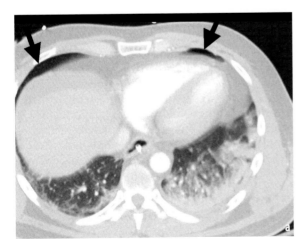

Fig. 3. Computed tomography (CT) of motor vehicle accident victim. Demonstrates bilateral pneumothoraces

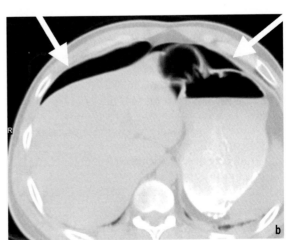

Fig. 4a, b. Motor vehicle accident victim with pneumoperitoneum. Demonstrates subphrenic air (*arrows*)

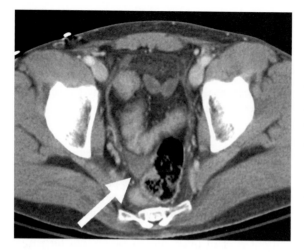

Fig. 5. Free intraperitoneal blood (*arrow*) in pelvis in blunt-trauma victim

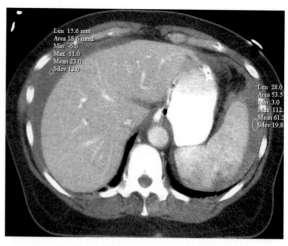

Fig. 6. Sentinel clot. Motor vehicle accident victim with splenic laceration. Perisplenic blood has higher density [61 Hounsfield units (HU)] compared with perihepatic blood (23 HU). Higher-density blood adjacent to the spleen is the "sentinel clot," helping to identify the source of bleeding. Lower-density blood adjacent to the liver is more serous in nature

hematoma is identified in the spleen or in any portion of an abdominal and pelvic CT, one should always search for active extravasation. Active extravasation of contrast material signifies arterial bleeding. Recognition of arterial bleeding or active extravasation has dramatically increased with the introduction of MDCT with rapid administration of high-concentration contrast media (Fig. 7). In 1989, Sivit et al. [5] reported the first demonstration of active intraabdominal arterial bleeding in a patient with splenic rupture from blunt trauma. Gavant et al. were among the first to describe the usefulness of detecting active bleeding in predicting the need for surgical intervention [3]. Jeffrey et al. [6] and later Federle et al. [7] further characterized and clarified the importance of active extravasation in helical CT. Detection of active extravasation on CT implies arterial bleeding and is usually considered an indication for splenic arteriography with possible embolization as alternative to surgery.

Traditionally, splenic injuries have been classified using a CT-based scoring or grading system [8]. Such grading systems may be misleading, as a minor injury may go on to a devastating delayed bleed:

- Grade 1: Subcapsular hematoma or laceration <1 cm
- Grade II: Larger subcapsular hematoma or laceration 1–3 cm
- Grade III: Capsular disruption or laceration >3 cm
- Grade IVA: Shattered spleen or active extravasation into spleen or subcapsular hematoma or pseudo aneurysm or arteriovenous fistula (Fig. 7)

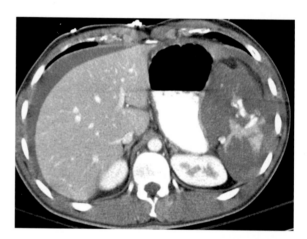

Fig. 7. Motor vehicle accident victim with splenic injury demonstrating active intrasplenic arterial bleeding

- Grade IVB: Active intraperitoneal bleeding (Fig. 8)

The severity predicted by traditional CT scoring systems for solid-organ injury using the American Association for the Surgery of Trauma (AAST) scoring system is controversial, with a number of authors finding them unhelpful [8–11], while others find them of use in patients with massive splenic injury, as most patients with Grades IVA or IVB splenic injury will require catheter embolization or surgery [12].

Liver Survey
The liver is the most frequently injured organ in trauma patients in general when both blunt and penetrating trauma is considered, while in blunt trauma patients, the spleen is the most commonly

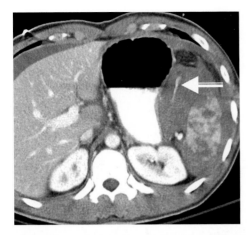

Fig. 8. Motor vehicle accident victim with severely injured spleen with active intraperitoneal bleeding (*arrow*) and evidence of a shattered spleen

injured organ. Survey of the liver is similar to that of the spleen, with an initial review of the deep hepatic parenchyma in the search for laceration or hematoma. A second review of each slice containing liver is performed to evaluate the margin of the liver in the search for subtle lacerations and perihepatic blood. Finally, one should evaluate the right paracolic gutter for small amounts of fluid. Occasionally in a patient with extensive respiratory motion, subtle hepatic injuries will not be detectable, but perihepatic blood, especially in the upper right paracolic gutter, will point to the site of injury.

With hepatic injuries, as with any solid organ injury, it is important to look for signs of active extravasation manifested as high-density contrast equivalent to arterial structures on the same slice (Fig. 9). But besides arterial injury, venous injury is of extreme importance in hepatic trauma. With liver injuries, it is essential to look for signs of hepat-

ic vein damage. Traumatic avulsion of the hapatic vein occurs in approximately 13% of liver injuries, often as a result of avulsion of the right hepatic vein from the inferior vena cava. Such vein damage is suggested on CT when lacerations extend around the inferior vena cava or into the porta hepatis (Fig. 10). With venous injuries, active extravasation is usually not detected. As the liver parenchyma itself compresses the laceration of the vein, no large hematomas are encountered. However, if the patient goes to the operating room and the surgeon elevates the liver, the tamponading effect of the liver parenchyma against the bleeding site is removed, and patients frequently exsanguinate on the operating room table. Therefore, if there is a detectable deep injury in the liver near the hepatic veins or the inferior vena cava (Fig. 11), the surgeon should be alerted to the finding prior to any operative intervention. With venous injuries, control of the inferior vena cava is obtained prior to elevating the liver in order to prevent exsanguination.

Pancreatic and Duodenal Injury
Duodenal hematomas may be subtle, with only mild thickening of the duodenal wall. Paraduodenal fluids often have a triangular, pointed shape and suggest a tear of the serosal surface of the duodenum (Fig. 12).

Pancreatic lacerations are often associated with duodenal injuries but can occur without CT-detectable duodenal hematoma. Pancreatic lacerations are often difficult to diagnose on the immediate trauma MDCT. Traumatic pancreatic injuries require time to produce edema within the pancreas. The initial CT may fail to show pancreatic injury unless a laceration within the pancreas is large enough to be visualized or there is peripancreatic

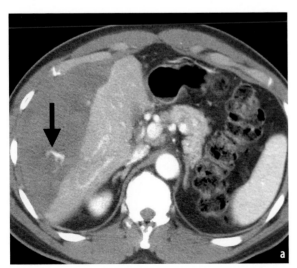
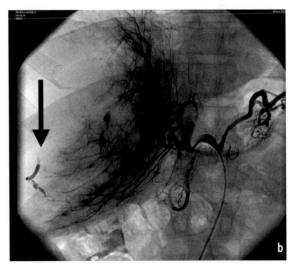

Fig. 9a, b. Large subcapsular hematoma with active arterial bleeding from hepatic injury. **a** Linear area of active extravasation (*arrow*) lateral to liver within subcapsular hematoma on axial computed tomography (CT). **b** Celiac artery angiogram demonstrates active extravasation (*arrow*) in subcapsular hematoma mimicking vessel

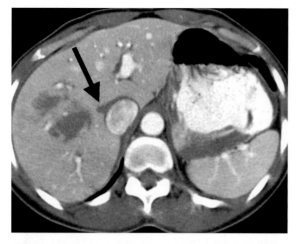

Fig. 10. Hepatic laceration with extension to inferior vena cava (*arrow*)

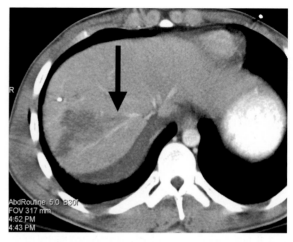

Fig. 11. Hepatic laceration extends along right hepatic vein and its branches (*arrow*)

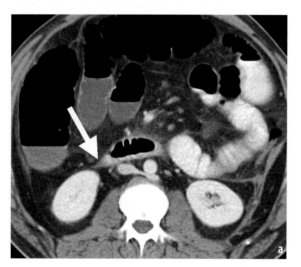

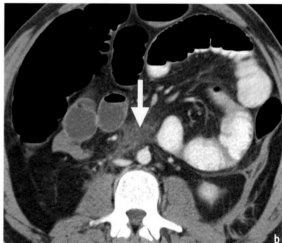

Fig. 12a, b. Periduodenal hematoma (*arrow*) with triangular shape (**a**). Retroperitoneal hematoma (*arrow*) (**b**)

bleeding. Always look for fluid density between the pancreas and the splenic vein (Fig. 13) Normally, only fat is found between the pancreas and the splenic vein. If fluid is visible, then either traumatic pancreatitis or actual bleeding on the posterior pancreatic surface is present. More obvious pancreatic injuries will be detected as a linear laceration extending through the tissue of the pancreas. Pancreatic injuries often occur slightly to the right or left of midline in locations where the pancreas is sheered against the side of the vertebral body. Therefore, lacerations typically occur either at the junction of the head and body of the pancreas to the right of the spine or within the body just to the left of midline (Fig. 14). The severity of a pancreatic injury is predominantly dependent upon the status of the main pancreatic duct. Bruises to the pancreas can often be treated conservatively. However,

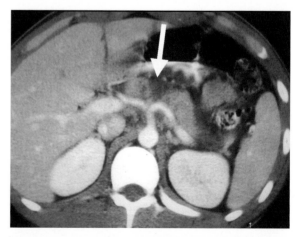

Fig. 13. Motor vehicle accident victim with pancreatic laceration (*white arrow*) through body of pancreas. This is a typical location for a deceleration injury due to shearing of the pancreas along side the vertebral body

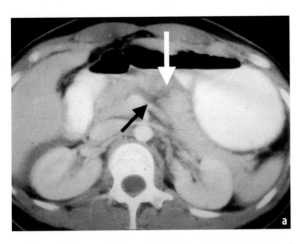

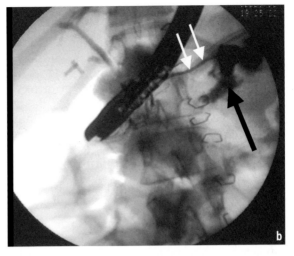

Fig. 14a, b. Motor vehicle accident victim with shearing injury of pancreatic body. **a** Laceration of posterior aspect of pancreas (*white arrow*) with blood separating pancreas from splenic vein (*black arrow*). **b** Endoscopic retrograde cholangiopancreatography (ERCP) demonstrates large area of extravasation (*black arrow*) from pancreatic duct (*white arrows*)

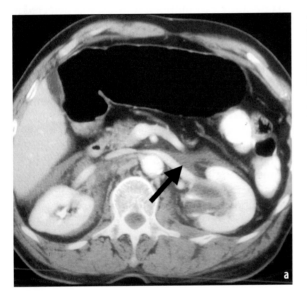

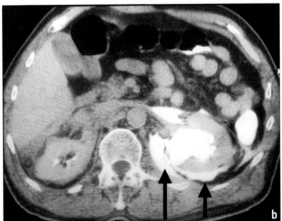

Fig. 15a, b. Left renal injury: patient status post motor vehicle accident. **a** Initial computed tomography (CT) study demonstrated fluid anterior to left kidney (*arrow*) and unusual fullness of renal pelvis. **b** Five-minute delayed image demonstrates urinoma (*arrows*). Fluid adjacent to the kidney and in the renal pelvis is extravasated urine, not blood

a laceration or transection of the main pancreatic duct usually requires a surgical repair.

Patients with duodenal or pancreatic injury should be monitored carefully for significant pancreatic injuries. Even if a patient has only mild swelling of the pancreas or inhomogeneity in blunt trauma, a follow-up CT is often warranted. Serum amylase may be used to detect change in amylase level suggesting traumatic pancreatitis, although the initial amylase obtained in the Emergency Room may be misleading. For instance, patients who have been subjected to head and neck injury may have an elevated amylase because of salivary gland injury. And the initial amylase in a pancreatic trauma patient may be normal while it may rise later.

In patients with questionable pancreatic in-

juries, especially with an elevating amylase on serial lab tests, a magnetic resonance cholangiopancreatography (MRCP) or occasionally an endoscopic retrograde cholangiopancreatography (ERCP) may be useful to better assess continuity of the main pancreatic duct (Fig. 14).

Kidneys

With renal trauma, CT findings include laceration, fracture, and perirenal blood or urine. Kidney analysis in the trauma patient is different from that of the liver or spleen. While perihepatic or perisplenic fluid is usually due to blood, perinephric fluid may represent either urine or blood. Therefore, when renal trauma is suspected, it is essential to obtain delayed CT images (Fig. 15) Generally, such delayed images should be obtained after a sufficient length of time for contrast to have been excreted into the renal collecting system, allowing for the detection of urinomas. Typically, a 3-min delay is adequate. Our routine includes initial evaluation of the abdominal CT prior to removing the patient from the CT table. If the patient demonstrates any abnormality in the kidney region, delayed imaging is obtained. If the patient is known to have hematuria prior to CT, then delayed images are protocoled in prior to initiation of the CT examination.

Retroperitoneal Structures

While adrenal injuries are often associated with renal injuries, solitary adrenal hematomas can occur without detectable renal injury. Adrenal injuries usually manifest as simple adrenal masses.

It is important to image the inferior vena cava in the detection of shock. Shock is identified on CT as a flat or slit-like inferior vena cava on at least three slices in the infrahepatic inferior vena cava. We typically look at the inferior vena cava at the level of the left renal vein (Fig. 16). Please note that a flat or slit-like inferior vena cava seen on one or two sections only may be simply due to a rapid inspiration of the patient, sucking blood out of the abdomen into the thorax if the patient gasps during CT examination. Therefore, one should see a narrowed inferior vena cava on three slices to increase specificity of this finding.

We recently reviewed our experience of shocked or hypotensive patients studied with CT in our Emergency Department and identified that a small spleen is an additional finding of hypotension (Fig. 17). In a series of patients who were hypotensive either in the ambulance during transportation to or on arrival in the Emergency Room, we found that mean spleen volume in hypotensive

patients was 142 cc. Following fluid resuscitation, the spleen in the same patients was noted to increase to a mean volume of 227 cc.

Hollow Viscus Injury

Identification of bowel injury in a blunt trauma patient is difficult. Bowel injury is often not detectable on clinical examination and can easily be overlooked on a CT study. Findings suggestive of bowel injury include free intraperitoneal air, free intraperitoneal fluid, and wall thickening of the bowel. Unfortunately, extraluminal gas has been reported to be detectable on CT, with a range of 46–63% [13–15]. When a loop of bowel that is fluid filled and does not contain air is ruptured, there will be no initial release of gas into the peritoneum. Therefore, a CT obtained soon after a bowel injury will often fail to detect extraluminal gas. Extraluminal contrast has been reported as a helpful finding in abdominal trauma CT. However, in one study, extraluminal contrast was detected in only 19% of cases [16]. In our experience, extraluminal contrast is infrequently identified. As CT scans are obtained more rapidly following abdominal trauma, the incidence of detectable extraluminal contrast has declined. Patients are scanned so quickly after arrival in the Emergency Room that administered contrast, either given orally or via nasogastric tube, often has not had time to reach the site of bowel injury. Reports from the radiology literature suggest an overall sensitivity for bowel injury ranging between 88% and 93% [16]. However, in the nonradiology literature there have been reports of significantly lower accuracy rates. In a 1998 study from a large trauma center in Texas involving 19,621 patients, CT missed hollow viscus injuries in 43% of children and 21% of adults [17].

Bowel injury has been studied in an experimental model by a group of English surgeons [18].

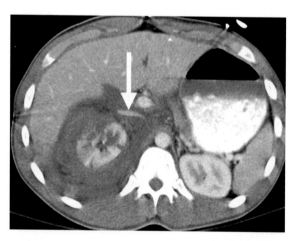

Fig. 16. Motor vehicle accident victim with hepatic and renal injuries and hypotension demonstrating slit-like inferior vena cava (*arrow*)

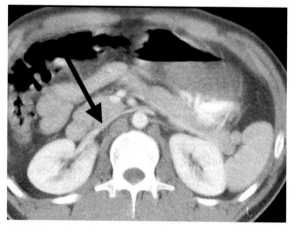

Fig. 17. Motor vehicle accident victim with bleeding into thigh from femoral fracture demonstrates slit-like inferior vena cava (*black arrow*) and small spleen due to hypotension

Their model used the pig and studied deceleration injuries. Their experiment consisted of anesthetized pigs thrown by a mechanical device into a solid object. They found that bowel injury occurred in 100% of the pigs when the speed at impact was 100 mph (161 kph) or greater. In a similar fashion to that of humans, they found that small-bowel injuries were twice as frequent as colonic injuries. Small-bowel injuries consisted of perforation or mesenteric avulsions while colonic injuries were usually serosal tears. The authors hypothesized that the increased frequency of small-bowel injuries was due to the fact that the small bowel is mobile and the colon is relatively fixed in the retroperitoneum.

Detection of intraperitoneal fluid is critical in the identification of bowel injury [19]. However, peritoneal fluid seen in the trauma patient can be either from traumatic or nontraumatic origin. Traumatic causes of intraperitoneal fluid include blood from a solid organ injury, blood from a bowel injury, bowel contents, and blood from a mesenteric injury but also can be due to bile from a ruptured gallbladder or biliary tree or urine from a ruptured bladder. Peritoneal fluid seen in the trauma patient can also arise from a combination of more than one injury. There are also nontraumatic causes of intraperitoneal fluid, which can be quite problematic. The most difficult cause is encountered in women of childbearing age who have a small amount of what is termed "physiologic fluid in the pelvis." In an ongoing study at our institution, we reviewed 175 CTs of women of childbearing age who were referred for evaluation of blunt trauma. Of those patients who had no evidence of injury on CT and required no operative management of abdominal injury, approximately 50% were identified to have at least a small amount of intraperitoneal fluid. In order to better characterize this fluid, density, volume, and location were analyzed. Using CT reconstruction at a 5-mm interval, of the 175 patients, only one had fluid seen on more than three slices in the pelvis with no evidence of injury. Therefore, identification of a "trace" amount of fluid seen on less than three slices seems likely to be an adequate predictor of a nontraumatic, physiologic fluid collection.

Fluid location is also extremely helpful in identifying the site of bleeding. As discussed above, the concept of a sentinel clot is quite useful. Since blood clots adjacent to the site of bleeding, when a higher density blood collection is encountered with a density that approaches that of adjacent muscles, the site of bleeding is likely to be adjacent to this clotted blood. More serous blood is seen further away from the bleeding site.

With solid-organ injuries initial bleeding occurs adjacent to the injured organ then extends down the pericolic gutters and into the pelvis. On-

ly after readily accessible potential spaces are filled, fluid will extend between the leaves of the mesentery. With a large amount of intraperitoneal blood from a solid organ injury "interloop" fluid will be detected. However, if bleeding occurs due to a bowel injury, the initial bleeding initially occurs into the interloop space. Therefore, if a patient has blood caught between the leaves of the mesentery and does not have blood in the pericolic gutters or pelvis, then bleeding is likely to be from a bowel injury.

Mesenteric or interloop fluid can be differentiated from the bowel by its shape [20], often manifesting as V- or triangular-shaped fluid collections between the leaves of the mesentery that are easily discerned from the more rounded shape of fluid within bowel loops (Fig. 18). The etiology of the V or triangular shape is simply that the mesentery leaves converge at the root of the mesentery, and any fluid caught between the leaves tends to have a point or apex of a triangle that points toward the mesentery root (Figs. 18 and 19).

Another sign of possible bowel injury on abdominal and pelvic MDCT is a group of "matted-together" bowel loops (Fig. 20). This matted-together appearance is due to blood extending between loops of unopacified bowel. This is a relatively nonspecific appearance and can occasionally be seen in normal unopacified bowel but should be considered a warning sign for possible bowel injury.

Bowel-wall thickening is an important finding in bowel injury. Since most small- and large-bowel loops are not opacified with contrast on a CT obtained in a trauma patient, one must be able to identify bowel-wall thickening without contrast. One useful trick is to remember that bowel-wall thickening is almost always circumferential in a trauma patient. Therefore, look at the anterior portion of a

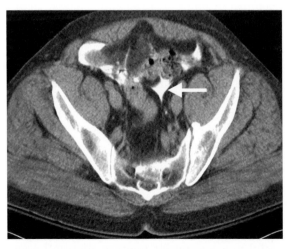

Fig. 18. Motor vehicle accident victim with extravasated urine from a bladder rupture: iodinated contrast caught between leaves of mesentery produces "V" shape (*arrow*) in upper pelvis

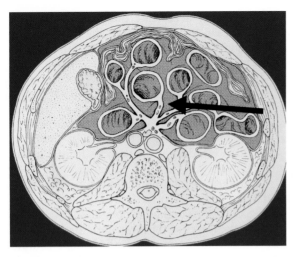

Fig. 19. Fluid caught between the leaves of the mesentery on this diagram demonstrates triangular shape (*arrow*)

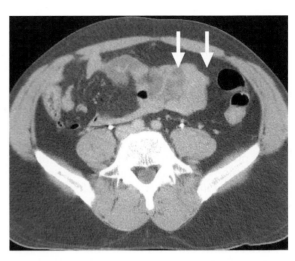

Fig. 20. Motor vehicle accident victim with bowel injury demonstrating "matted-together loop" appearance (*arrows*)

bowel loop. While bowel contents may make the bowel wall look thickened posteriorly, often, there is enough air or fluid in the lumen to identify whether or not there is anterior-wall thickening due to circumferential injury. An additional trick is to call bowel-wall thickening only when it is seen in the same bowel loop on two contiguous slices.

Identification of bowel injury is important. In our experience at San Francisco General Hospital, 46 patients with bowel injury had a delay in diagnosis resulting in more than 6 h from the time of injury to operative intervention [13]. There was a mortality rate of 4.3%, which corresponds to reports of mortality from bowel injury in the literature, which is up to 5.9%. One of the two deaths that occurred in our series was due to delayed diagnosis of a single jejunal perforation. Delay in diagnosis often occurred when the radiologist had identified an abnormality on the CT but the significance of the CT findings was not appreciated. For instance, a radiology report described colonic wall thickening with pericolonic soft tissue stranding, but the impression failed to mention "possible" or "probably colonic injury." In trauma patients with multiple problems, it is quite useful to be specific in reporting possible bowel injury. While the findings on CT may be subtle, the consequence of a delay in diagnosis can be severe.

Conclusion

Since almost any portion of the abdomen and pelvis can be injured in a trauma patient, it is quite useful to use a routine interpretation technique that ensures that the radiologist reviews all appropriate structures.

References

1. Novelline RA, Rhea JT, Rao PM, Stuk JL (1999) State-of-the-art. Helical CT in emergency radiology. Radiology 213(2):321–339
2. Halvorsen RA Jr, McCormick VD, Evans SJ (1994) Computed tomography of abdominal trauma; a step by step approach. Emerg Radiol 1:283–291
3. Gavant ML, Schurr M, Flick PA et al (1997) Predicting clinical outcome of nonsurgical management of blunt splenic injury: using CT to reveal abnormalities of splenic vasculature. AJR Am J Roentgenol 168(1):207–212
4. Orwig D, Federle MP (1989) Localized clotted blood as evidence of visceral trauma on CT: the sentinel clot sign. AJR Am J Roentgenol 153(4):747–749
5. Sivit CJ, Peclet MH, Taylor GA (1989) Life-threatening intraperitoneal bleeding: demonstration with CT. Radiology 171:430
6. Jeffrey RB Jr, Cardoza JD, Olcott EW (1991) Detection of active intraabdominal hemorrhage: value of dynamic contrast-enhanced CT. AJR Am J Roentgenol 156:725–729
7. Federle MP, Courcoulas AP, Powell M et al (1998) Blunt splenic injury in adults: clinical and CT criteria for management, with emphasis on active extravasation. Radiology 206:137–142
8. Mirvis SE, Whitley NO, Gens DR (1989) Blunt splenic trauma in adults: CT-based classification and correlation with prognosis and treatment. Radiology 171:33–39
9. Umlas SL, Cronan JJ (1991) Splenic trauma: can CT grading systems enable prediction of successful nonsurgical treatment? Radiology 178:481–487
10. Kohn JS, Clark DE, Isler RJ et al (1994) Is computed tomographic grading of splenic injury useful in the nonsurgical management of blunt trauma? J Trauma Mar 36(3):385–389; discussion 390
11. Becker CD, Spring P, Glattli A, Schweizer W (1994) Blunt splenic trauma in adults: can CT findings be used to determine the need for surgery? AJR Am J Roentgenol 162:343–347

12. Federle MP (2004) Splenic trauma. In: Federle, Jeffrey, Desser, Anne, Eraso (eds) Diagnostic Imaging: Abdomen. Amirsys, Salt Lake City, pp I:6:20–21
13. Harris HW, Morabito DJ, Mackersie RC et al (1999) Leukocytosis and free fluid are important indicators of isolated intestinal injury after blunt trauma. J Trauma 46:656–659
14. Mirvis SE, Gens DR, Shanmuganathan K (1992) Rupture of the bowel after blunt abdominal trauma: diagnosis with CT. AJR Am J Roentgenol 159:1217–1221
15. Sherck J, Shatney C (1996) Significance of intraabdominal extraluminal air detected by CT scan in blunt abdominal trauma. J Trauma 40:674–675
16. West OC (2000) Intraperitoneal abdominal injuries. In: West OC, Novelline RA, Wilson AJ (eds) Emergency and trauma radiology. American Roentgen Ray Society, Washington, pp 87–98
17. Allen GS, Moore FA, Cox CSJ et al (1998) Hollow viscus injury and blunt trauma. J Trauma 45:69–77
18. Cripps N, Cooper G (1997) Intestinal injury mechanisms after blunt abdominal impact. Ann R Coll Surg Engl 79:115–120
19. Dowe MF, Shanmuganathan K, Mirvis SE et al (1997) CT findings of mesenteric injury after blunt trauma: implications for surgical intervention. AJR Am J Roentgenol 168:425–428
20. Halvorsen RA Jr, McKenney K (2002) Blunt trauma to the gastrointestinal tract: CT findings with small bowel and colonic injuries. Emerg Radiol 9(3): 141–145

V.2

Role of MDCT in the Evaluation of Musculoskeletal Trauma

Sunit Sebastian and Hamid Salamipour

Introduction

Technical advances in the past decade have made computed tomography (CT) increasingly valuable in the early clinical management of patients with polytrauma. The development of multidetector CT (MDCT) has transformed CT from a simple, cross-sectional imaging technique to an advanced, three-dimensional (3-D) imaging modality, enabling excellent 3-D displays [1]. Multislice CT scanning is associated with a substantial gain in performance, decreased scan times, reduced section collimation, and reduction in scan length. The combined value of MDCT and 3-D reformations in assessment of the musculoskeletal system has been documented in the literature. The high contrast interface between bone and adjacent tissues in the musculoskeletal system makes it ideal for 3-D evaluation. The increased acquisition speed of MDCT with superior image resolution enables rapid diagnostic work up and institution of therapy in the setting of musculoskeletal trauma. This chapter will discuss the various techniques and applications of MDCT in orthopedic trauma. The use of 3-D reformations in the evaluation of musculoskeletal trauma will also be emphasized. The use of minimally invasive techniques such as CT angiography in the work up of a patient with skeletal trauma in appropriate indications will also be highlighted.

MDCT: Technical Considerations

MDCT significantly increases body coverage and thus reduces scanning time in most instances. Innovative detector arrays allow the acquisition of 0.5-mm-thick slices, with isotropic voxels [2]. This enables multiplanar reconstruction (MPR) images to be created in any plane with the same spatial resolution as the original sections without degradation of image quality.

MDCT in the Setting of Musculoskeletal Trauma

Extensive anatomic coverage is necessary in the evaluation of a patient with musculoskeletal trauma. MDCT is capable of acquiring multiple data sets simultaneously in each slice, leading to larger areas of scan coverage without correspondingly increasing the pitch and slice thickness [3]. This leads to longer scan ranges, near-isotropic imaging, better multiplanar reformatting, and 3-D rendering. Reduced scan times and motion artifacts are valuable in the evaluation of musculoskeletal trauma, especially in pediatric patients. MDCT can decrease artifacts related to metallic implant devices. Recently, automatic tube current modulation has been used to allow scanning of the musculoskeletal system with significantly less radiation [4].

MDCT Scanning Protocols

Technological advances in MDCT have led to the newer strategies to evaluate patients with orthopedic trauma. Radiation dose reduction is a significant issue that must be addressed in the evaluation of trauma patients in an emergent setting. Tables 1 and 2 present scanning protocols for facial and cervical trauma and extremity trauma, respectively, for a 16-slice MDCT scanner.

Table 1. Scanning protocol for facial and cervical trauma with AutomA technique on a 16-slice MDCT scanner (GE Healthcare)

Noise index	15–20
Tube current range:	
• Face	10–180 mA
• Cervical spine	10–270 mA
Gantry rotation time	0.5 s
Voltage	120 kVp
Beam pitch	0.938:1
Table speed	18.75 mm/rotation
Detector configuration	16×1.25 mm
Reconstructed slice thickness:	
• Face	1.25 mm
• Cervical spine	2.5 mm

Table 2. Scanning protocol for extremity trauma with AutomA technique on a 16-slice MDCT scanner (GE Healthcare)

Noise index	15–20
Tube current range	75–440
Gantry rotation time	0.5 s
Voltage	120 kVp
Beam pitch	0.938:1
Table speed	18.75 mm/rotation
Detector configuration	16×1.25 mm
Reconstructed slice thickness	1.25-2.5 mm (soft tissue & bone algorithm)

Indications for MDCT in Musculoskeletal Trauma

MDCT can be used to evaluate fractures of the spine, pelvis, and extremities. It has almost replaced plane radiography in the evaluation of skeletal trauma and is the standard of care in modern-day radiology practices. MDCT can also be used for the evaluation of soft tissue, tendons, and articular cartilage in conjunction with arthrography. Additional indications include postoperative evaluation of metallic implants. Complex intra-articular fractures of the extremities can also be evaluated thoroughly. Multiplanar reformatted images provide additional information regarding complex musculoskeletal injuries. Three-dimensional or volume-rendered images can play a crucial role in the further management of the patient.

Spinal Trauma

Traumatic injuries to the spine can cause permanent damage and are associated with high morbidity and mortality [5]. Spinal cord injuries are more common in males (75–85%), with the majority of the patients being younger than 30 years of age. The faster speed of acquisition and superior image resolution without significant patient manipulation has made MDCT the imaging method of choice for evaluation of a patients with of musculoskeletal trauma. Cervical spine injuries are associated with higher morbidity and mortality. Subtle fractures of the cervical spine may be difficult to diagnose on axial images alone. MPR images generated immediately after the scan in the sagittal and coronal planes can depict these fractures more precisely (Fig. 1). This serves as a roadmap for the surgeon and can prove to be a valuable guide for management of the patient.

The major mechanisms of spinal injury include hyperflexion, hyperextension, rotation, and vertical compression. Anterior wedge fractures of the thoracolumbar spine can be caused by flexion or compression injuries. These fractures can also cause posterior ligament injury with dislocation of facet joints.

The "seat belt" type injury is the most common type of injury associated with flexion distraction forces. Three patterns of seat belt injury described include:
- Type 1, or chance fracture: caused by disruption of posterior bony elements
- Type 2, or Smith fracture: caused by rupture of posterior ligaments
- Type 3: tear in annulus fibrosus causes subluxation injury

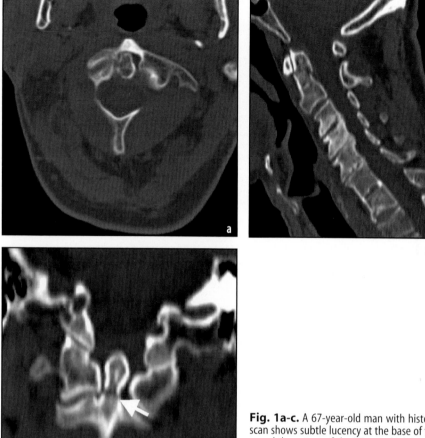

Fig. 1a-c. A 67-year-old man with history of motor vehicle crash. Axial CT scan shows subtle lucency at the base of the dens (**a**). Axial CT scan does not reveal the extent of the injury, which is perpendicular to the imaging plane. **b** Sagittal reformatted CT scan shows lucency through the dens just above the body of C2. (**c**) Coronal reformatted CT scan shows type II dens fracture in greater detail

The second cervical vertebra is the most common level of injury, involving the odontoid in 30% of the cases. The vertebral body is the most frequent site of fracture [6]. Spinal stability is crucial in determining the nature of injury and deciding the course of treatment. The most important determinant of spinal stability is the integrity of the middle column [7]. Instability of the spine is associated with inability to maintain normal alignment under normal physiological forces. The early detection of neurological injury associated with spinal instability is vital in preventing long-term disability.

Whiplash injuries result from a collision that includes sudden acceleration or deceleration. The person is often involved in a rear-end automobile collision or injured as a result of contact sports. The head swings backward, followed by a forward flexion, causing injuries to the cervical spine due to the relative weakness of the anterior longitudinal ligament. Tears or thrombotic obstruction of the vertebral artery and traumatic dissection of the extracranial part of the internal carotid arteries may occur even after moderate injury [8] .Whiplash injuries can cause significant morbidity

and impairment. A detailed history of the mechanism of trauma and thorough clinical examination can help make a diagnosis of whiplash injury. MDCT is useful to determine subtle fractures and facet lesions, which can be missed on plain radiography. MDCT is more sensitive than MRI in the detection of fractures of the posterior elements of the spine and to injuries of the craniocervical junction [9].

Screening helical CT has a sensitivity of 98.3%, a specificity of 100%, and an accuracy of 99.9% in the detection of clinically important fractures of the cervical spine [10]. Intravenous contrast should be administered to evaluate soft tissue and vascular structures in the region of trauma. Volume-rendered images can help detect subtle or hidden fractures that may have been missed on routine axial images. The 3-D images provide exact orientation of the fracture fragments and possible compression of the spinal cord by the displaced fracture fragments. This information is invaluable in planning treatment of the patient. MDCT allows improved imaging of orthopedic hardware by minimizing streak artifacts that traditionally plague CT in this setting.

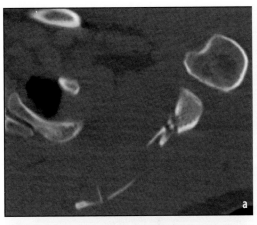
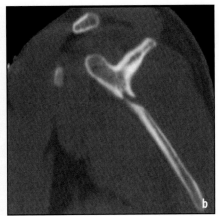
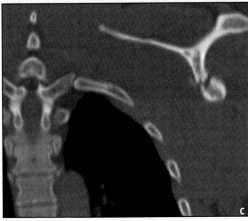

Fig. 2a-c. A 40-year-old man involved in a motor vehicle accident. Axial images show comminuted fracture of the body of the scapula (**a**). Sagittal (**b**) and coronal (**c**) reformatted images show the relationship of the fracture fragments to better advantage. There is minimal displacement of the fracture fragments

Upper Extremity Trauma

Sternoclavicular Joint

Blunt chest trauma, such as can occur in motor vehicle accidents, is usually associated with injuries to the sternoclavicular joint. Fractures of the ribs or shoulder joint are commonly associated with sternoclavicular joint trauma. Injury to the thoracic aorta and mediastinal vessels can occur with posterior displacement of the fracture fragments. CT angiography (CTA) must be performed if vascular injury is suspected. Complete obstruction of the brachiocephalic vein and impingement of the aorta can present with no clinical evidence of complication. A high index of suspicion is needed to prevent serious complications, which may appear insidiously in these injuries [11].

Shoulder Joint

MDCT has high sensitivity in the detection and evaluation of fractures of the shoulder with complex anatomical relationships. Scapular fractures can be difficult to detect on plain radiographs, but MDCT can demonstrate scapular fractures with a high degree of accuracy (Fig. 2). Fractures of the lesser tubercle and coracoid process are difficult to diagnose on plain radiographs and can present as occult fractures. MDCT in conjunction with MPR is proven to be useful in the evaluation of complex proximal humerus fractures where the extent of the fractures and alignment of fracture fragments is not adequately depicted on radiography [12] Additional information regarding injury to the lung, chest wall, clavicle, and axillary artery can also be attained. The number and relative rotation of fracture fragments can be accurately determined, especially with the use of 3-D reformatted images, thus proving valuable information when planning open reduction and internal fixation [13].

Elbow Joint

Acute elbow trauma is common in both adult and pediatric age groups. Plain radiographs can be equivocal, especially in children, and inadequate characterization may warrant the use of MDCT, with fractures being the most common finding.

Volume-rendered images can provide detailed information regarding the alignment of fracture fragments. Automatic tube-current modulation has been demonstrated to effectively minimize radiation from the MDCT examination of the elbow in pediatric patients [14].

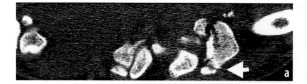

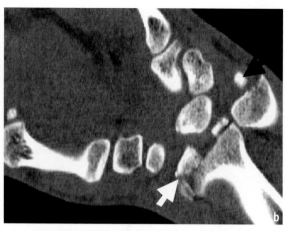

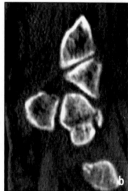

Fig. 3a, b. A 38-year-old man with history of fall on outstretched hand. Axial image shows comminuted fracture of the distal radius (**a**). Coronal reformatted images better demonstrate comminuted fractures of the distal radius involving the articular surface and fracture of the ulnar styloid process (*black arrowhead*) (**b**)

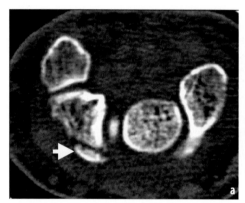

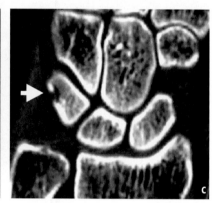

Fig. 4a, c. A 51-year-old man with history of industrial accident to the wrist joint. Triquetral avulsion fracture (*arrow*) on axial image (**a**) is better demonstrated on sagittal (**b**) and coronal (**c**) reformatted images

Wrist Joint

MDCT examinations are not dependent on the wrist position in the CT gantry due to its ability to generate 3-D reformatted images. Distal radio-ulnar joint injuries can occur independently or in unison with distal radius fractures and Galeazzi fractures. Diagnosis of stable, partially unstable (subluxation), and unstable (dislocation) patterns of injury can be based on MDCT evaluation. The early diagnosis and suitable treatment of an acute distal radioulnar joint injury is crucial to prevent development of a chronic disorder [15]. Complex fractures involving the distal radius and ulna can be accurately assessed with multiplanar reformats using MDCT (Fig. 3). Also, 3-D CT imaging is useful in evaluating extensor tendons proximal to the metacarpophalangeal joint. This method increases the accuracy of diagnosis and is useful in surgical planning and patient education [16]. Volume-rendered CT can be performed with cast material without significantly decreasing image quality. MDCT provides quick and accurate information in assessing complex wrist fractures [17]. Arthrography is superior to diagnose scapholunate ligament tears and ulnolunate and ulnotriquetral ligament defects [18]. Carpal bone avulsion injuries can be clearly assessed in the sagittal and coronal planes (Fig. 4).

Pelvis

Plain radiography has low sensitivity in determining if the pelvic injury is stable or not. Tile classification describes pelvic injuries as stable, rotationally unstable, or rotationally and vertically unstable [19]. MDCT with MPRs and 3-D reformats has greater sensitivity in detection of complex pelvic and acetabular traumatic injuries and is preferred as the imaging of choice in severe trauma in the emergency department [20]. Comminuted acetabular fractures can be better visualized on the multiplanar reformat images (Fig. 5). A vascular map of the abdominal aorta, iliac, and femoral vessels can be obtained after contrast administration, especially in the setting of penetrating trauma.

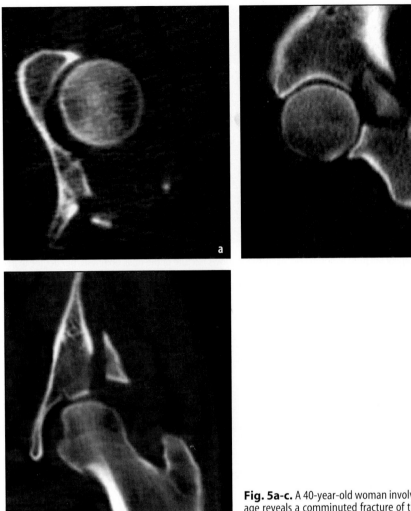

Fig. 5a-c. A 40-year-old woman involved in a motor vehicle accident. Axial image reveals a comminuted fracture of the posterior acetabulum (**a**). Sagittal (**b**) and coronal (**c**) images depict the fracture without dislocation of the hip joint

Lower Extremity Trauma

Knee Joint

Subtle fractures can be missed on plain radiography. Intra-articular extension of the fracture line can be depicted clearly using sagittal and coronal reformats (Fig. 6). This is critical in determining appropriate therapy. CT arthrography and virtual arthroscopy have shown good diagnostic accuracy in detecting anterior cruciate ligament and meniscal abnormalities [21]. Patellofemoral joint evaluation after arthroscopic stabilization can be assessed in various degrees of knee flexion [22].

Ankle Joint

On axial CT images alone, it can be difficult to interpret the complex anatomy of the ankle and foot. Comminuted fractures of the distal tibia and fibula can be accurately assessed using MDCT (Fig. 7). Articular facets of the subtalar joints may not be seen clearly depicted on routine axial scans. MPR images can significantly improve visualization of the subtalar joint anatomy. Talar and calcaneal injuries can also be easily assessed (Fig. 8). Volume rendering is useful for determining anatomic relationships between ankle tendons and underlying bones. Surface shaded display is valuable when fractures extend to the articular cortex and a disarticulated view is needed [23].

Summary

MDCT enables rapid and thorough evaluation of the musculoskeletal system. It has transformed an axial imaging modality to a multiplanar one in which reformations and 3-D reconstructions can be obtained routinely and at will [24]. Evolving techniques such as automatic exposure control have led to lower radiation doses in MDCT evalua-

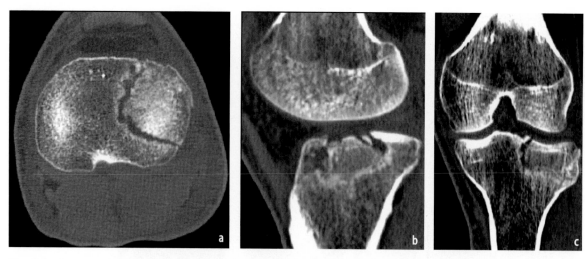

Fig. 6a-c. A 39-year-old man with history of fall from a motorcycle. Axial image shows fracture of the tibial epiphysis, but degree of depression is difficult to assess (**a**). Sagittal (**b**) and coronal (**c**) images reveal fracture involving the tibial plateau with extension to the articular surface of the knee joint. Degree of depression can be accurately determined

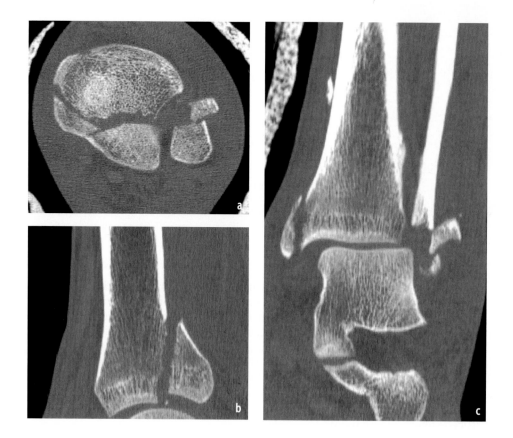

Fig. 7a-c. A 31-year-old man with fracture due to a motor vehicle accident. Fracture involves the distal tibia, as well as the fibula. Alignment is difficult to assess (**a**). Sagittal reformats demonstrate pilon fracture with displacement (**b**). Coronal reconstructions show complexity of fracture, with involvement of distal fibula (**c**)

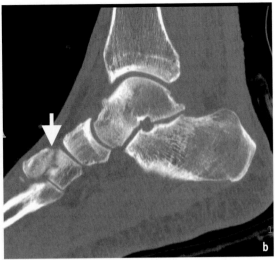

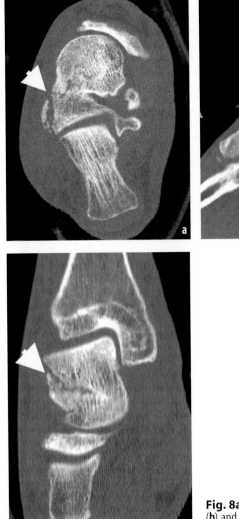

Fig. 8a-c. A 51-year-old man with talar neck fracture due to fall from height (**a**). Sagittal (**b**) and coronal (**c**) multiplanar reconstructions from MDCT images show that joint alignment is still maintained

tion of the musculoskeletal system. Appropriate scanning protocols should be tailored to incorporate these advances.

Acknowledge

We would like to acknowlege Jay Curtin for his valuable assistance in preparing the figures.

References

1. Prokop M (2003) General principles of MDCT. Eur J Radiol 45[Suppl 1]:S4–10
2. El-Khoury GY, Bennett L, Ondr GJ (2004) Multidetector-row computed tomography. J Am Acad Orthop Surg 12(1):1–5
3. Rydberg J, Buckwalter KA, Caldemeyer KS et al (2000) Multisection CT: scanning techniques and clinical applications. Radiographics 20:1787–1806
4. Dalal T, Kalra MK, Rizzo SM et al (2005) Metallic prosthesis: technique to avoid increase in CT radiation dose with automatic tube current modulation in a phantom and patients. Radiology 236(2):671–675
5. Harris JH Jr (2000) Spine, including soft tissues of the pharynx and neck. In: Harris JH Jr, Harris WH (eds) The radiology of emergency medicine. Lippincott Williams and Wilkins, Philadelphia, pp 137–298
6. Goldberg W, Mueller C, Panacek E et al (2001) Distribution and patterns of blunt traumatic cervical spine injury. Ann Emerg Med 38:17–21
7. El-Khoury GY, Moore TE, Kathol MH (1992) Radiology of the thoracic spine. Clin Neurosurg 38:261–295
8. Viktrup L, Knudsen GM, Hansen SH (1995) Delayed onset of fatal basilar thrombotic embolus after whiplash injury. Stroke 26: 2194–2196
9. Crim JR., Moore K, Brodke D (2001) Clearance of the cervical spine in multitrauma patients: the role of advanced imaging. Semin Ultrasound CT MRI 22(4):283–305

10. Ptak T, Kihiczak D, Lawrason JN et al (2001) Screening for cervical spine trauma with helical CT: Experience with 676 cases. Emerg Radiol 8:315–319

11. Mirza AH, Alam K, Ali A (2005) Posterior sternoclavicular dislocation in a rugby player as a cause of silent vascular compromise: a case report. Br J Sports Med 39(5):28

12. Haapamaki VV, Kiuru MJ, Koskinen SK (2004) Multidetector CT in shoulder fractures. Emerg Radiol 11(2):89–94

13. Jurik AG, Albrechtsen J (1994) The use of computed tomography with two- and three-dimensional reconstructions in the diagnosis of three- and four-part fractures of the proximal humerus. Clin Radiol 49(11):800–804

14. Chapman VM, Kalra M, Halpern E et al (2005) 16-MDCT of the posttraumatic pediatric elbow: optimum parameters and associated radiation dose AJR Am J Roentgenol 185(2):516–521

15. Nicolaidis SC, Hildreth DH, Lichtman DM (2000) Acute injuries of the distal radioulnar joint. Hand Clin 16(3):449–359

16. J Sunagawa T, Ishida O, Ishiburo M et al (2005) Three-dimensional computed tomography imaging: its applicability in the evaluation of extensor tendons in the hand and wrist. Comput Assist Tomogr 29(1):94–98

17. Kiuru MJ, Haapamaki VV, Koivikko MP, Koskinen SK (2004). Wrist injuries; diagnosis with multidetector CT. Radiol 10(4):182–185

18. Klein HM, Vrsalovic V, Balas R, Neugebauer F (2002). Imaging diagnostics of the wrist: MRI and arthrography/arthro-CT. Rofo 174(2):177–182

19. Pennal GF, Tile M, Waddell JP, Garside H (1980) Pelvic disruption: assessment and classification. Clin Orthop 151:12–21

20. Their ME, Bensch FV, Koskinen SK et al (2005) Diagnostic value of pelvic radiography in the initial trauma series in blunt trauma. Eur Radiol 15(8):1533–1537

21. Lee W, Kim HS, Kim SJ et al (2004) CT arthrography and virtual arthroscopy in the diagnosis of the anterior cruciate ligament and meniscal abnormalities of the knee joint. Korean J Radiol 5(1):47–54

22. Schroder RJ, Weiler A, Hoher J et al (2003) Computed tomography of the patellofemoral alignment after arthroscopic reconstruction following patella dislocation. Rofo 175(4):547–555

23. Choplin RH, Buckwalter KA, Rydberg J, Farber JM (2004) CT with 3D rendering of the tendons of the foot and ankle: technique, normal anatomy, and disease. Radiographics 24(2):343–356

24. Salamipour H, Jimenez RM, Brec SL et al (2005) Multidetector row CT in pediatric musculoskeletal imaging. Pediatr Radiol 35(6):555–564

Appendix
MDCT Protocols

From: *Kalra MK, Saini S*, Chapter I.1, page 5

Table 1. Important scanning parameters and contrast considerations that must be addressed during development of scanning protocols for a given diagnostic indication

CT scanning parameters	Contrast consideration
Scan area of interest	Contrast versus noncontrast
Scan direction	Route
Localizer radiograph	Concentration
Scan duration	Volume
Gantry revolution time	Rate of injection
Table speed, beam pitch, beam collimation	Trigger-fixed, automatic tracking, or test bolus
Reconstructed section thickness	
Extent of overlap	
Reconstruction algorithms	
Tube potential	
Tube current and automatic exposure control	
Radiation dose	

From: *Kalra MK, Saini S*, Chapter I.1, page 5

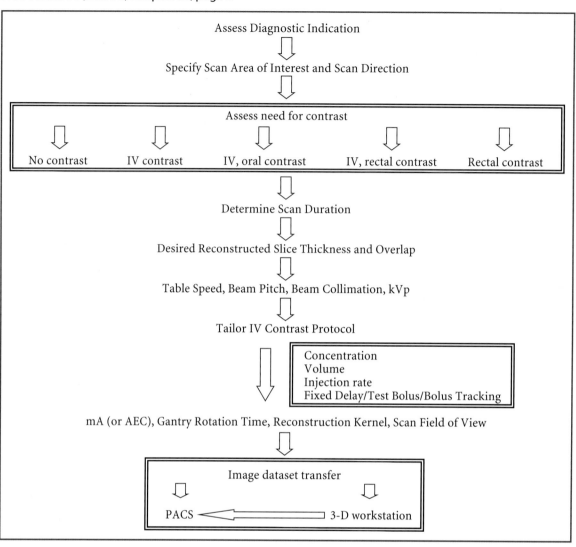

Fig. 1. Building blocks for scanning protocols

From: *Bae KT*, Chapter I.2, page 18

Table 1. Contrast enhancement times and proposed scan delays in different applications

	Pulmonary CTA	Coronary thoracic aorta CTA	Abdominal aorta/peripheral runoff	Hepatic parenchyma/portal vein
Contrast arrival time (s)[a]	$Tarr = 7$–10	$Tarr = 12$–15	$Tarr = 15$–18	30–40 ($Tarr = 15$–18)
Peak time (s)[a]	From 15 to ID (peak reaches a plateau rapidly)	$ID + (0$ to $5)$[b]	$ID + (5$ to $10)$[b]	$ID + (25$ to $40)$[b]
Fixed scan delay (s)	15 (20 for slow injection)	20	30 (20-25 for slow scan)	60–70
Variable scan delay (s)	15 (20 for slow injection)	$ID + 5 - SD/2$	$ID + 5 - SD/2$	$ID + 35 - SD/2$
Circulation-adjusted delay	$Tarr + 5$	$ID + (Tarr - 10) - SD/2$	$ID + (Tarr - 10) - SD/2$	$ID + (Tarr \times 2 + 5) - SD/2$

CTA computed tomography angiography, *Tarr* contrast arrival time, *ID* injection duration (s), *SD* scan duration (s)

For CTA, ID = "15 s + $^1/_2$ SD" (with saline flush) or "20 s + $^1/_2$ SD" (without saline flush) is suggested with the injection rate of 4 ml/s

For the liver, ID is determined by considering the total iodine load of 0.5 gI/kg

Peak time increases by 3–5 s with the use of saline flush

Tarr. **a** for pulmonary CTA, 100 HU threshold over the pulmonary artery with the first scan at 10 s after the start of the injection; **b** for aorta and hepatic phases, 50 HU threshold over the aorta with the first scan at 10 s after the start of the injection

[a]Assuming normal cardiac circulation, body weight of 60–80 kg, and the injection rate of 3–5 ml/s via the antecubital vein

[b]A larger number is used for a shorter injection duration

From: *Solomon R*, Chapter I.3, page 25

Estimated GFR/1.73 m² = 186 x Serum [creatinine]-1.154 x Age -0.203

x 0.74 if female x 1.21 if African American

Formula was empirically determined in a cohort of individuals (1628) (mostly white) with chronic kidney disease (determined by iothalamate clearance <55 m l/m in/1.73m²).

Evidence from other studies suggests that it underestimates GFR by 25-30% in subjects with "normal" renal function.

Fig. 1. MDRD or Levey Formula

From: *Solomon R*, Chapter I.3, page 26

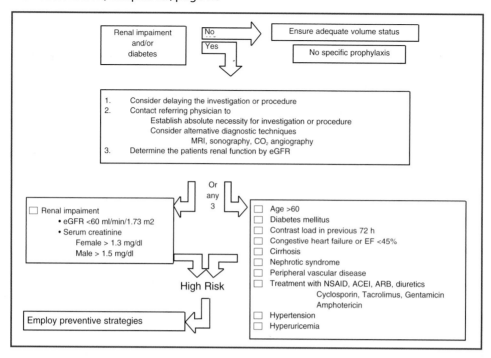

Fig. 2. Protocol (modified from [3])

From: *Sahani DV, Singh AH*, Chapter II.1, page 43

Table 2. Multidetector computed tomography (MDCT) liver protocols on different computed tomography (CT) scanners

Parameters	4 channel	16 channel	64 channel
DC (mm)	4×1.25	16×0.625	64×0.6
TS (mm/s)	15	18.75	38
Pitch	1.0–2.0	0.938	0.984
Slice thickness (mm)			
Arterial phase (CTA)	1.25	1.0	1.0
Arterial phase (liver)	2.5–5.0	2.5	2.5
Venous phase (CTA)	2.5	2.0	2.0
Venous phase (liver)	5.0	5.0	5.0
Arterial Delay (s)	Bolus tracking/automated trigger		
	Empirical delay:25–30 s		
Venous Delay (s)	65–70 s	60 s	50–60 s

DC detector collimation, *TS* table speed, *CTA* computed tomographic arteriography

From: *Schindera ST, Nelson RC*, Chapter II.2, page 50

Table 1. Scan parameter for PVP and HAP using 4-, 16-, and 64- slice MDCT (developed for GE scanners)

	4-slice MDCT		16-sclice MDCT		64-slice MDCT	
	HAP	*PVP*	*HAP*	*PVP*	*HAP*	*PVP*
Detector configuration(mm)	4×3.75	4×2.5	16×1.25	16×0.625	64×0.625	64×0.625
Pitch	1.5	1.5	1.38	1.75	1.38	1.38
Table speed (mm/rotation)	22.5	15	27.5	17.5	55.0	55.0
Rotation time (s)	0.8	0.8	0.6	0.5	0.5	0.5
kV	140	140	140	140	140	140
mA	220	220	300	380	450	450
Slice thickness (mm)	5.0	5.0	5.0	5.0	5.0	5.0
Axial slice thickness for MPR and 3D-reconstruction (mm)	2.5	2.5	1.25	0.625	1.25	0.625

From: *Sahani DV, Shah ZK*, Chapter II.3, page 68

Table 1. Multidetector computed tomography (MDCT) parameters for the pancreas: Protocols for GE Scanners at our institute

Parameters	4 channel	16 channel	64 channel
DC (mm)	1.25	0.625	0.6
TS (mm/s)	15	18.75	38
	Beam Pitch 1.0–2.0		
Slice thickness (mm)			
Arterial (CTA)	1.25	1.0	1.0
Arterial (liver)	2.5–5.0	2.5	2.5
Venous (CTA)	2.5	2.0	2.0
Venous (liver)	5.0	5.0	5.0
	Delay arterial bolus tracking empirical delay 25–30 s		
Venous Delay (s)	65–70	65–70	65–70

DC detector collimation, *TS* table speed, *CTA* computed tomographic arteriography

From: *Kavangh JJ et al*, Chapter III.3, page 130

Table 1. Computed tomography (CT) protocols: CT pulmonary angiography

Scanner type	4 slice	16 slice	64 slice
Collimation		16 × 0.75	64 × 0.6
Reconstruction (mm)	1.25	1.00	0.75
Rotation time (s)	0.8	0.5	0.33
Contrast volume (370 mgI/mL)	100 ml	100 ml	75–100 ml
Saline flush		50 ml	50 ml

From: *Shetty SK, Lev MH*, Chapter IV.2, page 168

Table 1. Sample acute stroke computed tomography (CT) protocol employed at the authors' institution, incorporating CT angiography (CTA) and CT perfusion (CTP). The protocol is designed to answer the four basic questions necessary for stroke triage described. Note the alteration in the kilovolt peak (kVp) for perfusion acquisition. Parameters are presented for illustrative purposes and have been optimized for the scanner currently employed (General Electric Healthcare Lightspeed 16) in our emergency department. Parameters should be optimized for each scanner

Scan series	Unenhanced	CTA head	CTA neck	Cine perfusion ×2
Contrast		Biphasic contrast injection: 2.5 cc/s for 50 cc, then 1.0 cc/s for 20 cc		7 cc/sec for 40 cc for each CTP acquisition
Scan delay		Delay: 25 s (35 s if poor cardiac output, including atrial fibrillation)		Delay: 5 s (each series is a 60-s cine acquisition)
Range	C1 to vertex	C1 to vertex	Arch to C1	Two CTP slabs
Slice thickness	5 mm	2.5 mm	2.5 mm	5 mm
Image spacing	5mm	2.5 mm	2.5 mm	N/A
Table feed	5.62 mm	5.62 mm	5.62 mm	N/A
Detectors configuration (mm)	16×0.625	16×0.625	16×0.625	16×1.25
Pitch	0.562:1	0.562:1	0.562:1	N/A
Mode	Helical	Helical	Helical	Cine 4i
kVp	140	140	140	80
mA	220	200	250	200
Rotation time	0.5 s	0.5 s	0.5 s	1 s
Scan FOV	Head	Head	Large	Head
Retrospective slice thickness/interval	None	1.25/0.625 mm	1.25/1.0 mm	None

Standard reconstruction algorithm is used for all image reconstruction
CTA computed tomography angiography, *CTP* computed tomography perfusion, *kVp* kilovolt peak, *mA* milliampere, *FOV* field of view

From: *Sebastian S, Salamipour H*, Chapter V.2, page 197

Table 2. Scanning protocol for extremity trauma with AutomA technique on a 16-slice MDCT scanner (GE Healthcare)

Noise index	15–20
Tube current range	75–440
Gantry rotation time	0.5 s
Voltage	120 kVp
Beam pitch	0.938:1
Table speed	18.75 mm/rotation
Detector configuration	16×1.25 mm
Reconstructed slice thickness	1.25-2.5 mm (soft tissue & bone algorithm)